Health Informatics

This series is directed to healthcare professionals leading the transformation of healthcare by using information and knowledge. For over 20 years, Health Informatics has offered a broad range of titles: some address specific professions such as nursing, medicine, and health administration; others cover special areas of practice such as trauma and radiology; still other books in the series focus on interdisciplinary issues, such as the computer based patient record, electronic health records, and networked healthcare systems. Editors and authors, eminent experts in their fields, offer their accounts of innovations in health informatics. Increasingly, these accounts go beyond hardware and software to address the role of information in influencing the transformation of healthcare delivery systems around the world. The series also increasingly focuses on the users of the information and systems: the organizational, behavioral, and societal changes that accompany the diffusion of information technology in health services environments.

Developments in healthcare delivery are constant; in recent years, bioinformatics has emerged as a new field in health informatics to support emerging and ongoing developments in molecular biology. At the same time, further evolution of the field of health informatics is reflected in the introduction of concepts at the macro or health systems delivery level with major national initiatives related to electronic health records (EHR), data standards, and public health informatics.

These changes will continue to shape health services in the twenty-first century. By making full and creative use of the technology to tame data and to transform information, Health Informatics will foster the development and use of new knowledge in healthcare.

More information about this series at http://www.springer.com/series/1114

Pamela Hussey • Margaret Ann Kennedy
Editors

Introduction to Nursing Informatics

Fifth Edition

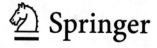 Springer

Editors
Pamela Hussey
School of Nursing
Psychotherapy and Community Health
Center of eIntegrated Care
Dublin City University
Dublin
Ireland

Margaret Ann Kennedy
Center of Excellence
Gevity Consulting Inc and Kennedy Health
Informatics Inc
Halifax, NS
Canada

ISSN 1431-1917   ISSN 2197-3741   (electronic)
Health Informatics
ISBN 978-3-030-58742-0   ISBN 978-3-030-58740-6   (eBook)
https://doi.org/10.1007/978-3-030-58740-6

This Springer imprint is published by the registered company Springer Nature Switzerland AG
The registered company address is: Gewerbestrasse 11, 6330 Cham, Switzerland

We dedicate this new edition to frontline healthcare workers around the world. For those who are managing care delivery in the midst of the COVID-19 pandemic. We thank them for their dedication, commitment, and unwavering efforts. By focusing our minds not on fear but on creating knowledge in the design of digital health services we can expand thought and targeted action for positive societal impact.

Preface

The publication of this fifth edition of an *Introduction to Nursing Informatics* is timely. Its core purpose is to act as primer for nurses searching for basic information on the topic of nursing informatics and to act as a resource for nursing education in informatics. Interest in health informatics and its relevance to digital health is expanding. The World Health Organization recently published State of the Worlds Nursing Report which calls for a massive acceleration in nurse education which needs to respond to changing technologies and advancing models of integrated health and social care.

As a profession, nursing is accountable for a significant contribution to healthcare service provision. Contemporary nursing practice is changing, and at the same time, facing a number of critical challenges. For example, two global issues that the profession is striving to address include a high staff turnover and nursing skill mix shortages. Articulating the nursing contribution to self-management support and design of systems for new models of care delivery is a key priority. Nursing informatics continues to be an essential aspect in which to inform not only the profession but also nurse leaders in their quest for the expansion of nursing knowledge and theory development.

Twenty-first century medicine offers exciting opportunities for the nursing profession to engage with and develop within. One example includes the increasing diffusion of artificial intelligence and machine learning within health and society. Additionally, concepts relating to health ecosystems which can be used to transform and enhance health and social care delivery in context are seeking nurse's expertise and imagination. There is a need to ensure that resources such as the Electronic Health Records and Telehealth applications are pragmatic and fit for purpose. Nurses often described as context experts, understand the care flow of healthcare processes, and are key agents for design, requirements identification, and benefit realization of systems deployment to progress integrated care.

In this fifth edition of *An Introduction to Nursing Informatics*, the editors have collected the best available evidence to inspire and support nurses to think critically about both current and future practice. This book is presented in such a manner as to encourage the reader to pause and reflect upon key concepts presented from the perspective of their existing practice domain. Starting with the fundamental concepts of nursing practice, and exploring the nursing contribution on digital health and integrated care, the chapters illustrate their relationship to informatics. This edition includes a number of contributions from leading experts, who have practiced in the field of informatics over a number of years. Preparing nurses for engagement with initiatives relating to eHealth transformational programs locally, regionally, or nationally is supported with additional files for downloading from extras.springer. com. There is a strong emphasis on both education and continuous professional development, and the pedagogical framework used to devise the core learning activities is explained in Chap. 1. This book builds on previous editions and provides readers with a basic primer for searching information on the topic of nursing informatics and accelerating nursing education on informatics. It includes online resources and tools to support the acquisition of informatics skills for future professional development. We hope you enjoy this fifth edition.

Dublin, Ireland   Pamela Hussey
Halifax, NS, Canada   Margaret Ann Kennedy

Acknowledgments

Dr Pamela Hussey and Dr Margaret Anne Kennedy would like to acknowledge the following individuals for their contribution to this new edition: Dr Kathryn Hannah for her unshakeable support to us both over the years in advancing our respective careers, Prof Nick Hardiker for his contribution to editing Chap. 6 of this fifth edition, and Ms Anne Casey who originally authored this chapter in the fourth edition.

Contents

About the Editors and Contributors

About the Editors

Pamela Hussey is an Associate Professor in the School of Nursing Psychotherapy and Community Health and Director of the Center for eIntegrated Care at Dublin City University, Ireland. Her current research activity relates to testing, deployment, and reporting on health informatics standards. She acts as an advisor to different agencies on topics relating to semantic and syntactic interoperability on integrated care. Dr. Hussey's teaching interests include health informatics, concepts, and terminology, as well as the creation and use of technology enhanced learning in undergraduate and postgraduate education.

Margaret Ann Kennedy is Chief Nursing Informatics Officer based in Gevity's Center of Excellence. She holds a PhD in Nursing from the University of South Australia, a Master of Nursing from Dalhousie University (Canada), a Bachelor of Science in Nursing from St. Francis Xavier University (Canada), and a Post Graduate Certificate in Standards for Health Informatics from the University of Sherbrooke (Canada).

Contributors

Alexander Berler IHE-Europe, Brussels, Belgium

Richard Booth Arthur Labatt Family School of Nursing, Western University, London, ON, Canada

Karima Bourquard IN-SYSTEM, IHE-Europe, Brussels, Belgium

Rosanne Burson University of Detroit Mercy, CHP/MSON, Detroit, MI, USA

Ryan Chan Arthur Labatt Family School of Nursing, Western University, London, ON, Canada

Dianne Conrad Grand Valley State University, Grand Rapids, MI, USA

Samantha Cooke Arthur Labatt Family School of Nursing, Western University, London, ON, Canada

Catherine Corrigan School of Nursing Psychotherapy and Community Health, Dublin City University, Dublin, Ireland

Kendra Cotton Arthur Labatt Family School of Nursing, Western University, London, ON, Canada

Subhashis Das School of Nursing Psychotherapy and Community Health Adapt Research Center, Dublin City University, Dublin, Ireland

G. Doleman School of Nursing and Midwifery, Edith Cowan University, Perth, WA, Australia

C. Duffield School of Nursing and Midwifery, Edith Cowan University, Perth, WA, Australia

Faculty of Health, University of Technology Sydney, Sydney, NSW, Australia

Orna Fennelly ICHEC, Irish Centre for High-End Computing, Dublin, Ireland

Ross Fraser Sextant Inc., Toronto, ON, Canada

Loretto Grogan Health Service Executive, Dublin 8, Ireland

Five Country Nursing and Midwifery Digital Leadership Group, Belfast, Ireland

Simon Hagens Canada Health Infoway, Toronto, ON, Canada

K. J. Hannah Professor (Adjunct), School of Nursing, University of Victoria, Victoria, BC, Canada

Christopher Henry FINEOS, Dublin, Ireland

Pamela Hussey School of Nursing Psychotherapy and Community Health, Dublin City University, Dublin, Ireland

Margaret Ann Kennedy Centre of Excellence, Gevity Consulting Inc., Vancouver, BC, Canada

Ulla-Mari Kinnunen Department of Health and Social Management, University of Eastern Finland, Kuopio, Finland

Shelagh Maloney Canada Health Infoway, Toronto, ON, Canada

Josephine McMurray Business Technology Management/Health Studies, Wilfrid Laurier University, Waterloo, ON, Canada

Katherine Moran Grand Valley State University, Grand Rapids, MI, USA

Lynn M. Nagle Director of Digital Health and Virtual Learning, Faculty of Nursing, University of New Brunswick, Fredericton, New Brunswick, Canada

Lawrence S. Bloomberg Faculty of Nursing, University of Toronto, Toronto, Canada

Arthur Labatt Family School of Nursing, Western University, London, Canada

Angela Reed Northern Ireland Practice and Education Council for Nursing and Midwifery, Belfast, UK

Five Country Nursing and Midwifery Digital Leadership Group, Belfast, UK

Tracie Risling College of Nursing, University of Saskatchewan, Saskatoon, Saskatoon, SK, Canada

Kaija Saranto Department of Health and Social Management, University of Eastern Finland, Kuopio, Finland

Diane J. Skiba College of Nursing, University of Colorado, Aurora, CO, USA

Anne Spencer St Michael House, Ballymun, Dublin, Ireland

Gillian Strudwick Centre for Addiction and Mental Health, Toronto, Ontario, Canada

Institute of Health Policy, Management and Evaluation, University of Toronto, Toronto, ON, Canada

Chapter 1
Introduction to Nursing Informatics

Pamela Hussey

Abstract This chapter introduces the reader to the structure and content of this new edition. As with the fourth edition, this next edition is designed as an ebook. This fifth edition describes how the acronym CARE originally introduced in early editions by Hannah and Ball and used in the previous editions has evolved and presents content in four discrete sections. Educational tools devised to support the reader are also presented in this chapter, and 3 distinct learning approaches; assimilative, productive and interactive/adaptive styles are explained. Each chapter has an associated learning template that can be downloaded at the end of the resource. In this chapter the structure and presentation of the learning templates is also presented.

Keywords Introduction to 5th edition structure · Supporting educational resource tools · Learning approaches explained · The revised CARE acronym

Learning Objectives for the Chapter
1. Introduce the reader to the 5th Edition of An Introduction to Nursing Informatics
2. Explain the acronym of CARE
3. Describe the Educational approach devised by the editors to support the reader of this 5th edition

The 5th edition of An introduction to Nursing Informatics, is designed for use with practicing nurses and students in undergraduate and post graduate programmes of study. It presents the fundamental concepts of nursing informatics and considers

Electronic Supplementary Material The online version of this chapter (https://doi.org/10.1007/978-3-030-58740-6_1) contains supplementary material, which is available to authorized users.

P. Hussey (✉)
School of Nursing Psychotherapy and Community Health, Faculty of Science and Health, Dublin City University, Dublin, Ireland
e-mail: pamela.hussey@dcu.ie

© Springer Nature Switzerland AG 2021
P. Hussey, M. A. Kennedy (eds.), *Introduction to Nursing Informatics*, Health Informatics, https://doi.org/10.1007/978-3-030-58740-6_1

how the theory of health informatics informs service improvements for citizens in an evolving digital society.

The text includes a number of contributions from leading experts who have practiced in the field of informatics over a number of years. This fifth edition provides insights into current and future leader's visions, it demonstrates how nurses are using informatics competencies to play an influential role in health policy formulation in addition to contributing to the effectiveness of health and social care systems globally.

We revisit in this new edition the CARE acronym and the associated Fig. 1.1 considering key concepts, which underpin the material, reflect our understandings and insights based on the evidence reviewed and our experiences. We start with core questions such as what the role of a nurse is and how this role expands in a digital enabled society. We reflect and consider how as a profession we can empower individuals to use digital health to maintain good quality of life for optimal health and wellbeing. Democratisation of health care is increasingly evident, it brings with it challenges and opportunities of dealing with newly acquired data and information (Topol 2016). Nursing leadership is now more than ever a priority and informatics a core competency to optimise the nursing professions contribution. As you will read in Chap. 8, there is a need to deliver at least 6 million new nursing jobs by 2030, primarily in low- and middle-income countries. Nursing as a profession needs to accelerate its impact through the expansion of effective nurse-led models of care to meet population health needs and improve access to primary health care.

In Connecting Health Immersion of Digital into eHealth (Chap. 2), we will delve deeper in to the evidence and policy debate to see what nursing activity is shaping effective and efficient systems design and development. This chapter explores where the profession of nursing is situated, within the intersection of data, devices and AI. In Chap. 16 the authors will describe what nursing care practice will

Fig. 1.1 CARE diagram

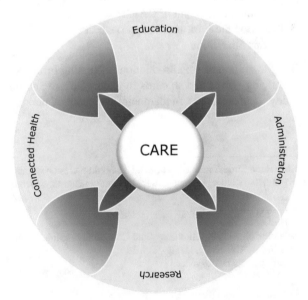

potentially look like in the future? We discuss the evolving role of the nurse as an under utilised resource in the design and deployment of new models of care. In Nursing Informatics: A Core Competency for the Profession Chap. 3, we provide examples of where nursing as a profession is drawing on traditional and contemporary nursing theory to inform and generate new knowledge. Specifically we include the focus on visualization of data and measurement of impact on patient outcome and experiences for new integrated care delivery. Health information is no longer delivered solely in a top down fashion from doctor to patient through a medical model. Nowadays we see an increasing bank of self-generated health data owned by individuals and which is challenging existing traditional power structures in medical models of care. Nurses will not disappear in the future, but their roles and responsibilities are evolving to meet the needs of the digital enabled patient.

We start with fundamental concepts in part one of the book, and then progress on to core concepts and practice applications in sections two through four. The content is linked with case based examples to contextualise the theory presented by authors. A content map, which demonstrates the overall structure of the book is presented in Fig. 1.1, and this map will be explained in greater detail through chapters and associated sections. Briefly, the word CARE is presented as an acronym for Connected Health, Administration, Research and Education and the book is organised sections into these sub themes. Part one is included as an introductory section. The main changes from earlier editions is the manner in which administration as a concept within nursing is considered. Adopting the Cambridge definition, we reshape the material on this administration section of this new edition. We define Administration not from an acute model of nursing care, in a tightly bound set of nursing information systems but rather consider the concept of administration in the widest context of care delivery. Briefly considering administration as a set of core arrangements and tasks needed to control the operations of a plan (Cambridge University Press Dictionary 2019). We believe this approach is important as we enter a period of professional reflection on redefining roles and responsibilities within the profession This plan for example can include administration of integrated care across service providers or administrator of action plans for self-management support underpinned by Smart and Internet of Things IoT using connected devices.

In the year of the Nurse 2020, our goal is to empower nursing, to build capacity within the profession to use Informatics as an enabler to cultivate digital leaders for health and social care transformation. The State of the Worlds Nursing Report published in April 2020 recommends the nurse education and training programmes must graduate nurses who drive progress in primary health care and universal health coverage. They contend that graduate nurses should emerge as a career choice grounded in science, technology, teamwork and health equity, and that curricula must be aligned with national health priorities as well as emerging global issues to prepare nurses to work effectively in interprofessional teams and maximize graduate competencies in health technology (State of the World's Nursing Report 2020).

We will support the evidence in this fifth edition with examples from international leaders in the field of informatics who are demonstrating initiatives which are

Introduction to Nursing Informatics 5th Edition

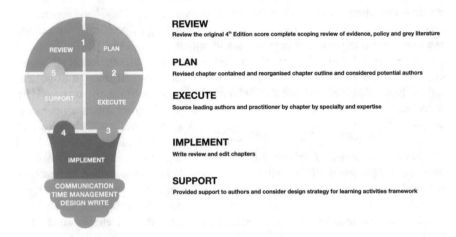

REVIEW
Review the original 4th Edition score complete scoping review of evidence, policy and grey literature

PLAN
Revised chapter contained and reorganised chapter outline and considered potential authors

EXECUTE
Source leading authors and practitioner by chapter by specialty and expertise

IMPLEMENT
Write review and edit chapters

SUPPORT
Provided support to authors and consider design strategy for learning activities framework

Fig. 1.2 Methods adopted

driving this change. Figure 1.2 provides an overview of the methods adopted to draft this latest edition of the text.

As an eBook, it is important that you have an opportunity to view a site map of the content in order to synthesize the material in a structured and systematic way. There is a number of associated learning activities presented at the end of each chapter in a template format. An example of the structure of the template is explained at the end of this introductory chapter (Fig. 1.3). In each chapter, a signpost will direct you to a set of learning activities designed to assist you to meet your personal learning objectives. Drawing on years of lecturing and teaching informatics in both face-to-face and online programmes, we advocate this as an effective way to maximise potential learning and gain a deeper understanding of the topic.

Adopting Conole's (2013) work, three specific activity profiles are presented to assist you to learn. The first and largest activity profile is to review the material presented in this ebook by reading, watching, accessing and thinking about the informatics material presented. This process is known as assimilative activity. The second activity is to produce, list create, construct, compose, draw or write what you read and are assimilating, this process is called a productive activity. Finally, we would ask you to consider completion of the assimilative and production activities by engaging with interactive or adaptive activities. Such activities involve you exploring newly acquired information by experimenting, and simulating the information using design patterns with a view to you enhancing your practice. The blending of these three activities, with your practice experience in association with reading this text offer you as a practicing nurse or informatics student, a fundamental understanding of what nursing informatics is. In this way informatics and it role can be located and understood

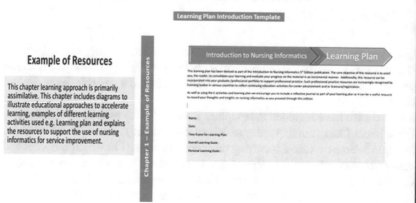

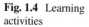

Fig. 1.3 Example of learning template

Fig. 1.4 Learning activities

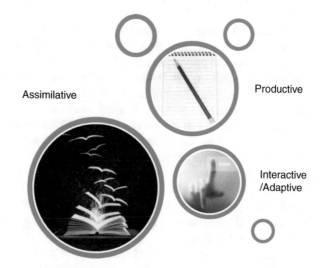

within the profession of nursing. Figure 1.4 offers a summary diagram of this process.

Each of the learning approaches identified in Fig. 1.4 can be used as scaffolding by educators and trainers with different design tools to assist the student or practitioner to contextualise the material within the individual chapters as part of a module or set of learning outcomes. Drawing on early work of Conole in 2008 and 2013 (Conole 2008, 2013), specific learning activities can be used to abstract and transfer key learning material which can be cognitively processed by you and then applied to differing contexts. The following summary provides some examples of the tools that we have included within this ebook.

1.1   Summary of Learning Tools and Supporting Resources Included In This Book

Case studies are useful for developing and testing problem-solving skills. They are used in this text to demonstrate a particular challenge relating to informatics within the nursing context that the student must overcome in order to achieve the desired outcome.

Rationale We have included case studies in this book to assist you to reflect on pertinent issues facing nursing today which informatics may have a direct impact on.

Design Patterns capture a recurring problem, the context in which it occurs and a possible method of solution derived from experience and backed up by theory. Design patterns often include an interactive learning pattern which is described by Conole in 2013 (Conole 2013) as creating an interactive space for team work as well as interpersonal reflection. The pattern usually includes: lectures, keeping a diary, elaboration of a team project, self and or peer evaluation and summative assessment (Conole 2013). Design patterns are also used in design science for development of information systems (Vaishnavi et al. 2004/2019).

Rationale Nursing as skill-based profession has a core role to play in problem solving and design science of new models of care. Considered context and domain experts, nurses can provide key insights in mapping process models of existing and proposed care delivery mechanisms. Design patterns will assist you to achieve key attributes for self-development on informatics tools and their overall impact upon service improvement activity and patient outcomes.

Scenarios which can offer more current and future challenges facing practitioners can be used as test cases to demonstrate the validity and utility of patterns within the informatics domain (Conole 2008).

Rationale healthcare operates within a dynamic environment and the pace of progression with topical issues such as the eHealth and Digital agendas requires that the nursing profession can adopt and adapt to this changing environment. Using scenarios will assist nurses to recognise future nursing informatics requirements in their practice domain.

Visual representations such as mind maps or formalised diagrams to summarise or outline key points noted in the material reviewed.

Rationale Using mind maps will assist you to generate and link core concepts assimilated in the text. The process of mind mapping may include an associated hierarchy using images lines and links as well as random associations.

Role play often linked with visual representations such as mind maps or web searches to design discuss or report on material reviewed within a chapter (Vaishnavi et al. 2004/2019; Mor et al. 2012).

Rationale Presents to you a learning opportunity to develop a greater awareness of the issues raised in a particular setting and can develop a more focused approach on the specific knowledge presented in a chapter. Role play demonstrates how well the learner understands the topic e.g. motivational interviewing (Health Services Executive Making Every Contact Count 2019) and provides dedicated time to apply what is learned to practice in a safe environment removed from the practice setting.

A Reflective practitioner exercise which encourages you to answer a question, make a judgement, or react to the material presented in the chapter. Whilst this exercise can be completed as a stand-alone activity it is useful to complete this activity as part of a peer review exercise.

Rationale The advantages of reflection in practice and on reflective practice within the profession of nursing are well documented and are recognised as a credible educational tool (Bradbury-Jones et al. 2009).

In addition to the learning tools in this text we have also included some support resources to accompany the text. These include website links, video links, a glossary, and PowerPoint presentations. A brief description for these supporting resources is included in the following section in addition to an example of a learning plan which can be used listed as an appendix to this introductory chapter.

1.2 Glossary

The glossary of key terms frequently used within the domain of nursing informatics has been included.

1.3 Powerpoint Presentations

The purpose of including PowerPoint presentations with some of the chapters is to offer you the key points identified in the chapter in a short summarised format.

1.4 Online Resources

In some of the chapters we have included website links and links to video which are available to download from the related websites.

Glossary

Administration The process of running a business or organisation
Assessment An evidence based approach used to generate data which will inform interpretations about the level of knowledge, skills or capabilities of a person or group for a specific purpose

Assimilative Activity An intervention that includes reading watching assessing and thinking about resources provided to enhance learning about a specific topic

Case Study An activity which involves a thorough analysis of an individual or group or other social unit

Concept An abstraction based on observations of behaviours or characteristics

Conceptual model A representation of a specific idea or product, illustrated through inter-related concepts or abstractions and presented in a rational scheme by virtue of their relevance to a common theme; also referred to as a conceptual framework

Connected Health Connected Health is a term used to describe a model for health-care delivery that uses technology to provide healthcare remotely, and to allow patients more freedom to lead their own lives.

Design Patterns An approach to identify and document a recurring problem, the context in which it occurs and a possible method of solution derived from experience and backed up by theory

Digital Digital Health is used as an umbrella term for areas including eHealth, telehealth, mHealth and more. Digital Health is the integration of all information and knowledge sources involved in the delivery of healthcare via information technology (IT)-based systems. This includes information created by caregivers, often within electronic health record systems at a hospital or GP practice, and information created by patients using apps, monitoring devices and wearable sensors. Digital health information also includes management and administrative information needed to co-ordinate and manage activities within the healthcare system

Education The process of giving or receiving systematic instruction

Glossary Key terms frequently used within the subject domain

Interactive Activity A process which involves exploring newly acquired information by experimenting, and simulating the material reviewed using design patterns with a view to you enhancing your practice

Podcast A digital audio or video file or recording that can be downloaded from a Web site to a media player or computer

Productive Activity A learning strategy which aim is to improve the quality of learner achievement against the learners time. Productive activities usually involve an output from task related activities such as an assignment or critical review exercise that can be posted to a journal

Productive Activity An action orientated process which can include composing drawing writing or constructing reflections on a particular topic usually completed following an assimilative activity

Quicktime A multimedia platform and media player that allows you to view internet video

Reflective Practitioner Exercise which encourages you to answer a question, make a judgement, or react to the material presented often in tandem with your personal experiences, practice and pre conceptions

Research Systematic inquiry that uses a variety of methods to answer questions or solve problems

Role Play Exercises often linked with visual representations such as mind maps or web searches to design discuss or report on material reviewed within a chapter

Scenario Exercise which present challenges facing practitioners which can be used as test cases to demonstrate the validity and utility of patterns within a specific domain or context

Appendix

Example of Learning Plan

Introduction to Nursing Informatics	Learning Plan

This learning plan has been devised as part of the Introduction to Nursing Informatics 5th Edition publication. The core objective of this resource is to assist you, the reader, to consolidate your learning and evaluate your progress on the material in an incremental manner. Additionally, this resource can be incorporated into your graduate/professional portfolio to support professional practice. Such professional practice resources are increasingly recognised by licensing bodies in various countries to reflect continuing education activities for career advancement and or licensure/registration.

Name:
Date:
Time frame for Learning Plan:
Overall Learning Goals:
Personal Learning Goals:

As well as using the E-activities and learning plan we encourage you to include a reflective journal as part of your learning plan as it can be a useful resource to record your thoughts and insights on nursing informatics as you proceed through this edition.

Introduction

Chapter 1 Introduction
Chapter 2 Connected Health Immersion of Digital into eHealth

Section-1 Connected Health

Chapter 3 Nursing Informatics: A Core Competency for the Profession
Chapter 4 The Mechanics of Technology & Digital
Chapter 5 Health Information Exchange
Chapter 6 Health Informatics Standards
Chapter 7 Nursing Documentation in Digital Solutions
Chapter 8 Connected Health and the Digital Patient

Section 2 Administration

Chapter 9 Administration Applications
Chapter 10 Data Privacy & Security
Chapter 11 The Role of the Informatics Nurse

Section 3 Research

Chapter 12 Researching Nursing Informatics in the Digital Age
Chapter 13 Applied Informatics Research in Nursing for eHealth

Section 4 Education

Chapter 14 Knowledge Networks in Nursing
Chapter 15 Technology Enabled Learning in Nursing
Chapter 16 The Future of Nursing Informatics in a Digitally Enabled World

Introduction

Introduction				
Learning Goals What do I need to accomplish to achieve my learning goals? (Must be a SMART objective, i.e. specific, measurable, achievable, realistic, time-oriented)	**Learning Strategies** What exercises can I use to reach this learning goal	**Required Resources** What resources do I need to achieve this learning goal?	**Learning Outcomes** How can I demonstrate to myself and others that I have achieved this learning	**Target Date for Completion** When do I want to achieve this by?

Section 1 - Connected Health

Section 1 Connected Health				
Learning Goals What do I need to accomplish to achieve my learning goal? (Must be a SMART objective, i.e. specific, measurable, achievable, realistic, time -oriented)	Learning Strategies What exercises can I use to reach this learning goal	Required Resources What resources do I need to achieve this learning goal?	Key Performance Indicators How can I demonstrate to myself and others that I have achieved this learning	Target Date for Completion When do I want to achieve this by?

Section 2 - Administration

Section 2 – Administration				
Learning Goals What do I need to accomplish to achieve my learning goals? (Must be a SMART objective, i.e. specific, measurable, achievable, realistic, time-oriented)	Learning Strategies What exercises can I use to reach this learning goal	Required Resources What resources do heed to achieve this learning goal?	Key Performance Indicators How can I demonstrate to myself and others that I have achieved this learning	Target Date for Completion When do I want to achieve this by?

Section 3 - Research

Section 3 – Research

Learning Goals What do I need to accomplish to achieve my learning goals? (Must be a SMART objective, i.e. specific, measurable, achievable, realistic, time-oriented)	Learning Strategies What exercises can I use to reach this learning goal	Required Resources What resources do I need to achieve this learning goal?	Key Performance Indicators How can I demonstrate to myself and others that I have achieved this learning	Target Date for Completion When do I want to achieve this by?

Section 4 - Education

Section 5. – Education

Learning Goals What do I need to accomplish to achieve my learning goals? (Must be a SMART objective, i.e. specific, measurable, achievable, realistic, time-oriented)	Learning Strategies What exercises can luse to reach this learning goal	Required Resources What resources do I need to achieve this learning goal?	Key Performance Indicators How can I demonstrate to myself and others that I have achieved this learning	Target Date for Completion When do I want to achieve this by?

Learning Plan   **Reflective Journal**

When writing your reflective journal you may find the following key points useful.

In the learning exercises devised in this 5th edition we have included three sets of activities:

1. Assimilative
2. Productive
3. Interactive or adaptive

In your journal it may be useful to write some reflections about each of these activities using the following questions to assist you in the process.

- What have I learned from completing this particular activity?
- How well have I completed this particular activity?
- If I were to complete this activity again what if anything would I do differently?

Evaluating your performance can assist you in enhancing your knowledge and build a deeper insight into focusing your learning objectives.

References

Bradbury-Jones C, Hughes SM, Murphy W, Parry L. A new way of reflecting in nursing: the Peshkin approach. J Adv Nurs. 2009; 65(11):2485–2493. Online Resource Available from http://www.ncbi.nlm.nih.gov/pubmed/19832751

Cambridge University Press Dictionary. 2019. Online Resource Available from https://dictionary.cambridge.org/dictionary/english/administration Accessed 9 Dec 2019

Conole G. Capturing practice; The role of mediating arte facts in learning design. In: Lockyer I, Agostinho SBS, Harper B, editors. Handbook of learning designs and learning objects. Hershey: IGI Global; 2008.

Conole G. Designing for learning in an open world, explorations in learning sciences, instructional systems and performance technologies. 4th ed. New York: Springer; 2013.

Health Services Executive Making Every Contact Count. 2019. Online Resources Available from https://www.hse.ie/eng/about/who/healthwellbeing/making-every-contact-count/ Accessed 9 Dec 2019

Mor Y, Warburton S, Winters N. Practical design principles for teaching and learning with technology: a book for sense publishers technology enhanced learning series, London: Sense Publishers; 2012. Online Resource Available from http://www.practicalpatternsbook.org/ Accessed 28 Feb 2013

State of the World's Nursing Report. 2020. [Internet]. [cited 2020 Apr 8]. Available from: https://www.who.int/publications-detail/nursing-report-2020

Topol E. The Patient will see you Now. New York: Basic Books; 2016.

Vaishnavi V, Kuechler W, Petter S, editors. Design science research in information systems, January 20, 2004 (created in 2004 and updated until 2015 by Vaishnavi, V. and Kuechler, W.); last updated (by Vaishnavi, V. and Petter, S.), June 30, 2019; 2004/2019. Online Resource Available from: http://www.desrist.org/design-research-in-information-systems/

Chapter 2
Connecting Health Immersion of Digital into eHealth

Pamela Hussey

Abstract Globally, in most countries the deployment and integration of national eHealth programmes is at an advanced stage. Digital progression in society is recognised as inevitable. Consequently, there is a growing awareness amongst nurse leaders for prioritisation of strategies relating to digital leadership and use of informatics competencies within the profession. As artificial intelligence, machine learning and robotics progress at an accelerated rate in society, thought leaders and policy makers turn their attention to consider how such technology can support healthy behaviors and health care delivery. Considerable efficiencies have been realised by deployment of digital in specific business domains such as fast food outlets, the hospitality and transport industries. Automation of passenger check in for example through air travel security has realised better use of staff time in processing of routine tasks and functions. The natural question is can such efficiencies be realised in the domain of healthcare? Large-scale deployment of digital within the health care domain lags somewhat behind other industries. Health administrations engaged with strategic business cases are deliberating on how the digital transformation can assist with planned service improvements from a macro, meso, and micro systems perspective. A key enabler in targeted service planning is the need to advance shared patient centric integrated care through interdisciplinary care service delivery. In this chapter we consider from a practical perspective the seismic impact of digital health, and how it will influence contemporary nursing practice.

Keywords eHealth · Digital · Reorientation health care models · Artificial intelligence · Machine learning · Nursing and technology

Electronic Supplementary Material The online version of this chapter (https://doi.org/10.1007/978-3-030-58740-6_2) contains supplementary material, which is available to authorized users.

P. Hussey (✉)
School of Nursing Psychotherapy and Community Health, Dublin City University, Dublin, Ireland
e-mail: pamela.hussey@dcu.ie

© Springer Nature Switzerland AG 2021
P. Hussey, M. A. Kennedy (eds.), *Introduction to Nursing Informatics*, Health Informatics, https://doi.org/10.1007/978-3-030-58740-6_2

Learning Objectives for the Chapter
1. Understand the nursing role in future health care delivery requirements.
2. Explain the principles underpinning change management in the implementation of the electronic health record and its variants.
3. Determine how information relating to patients can be used responsibly and ethically particularly in relation to Data Protection.
4. Understand the need for nursing engagement in design of systems and recording patient outcomes for self-management support.
5. Understand system theory agenda from the macro meso and micro context and explain where nursing can assist in advancing patient centered care.

2.1 Introduction

This chapter will introduce the reader to the topic of Connecting Health and using E-Health Systems and Digital. It will define key concepts used in digital and connected health in order to assist nurses to contextualise the role and use of eHealth in practice. The subject area is broad in scope, diverse in nature, and rapidly expanding. Globally, the context in which health and social care delivery processes occur varies widely. eHealth systems are at different stages of deployment internationally, and no country has achieved a fully interoperable Electronic Health Record across both community and acute services (Fennelly 2019a). There is however significant pressure to achieve fifth generation computing globally to advance interoperable Electronic Health Records and their variants. Fifth generation computing relates to using smart technologies such as artificial intelligence to have access to share and mine Internet data on platforms. This generation of computing is facilitating a surge of applications to support smart and mobile devices (Tutorialspoint 2020). Clinical opinion on the design of such devices is needed to align with the health domain and ensure what is implemented is ethically appropriate and safe. Health care strategic planning and revision on how we deliver health care has moved beyond acute episodic care. Increasingly a whole system approach to implementation of self-management support considers key actions are required across one to many service providers. Thus thinking and designing at a system level, which spans across the wider system, to the Organisation, and the health care professional and of course to the patient is required (Mullaney et al. 2016, p. 14). For this reason, in this chapter we use the wider and whole systems approach to present the evidence. Primary and ambulatory care is the foundation and the key to high-performing, sustainable and resilient health systems. Most health activity takes place in this setting with over eight billion encounters each year in OECD countries alone (Auraaen and Slawomirski 2018). In this chapter, we present the material from the three system levels and present with examples where appropriate. This approach provides a background context to unpack key insights required to explore and exploit eHealth and Digital in the connected health and social care domain.

2.2 The Wider System

There are many definitions of systems in the literature but core attributes of the definition is that a system involves a group of structures that together provide a function. From the perspective of informatics a system can be described as an ordered composition of inter related elements separated from and interfacing with its environment (Blobel 2019). Interfacing with the environment is important as it involves communicating with a number of actors such as organisations, people and technology. Each of these actors needs to be involved in designing and defining any changes in the existing system.

To understand systems in the domain of health care it is important to consider the concept of health, and how we define health globally. From as far back as 1948 the World Health Organisation defined health as a state of complete physical, mental and social wellbeing, and not merely the absence of disease and infirmity (World Health Organisation 1986). In 1986 at the First International Conference on Health Promotion, the World Health Organisation stated that health is a resource for everyday life and not just an objective for living. As a resource health is therefore important to monitor, and important to maintain for each individual in communities and within wider populations. Important dimensions in the quality of life of individuals include a number of contributory factors not only on the physical state of citizens, but also on the state of their mental and social well-being. Perceiving health maintenance and promotion activity as enabling processes can assist with maintaining or enhancing independence and self-efficacy (Mullaney et al. 2016). Increasingly national policy centres are using indicators to guide and evaluate quality improvements for population health. Both the population and individual system perspectives are now briefly expanded upon.

2.2.1 Population Health Perspective

Research and policy analysts in population health rely on health indicators to provide insights in tracking overall health and wellbeing of populations and monitoring of service requirements now and in the future. Patient Reported Experience Measures (PREM) and Paitent Reported Outcome Measures (PROMs) at the population level provide core metrics to drive quality and service improvements and are considered important metrics to signpost global health evaluation on quality of care and service delivery. For example reports from the Australian Health Services Research Institute informed the Australian Commission on Safety and Quality in Health Care (ACSQHC) by providing guidance on how reporting of PROMS and PREMS should be completed (Thompson et al. 2016). In this report they recommend that PREMS can guide service and quality improvements by capturing both experience and satisfaction measures. Collecting both types of measures they maintain is important as it offers the opportunity to identify particular aspects of patients' experiences, which have the strongest influence on their satisfaction. Collecting satisfaction measures solely without experience measures has potential to lead to subjective metrics influenced by outside factors such as patient expectations and personal characteristics. Examples of PREMs include time spent waiting, access and ability to navigate services, involvement in decision making, knowledge of care plan and pathways and support to manage long term condition (Thompson et al. 2016, p. 4). Patient reported outcome measures (PROM) or Patient-reported outcomes (PROs) are described as a directly reported outcome by the patient without interpretation of the patient's response by a clinician or anyone else. They pertain to the patient's health, quality of life, or functional status associated with health care or treatment (Food and Drug Administration 2009). As a specific domain, analysts are spending time turning their attention to consider just what and how to measure wellbeing in the society of the digital age. A key focus of this attention relates to patient safety, whereby figures from OECD report that half the global disease burden arising from patient harm originates in primary and ambulatory care (Auraaen and Slawomirski 2018).

Generally focusing on outcomes of care examples include, patients reporting on their symptoms, functional status and health-related quality-of-life (HRQoL) during and after their treatment. Outcomes can be generic and measure 'general' health status (generic PROMs) or disease-specific (for example, for asthma or diabetes) or condition-specific whereby the PROMs do not focus on a particular disease but on a broader health condition or state, for example mental health. PROMs include varied assessments and measures and include health status assessment, the HRQOL, Symptom reporting measures and satisfaction with care and treatment. There are also PROM instruments for assessing dimensions of patient experience such as a depression and anxiety. An interesting resource is available to view by Chen who conducted a scoping review on the topic (Chen 2015).

Studies in Wales also provide a good case example of a large-scale national electronic PROM data collection programme that was published in 2018 as part of an effectiveness programme. This study found that implementation of an electronic PROM resulted in most questions being understood and easy to answer by patients within the study, however clarity on questions relating to alcohol and exercise warranted editing and refinement for future studies (O'Connell et al. 2018).

At an individual person centric level there is much evidence on the importance for citizens to possess control over, and maintenance of one's health. Some describe the patient centric approach where citizens monitor and make decisions on their health as shifting the locus of power to the individual as the *democratisation of care* (Topol 2016). Traditionally, the medical model has not recognised well the expertise of the individuals being treated in our services. Individuals have been positioned as passive clients of care whose role it was to be diagnosed, investigated and adhere to treatment as prescribed without any active participation in decision making of care planning. Contemporary health and social care policy reject this model and recommend a Self Management Support (SMS) approach to care delivery. Self-management as a support approach can be described as follows.

The systematic provision of education and supportive interventions, to increase patients' skills and confidence in managing their health problems, including regular assessment of progress and problems, goal setting, and problem solving support. It is an important element of person centred care, acknowledging patients as partners in their own care, supporting them in developing the knowledge, skills and confidence to make informed decisions (Mullaney et al. 2016, p. 6).

Self-Management Support as an approach therefore draws on social cognitive theory. Considering an individual's biography and specific characteristics as important factors to take in to consideration when building a plan of care for an individual citizen. Over their lifetime, this SMS approach takes into consideration the individual's knowledge, which they have acquired over time, who they are interacting with for example the context of social interactions, experiences, and outside media influences which will have a potential impact on their ability to manage their conditions. They can be summarised under four core elements, self-evaluation, self-observation, self-regulation and self-efficacy, however the promotion of self-efficacy is considered a cornerstone of self-management support. If individuals have relevant knowledge and skills, they are more likely to accept responsibility for, and have confidence in, managing their own health. In addition, they will have an increased ability for solving future health problems with supporting evidence-based information. An example of a self-management support guidance and information resources from the Irish National Health Service are available to view online (Health Service Executive 2020). Figure 2.1 provides a summary of what self-management support framework looks like from recent published policy reports in Ireland (Mullaney et al. 2016, p. 20).

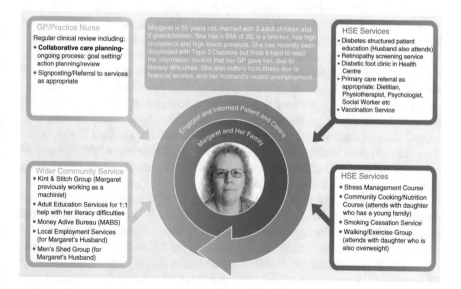

Fig. 2.1 Self-Management Support Framework (Mullaney et al. 2016)

The overall impact of this change for systems delivery is that individual patients play a more active role in self-management of health over the trajectory of their life course. This role includes emotional support, needs to consider the patients resilience and self-efficacy and includes a number of activities. These activities include but are not restricted to problem solving, shared decision making, action planning, and strong supports from health care professionals to access resources and provide supporting relationships.

Both the population and individual patient centered approaches to care delivery as outlined above are supported at policy level as global population trends predict that people are increasingly living longer and living with rather than dying from chronic illness (McEvoy 2014). Increasing our collective understanding that systems we currently use cannot continue without radical transformation is important. Digital and eHealth resources provide supports for transitioning to new models of care by providing a number of different networks.

2.2.2   eHealth and Digital

Two key international organisations drive the policy agenda for eHealth and digital globally.

State side the Pan American Health Organisation (PAHO) is an international public health agency working to improve health and living standards of the people of the Americas. Founded in 1902 with its headquarters in Washington it has a dedicated web portal for eHealth to promote the use of information and communication technologies (ICT) for health, and thereby foster universal access to health in the Americas (Regional Office of the Americas World Health Organisation 2020). Since 2011 in association with the World Health Organisations PAHO has endorsed a strategy urging the Organization to work to improve health service accessibility and quality using ICTs. Primarily this strategy focuses its energies under seven key areas. These include, governance for co-ordination for eHealth at regional and global level, supporting national strategies across the region, promoting standards and interoperability in addition to deployment of electronic health records, telehealth, mHealth and digital literacy. A recent Global Survey on eHealth in the Americas provides insights on progress from 2016 in nineteen of the region's 38 countries and is now available to view on the PAHO website (Regional Office of the Americas World Health Organisation 2020).

From the perspective of the European Union, in 2020 a new digital strategy is proposed across Europe. The European Commission is creating a new Digital European Wide programme, with €9.2 billion allocation of funding, the objective of which is to align the EU's next long-term budget for 2021–2027 with the growing challenges in the digital field. Building on the earlier strategy a Digital Agenda for Europe, the EU's programme 2021–2027 will focus on building the strategic digital capacities of the EU and on facilitating the wide deployment of digital technologies, to be used by Europe's citizens and businesses. Core areas of investment include supercomputing, artificial intelligence, cybersecurity, advanced digital skills, and ensuring a wide use of digital technologies across the economy and society. Its goal is to improve Europe's competitiveness in the global digital economy and increase its technological autonomy. Specifically investing in broadening the use of super-computing in areas of public interest such as health, environment and security, and in industry and engaging with small and medium-sized enterprises is part of the new strategic plan. The new digital Europe plan commences on January 2021 and detail of this Progamme is available from the European Commission Website and associated fact sheet (EU Commission 2019; OECD 2020a).

In November 2019, the Organisation for Economic Co-operation and Development (OECD) an international Organisation that works to *build better policies for better lives* published a report on digital transformation defining indicators on a roadmap for the future. This report provides an interactive toolkit and seven key policy dimensions. These policy dimensions relating to advancing digital include key concepts relating to market openness, access, use, innovation, job, society, trust and growth and wellbeing (OECD 2020b). OECD indicate that in the policy dimension relating to growth and wellbeing that the ongoing digital transformation of the economy and society holds many promises to spur innovation, generate efficiencies and improve services. It can therefore boost growth in addition to empowering people by increasing access to information and enabling new forms of social engagement. OECD suggest however, that such benefits come with challenges. Digital transformation changes the nature and structure of health care organisations, markets and communities, potentially raising concerns about equity and inclusion in society. Offering guidance, this OECD report linking to articulated policy dimensions, list key themes with specific indicators one of which relates to skills.

Defined as foundational, ICT and complementary skills, OECD stresses the attainment of skills as important for both quality of work and life. Additional publications from the nursing perspective report that a large number of OECD countries are implementing educational, regulatory and/or payment specific reforms to expand the practice profile of nurses. Suggesting that advancement of the nursing role incorporates two concepts. First, task shifting (a concept also referred to as 'substitution') whereby nurses—after additional training—take up activities formerly performed by physicians to alleviate shortages, reduce physician workloads and/or improve access. Second, nurses can also take on new complementary roles in clinical areas (often referred to as 'supplementation'), such as case managers, liaison roles. Such roles they suggest include interventions relating to eHealth monitoring and providing lifestyle advice. OECD suggests that the boundaries between these two types of advanced roles are not always evident and in some instances, they can overlap. One commonality within the profession is the advancement of nurse education, particularly focusing on the expanding role of nursing which is extending beyond the traditional scope of practice of registered nurses (Maier et al. 2017, p. 8). A discussion on the topic of nurse education skills knowledge and competency attainment is progressed further in Chaps. 11 and 15. Here in this chapter we suggest that for the profession of nursing stressing that the right mixture of skills is important in a fast-moving digital landscape, and that there is scope to review practice roles. Core to these new roles will be understanding the shifting models of care and in particular how eHealth and digital competencies within the profession of nursing need to considered as an important core competency. To look at set themes or indicators by country see OECD (2019) Measuring the Digital Transformation: A Roadmap for the Future which illustrates country indicators and themes in the following online resource http://goingdigital.oecd.org/en/themes/.

OECD (2019), measuring the Digital Transformation: A Roadmap for the Future, OECD Publishing, Paris.

Considering health and systems for delivery of care in the wider context, it is important to recognise that the domain of health does not operate in a vacuum. Just as social care determinants of health as defined in population demographic are important for the dimensions in management of illness so too is the attainment of the specific environmental goals. Delivery of the Sustainable Development Goals (SDG) by 2030 is the flagship policy of the United Nations (United Nations D of E and SA 2019). There are 17 goals, which are listed in the Table 2.1 and which were published in 2015.

Table 2.1 Sustainable Development Goals

1.	No poverty: End poverty in all its form everywhere
2.	Zero Hunger: End hunger, achieve food security and improved nutrition and promote sustainable agriculture
3.	Good Health and Wellbeing: Ensure healthy lives and promote well-being for all at all ages
4.	Quality Education: Ensure inclusive and equitable quality education and promote lifelong learning opportunities for all
5.	Gender Equality: Achieve gender equality and empower all women and girls
6.	Clean Water and Sanitation: Ensure availability and sustainable management of water and sanitation for all
8.	Decent Work and Economic Growth: Promote sustained, inclusive and sustainable economic growth, full and productive employment and decent work for all
9.	Industry Innovation and Infrastructure: Build resilient infrastructure, promote inclusive and sustainable industrialization and foster innovation
10.	Reduced Inequalities: Reduce inequality within and among countries
11.	Sustainable Cities and Communities: Make cities and human settlements inclusive, safe, resilient and sustainable
12.	Responsible Consumption and Production: Ensure sustainable consumption and production patterns
13.	Climate Action: Take urgent action to combat climate change and its impacts
14.	Life Below Water: Conserve and sustainably use the oceans, seas and marine resources for sustainable development
15.	Life On Land: Protect, restore and promote sustainable use of terrestrial ecosystems, sustainably manage forests, combat desertification, and halt and reverse land degradation and halt biodiversity loss
16.	Peace Justice and Strong Institutions: Promote peaceful and inclusive societies for sustainable development, provide access to justice for all and build effective, accountable and inclusive institutions at all levels
17.	Partnerships for the Goals: Strengthen the means of implementation and revitalize the global partnership for sustainable development

For a full review of the MDG see the UN website (United Nations D of E and SA 2019).

Health and social care providers are primarily focused on SDG 3. This sustainable goal is to ensure healthy lives and promote wellbeing for all at all ages. Also to note target 9.1 of SDG 9 focuses on innovation and infrastructure and seeks to develop quality, reliable, sustainable and resilient infrastructure, including regional and transborder infrastructure, to support economic development and human wellbeing, with a focus on affordable and equitable access for all. An example of an EU project which links to SDG 3 and SDG 9 is provided here as an example of how the millennium goals are being actioned through the Connecting Europe Facility (CEF) (Connecting Europe Facility 2015).

The CEF benefits people across all European Member States, as it makes travel easier and more sustainable, it enhances Europe's digital infrastructure by facilitating cross-border interaction between public administrations, businesses and citizens. Since 2011, the European institutions have been engaged in cross-border health services which are being progressively introduced in all EU Member States. The cross border health services provides access to two core services. Firstly, ePrescription and eDispensation which allows any EU citizen to retrieve his/her medication in a pharmacy located in another EU Member State. This occurs through the electronic transfer of their prescription from his/her country of residence to the country of travel via the CEF services EU portal. Secondly, access to a Patient Summaries which provides background information on important health-related aspects such as allergies, current medication, previous illness, surgeries, etc., making it digitally accessible in case of a medical (emergency) visit in another country (EUR-Lex 2020; BELLERIN MLS 2019).

2.2.3 Progress on Health and Social Care Delivery Goals 2010–2020

A report published in 2018 by the UN provides concerning insights in relation to progression and status of the Millennium Goals using available data from 2013 to 2018. The report indicates that close to 40% of all countries had fewer than 10 medical doctors per 10,000 people, and more than 55% had fewer than 40 nursing and midwifery personnel per 10,000 people. In addition, this report indicates that all least developed countries are reported to have had fewer than 10 medical doctors and fewer than 5 dentists and 5 pharmacists per 10,000 people, and 98% had fewer than 40 nursing and midwifery personnel per 10,000 people (United Nations Economic and Social Council 2019, p. 10).

Predictive models published in 2017 through The Lancet Journal provides a framework for projecting health systems strengthening for population-level and individual-level health service coverage from 2016 to 2030 was devised. This paper estimated the associated costs and health effects projecting available funding by country and year. The study found that an additional $274 billion spending on health is needed per year by 2030 to make progress with SDG 3 targets. Despite projected increases in health spending, a financing gap of $20–54 billion per year is projected when specific factors were taken into account. Should funds be made available and used as planned, the ambitious scenario would save 97 million lives and significantly increase life expectancy by 3.1–8.4 years in accordance with the country profile. This report recommended that all countries will need to strengthen investments in health systems to expand service provision in order to reach SDG 3 health targets (Stenberg et al. 2017). This prediction predates the Covid 19 pandemic of 2020.

Following on with the global policy agenda the publication of the World Health Organisation National eHealth Strategy Toolkit in 2015 (World Health Organisation 2012), reporting on global diffusion of eHealth in 2016 offers additional evidence from its third global survey on eHealth. Reports suggest the process of embedding eHealth everywhere still has a long way to go, in terms of both coverage and functionality. Suggesting a mixed picture, progress is reflected in different countries based on national and local priorities. Key anticipated enablers to drive developments over the next 5–10 years include the advancement of low cost smart phones, social media and big data. The potential over the next 10 years for low-cost smartphones to enable virtually everyone everywhere to have access to audio-visual examples of best (global and local) practices could impact on improving health behaviors and represent a paradigm shift in health care. Such advancements depend however on learning, vision, sharing and comparing experiences across communities (WHO 2020, p. 7). Later, in a 2018, the WHO published The Classification of Digital Health interventions (DHIs) which categorizes the different ways in which digital and mobile technologies are being used to support health system needs (World Health Organisation 2018). Targeting primarily public health audiences, this report reflects emerging uses of digital health interventions providing a set of overarching groupings for leveraging mobile health categorisations. These include Interventions for clients, interventions for health care providers, interventions for health system to resource managers, interventions for data services. Each digital health intervention represents a discrete functionality of the digital technology to achieve a health sector objective. Within the health system challenges the digital health intervention are listed in Fig. 2.2.

2.3   The Organisation

In the previous section, we presented the systems wide perspective and considered progress towards achieving SDG3 health and wellbeing for all. In order to move towards ensuring that all people and communities have access to health services, the organisational culture of organisations needs to consider impact of connected health and transformative use of digital and eHealth. Having a shared understanding at an organisational level of core concept definitions is important Boxes 2.1 and 2.2 provide the definitions adopted for this fifth edition of this text to explain key concepts Digital and eHealth.

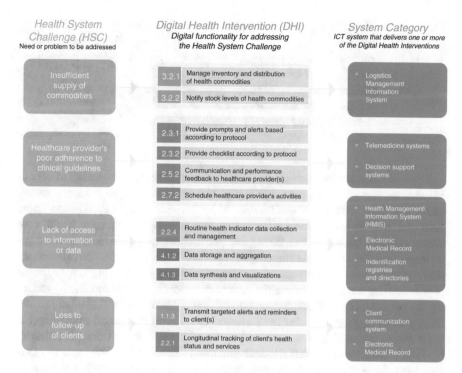

Fig. 2.2 Health System Challenges and Digital Health Interventions (World Health Organisation 2018)

Box 2.1 Definition of Digital Health

Digital Health is used as an umbrella term for areas including eHealth, tele-health, mHealth and more (see explanations below). Digital Health is the integration of all information and knowledge sources involved in the delivery of healthcare via information technology (IT)-based systems. This includes information created by caregivers, often within electronic health record systems at a hospital or GP practice, and information created by patients using apps, monitoring devices and wearable sensors. Digital health information also includes management and administrative information needed to co-ordinate and manage activities within the healthcare system cited from the Irish Platform for Patient Organisations, Science and Industry (IPPOSI 2020).

> **Box 2.2 Definition of eHealth**
> eHealth is the use of information and communication technologies that support the remote management of people and communities with a range of health care needs through supporting self-care and enabling electronic communications between health care professionals and patients. Source World Health Organisation eHealth Web (WHO 2020).

Organisations are increasingly seeking to collect indicators on quality of care to advance service improvement using digital and eHealth strategic transformational plans. The three indictors of quality defined by Berwick et al. in 2008 as the Triple Aim of Care has been widely accepted as foundational for effective health care system delivery (Berwick et al. 2008), and needs consideration in tandem with digital transformation. The triple aim proposes that health care organisations simultaneously pursue three dimensions of performance. Firstly improving the health of populations, secondly enhancing the patient experience of care, and thirdly reducing the per capita cost of health care. Subsequent publications by Bodenheimer and Sinsky in 2014, recommended the inclusion of a fourth dimension expanding the triple aim to the quadruple aim with a fourth goal improving the work life of health provider's clinicians and staff (Bodenheimer and Sinsky 2014). The topic of clinician work force planning and burnout is discussed further in Chap. 9. From a systems perspective for this chapter it is however useful to consider interventions and consider how they interface with the quadruple aims particularly for service improvement initiatives. For example, is it important that such initiatives include locally developed and context specific designed requirements to realise anticipated benefits and ensure clinicians and staff in organisations guide the development process. This approach supports the value proposition and is in line with good design for sustainable adoption (Berwick et al. 2008; Bodenheimer and Sinsky 2014; Greenhalgh et al. 2017).

An example of a framework which evaluates systems for health and social care technologies is presented in a research paper entitled the NASSS A New Framework for Theorizing and Evaluating Non adoption, Abandonment, and Challenges to the Scale-Up, Spread, and Sustainability of Health and Care Technologies published by Greenhalgh et al. (2017). This large study reviewed 28 technology implementation frameworks and included over 400 hours of ethnographic observation. The net result of this was a matrix of a requirements analysis framework, which can be used for analysis on any technological innovations in health and social care. This analysis can provide insight on informing the design of a new technology; identifying technological solutions and gauging their chance of achieving large-scale, sustained adoption, or to plan the implementation, scale-up, or rollout of a technology program. The framework can also be used retrospectively to explain and learn from program failures. The framework includes seven domains and classifies each project as simple (straightforward, predictable, few components), complicated (multiple interacting components or issues), or complex (dynamic, unpredictable, not easily disaggregated into constituent components). The seven domains used in the NASSS framework include the condition or illness, the technology, the value proposition, the adopter system (comprising professional staff, patient, and lay caregivers), the organization(s), the wider (institutional and societal) context, and the interaction and mutual adaptation between all these domains over time. In the domain of organisational management there is much literature published. In NASSS the organisational domain lists some key facilitators, which are critical as follows; the need for leadership with a capacity to innovate and the degree of the organisations readiness for the proposed change the system will necessitate. Finally, the nature of the adoption and extent of the change and work required to implement the change including any modifications to routine practices, which can cause additional burden (Greenhalgh et al. 2017, p.11).

Organisational theory stresses the need for strong leadership and recognition that staff in organisations provides the cultural glue to guide behaviors, create an overall sense of purpose and personal connection for digital transformation in healthcare (Organizational Change 2020, Kerr 2013). This process includes four stages for organisational change as defined by Hogg (World Health Organisation 2016).

- Building a case for change
- Building a compelling picture of the future
- Providing a sustained capability to change
- Providing a credible plan to execute

To achieve this target organisations need to advance patient centred integrated care services. WHO in 2016 published the Framework on integrated, people-centred health services (World Health Organisation 2016) which highlights that interventions need to be locally developed and negotiated. Each specific context dictates the mix of strategies to be used in response to local circumstances, values and preferences. There are five key strategies to achieve integrated care, which are expanded upon in the following section under Health Care Practitioner (HCP) and The Patient.

- Strategy 1: Empowering and engaging people and communities
- Strategy 2: Strengthening governance and accountability
- Strategy 3: Reorienting the model of care
- Strategy 4: Coordinating services within and across sectors
- Strategy 5: Creating an enabling environment

2.4   The Health Care Professional and Individual

Each of the five strategies listed in this framework has a key role to play in advancing connected health and realising people centred health services aligning with global policy on new models of care. Each one is briefly now expanded on in the following Sects. 2.4.1–2.4.4 with some related examples.

2.4.1 Strategy 1: Empowering and Engaging People and Communities

In Strategy 1 the WHO states, a call for change is urgently needed and indicates that it is essential to better respond to and prepare for health emergency crises providing examples such as the Ebola Virus Disease Outbreak (World Health Organisation 2016, p. 9). The purpose of Strategy 1 is to unlock community and individual resources for action at all levels. Empowering and engaging individuals to make decisions about their own health and to become co-producers of their own health. Over time, such strategic action will enable citizens to empower communities to co-produce healthy environments support the voice of minority populations and contribute to healthy public policy (World Health Organisation 2016, p. 21). Examples on how digital and connected health can advance Strategy 1 are illustrated here in the Nex project with some examples of digital devices in use in a feasibility study in Ireland. Further information on Strategy 1 is available from the following link:

https://apps.who.int/iris/bitstream/handle/10665/155002/WHO_HIS_SDS_2015.6_eng?sequence=1.

Case Study for Strategy 1: The NEX Digital Transformation Feasibility Study

The Nex research programme is conducting a feasibility study with a software company entitled Davra to determine how digital health devices can assist individual citizens to live independently in their home supported by appropriate digital health supporting services. Implementation research in Dublin City University (DCU), Dublin in Ireland with a team of academics and the industry partner Davra are testing digital resources using cross platform access to assist people to self-manage their own illnesses and co-produce design changes in their living environments to empower and make choices about care and treatment options. Figure 2.3a demonstrates health monitoring for the individual client using wearable personalized sensors. Figure 2.3b demonstrates how a home can be equipped with digital sensors to promote safety and wellness in the home. Providing structures to support reciprocal relationship between clinical and non-clinical professionals and the individuals using care services, their families, carers and communities (Organizational Change 2020; World Health Organisation 2016). Box 2.3 provides a case study and an example of a scenario used in the Center for eIntegrated Care (CeIC) in DCU to test health monitoring devices with a dedicated nursing scholarship group. Addtional examples of scenarios created in this case study are also included in Appendix 1 of this chapter. The focus of this learning activity exercise is to test and define requirements for continuity of care in the home for older adults with experienced nursing practitioners using digital health sensors.

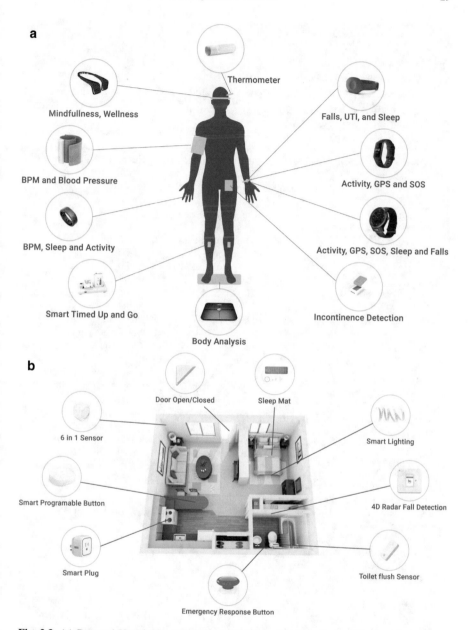

Fig. 2.3 (**a**) Personal Health Monitoring Suite Wearable The Nex Project; (**b**) Personal Health Monitoring Suite The Nex Project

Box 2.3 Case Example (Davra 2020; CeIC 2020) Example 1: The Nex Project

In this case based example a scenario is provided of how ambient and wearable sensors can be used in the home as illustrated in Figure 2.3a and Figure 2.3b.

Scenario A—Introducing John CEIC Simulation Case Study Service User Background

Scenario 1 Introducing John CeIC Simulation Case Study	Health Management	Current Medical Problems
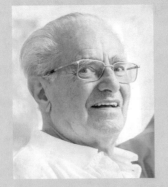 **About John** John is 72 year old widower, he lives in a residential complex with a mild cognitive decline. He has limited hearing and wears hearing aids in both ears. He also wears varifocal glasses for short and long vision. In 2018, John was diagnosed with Parkinson's disease and although he manages to mobilise in his residential home with the support of a walking stick, he is anxious about falling. He has a son Christopher and a daughter Mary who visit once a week and at the weekends, he often goes out to his family's home for lunch	His son Christopher manages his appointments and currently John is under the care of Three consultants: 1. Urologist 2. Neurologist 3. Gerontologist **Use of Technology— Dexterity** John can answer a mobile phone but cannot text; increasingly the television remote control is a problem for him to manage in his single room in which he resides. He does not use any other technology and needs help with his hearing aid remote control, which he finds difficult to operate with his tremor	Recurrent urinary tract infections × 3 in the past 12 months have led John to spend a lot of time in the toilet. **Activities of Daily Living** John is anxious about his increasing episodes of incontinence. He has fallen twice in the past 3 months once during the day when rushing to the toilet, and once at night mobilising from bed to the bathroom. In the past year, he finds eating meals difficult, his dietary and fluid intake are down, and his family have noticed that he has lost weight

Scenario Background 1—The setting is a residential community unit there is one member of staff available at night—they sleep from midnight to 0630 h.

John usually retires to bed at 22.30 h and sleeps for short periods only, he doesn't sleep well primarily because of the need to go the bathroom overnight—usually three times a night and he is anxious that he may be incontinent. He also has restless legs which impede his mobility and is partly attributable to his Parkinson's disease.

Day of week and time	Location	Activity—patient	Monitoring/sensors in place in location	Action from sensor	Nurse/carer activity
Saturday Morning 00:30 h	John's bedroom Single bed Light bed linen Height of the bed is ideal for his height and does not impact on his mobility/falls risk. He uses a Zimmer frame to mobilise. This is usually left adjacent to his bed at night. There are no other obstacles in the room which could present a slip/ trip or fall hazard	• Sleeping for short periods waking to go to the toilet. • Turning in bed from side to side. • Restless legs	1. Motion sensor—bedroom 2. Plug paired with strip light 3. Sleep Tracking Mat 4. Fit Bit watch 5. Toilet sensor	Status—all sensors monitoring	Carer in other part of house checking other service users before they go to bed
Saturday Morning 00:40 h	John's bedroom	John sits up in the bed and begins to get out of the bed John places his feet onto the floor and he attempts to put on his slippers and find his Zimmer frame	1. Motion sensor 2. Plug paired with strip light 3. Fit Bit Watch tracking 4. Sleep Tracking Mat 5. Toilet sensor	Status—monitoring 1. Motion sensor activated to alert carers that he is out of bed and moving 2. Light strip activated 3. Fit Bit Watch tracking 4. Toilet Flush sensor	Carer alerted by alarm from motion sensor Carer responds to alarm, enters John's room and escorts to bathroom

Day of week and time	Location	Activity— patient	Monitoring/sensors in place in location	Action from sensor	Nurse/carer activity
Saturday Morning 00:55 h	John's walks with carer to bathroom using his Zimmer frame wearing his slippers	John walks/ shuffles to bathroom	1. Motion sensor in bathroom activated 2. Plug paired with strip light 3. Toilet Flush sensor activated 4. Fit Bit Watch tracking	Status— monitoring 1. Room motion sensors activated 2. Light strip activated 3. Toilet Flush sensor 4. Fit Bit Watch tracking	Carer escorts John to bathroom and returns John to bed, ensures he is comfortable and a drink given. Zimmer frame and slippers are placed appropriately by the carer in case he needs to get out of bed again

Physical props required for Scenario 1	Actors required for Scenario 1	Technology IT props required
All sensors active as listed Links to Hub working Curtains/blind closed Slippers Pyjamas Zimmer frame Drink at bedside	John (service user) Carer Observer	• All sensors active as listed • Links to Hub working • Messaging device to alert carer to motion sensor being activated—*mobile phone send text message*—carer located in reception area of Clinical Skills Centre

Evaluation	

2.4.2 Strategy 2: Strengthening Governance and Accountability

Strategy 2 strengthening governance and accountability relates to effective governance and accountability in health systems. Recommending a need to promote transparency in decision-making and for health organisations to generate robust systems for the collective accountability of health providers and health system managers through aligning governance, accountability and incentives (World Health Organisation 2016, p. 24). Firstly that the report lists three characteristics for effective governance and accountability structures. Secondly, that mechanisms are established through which service providers are held accountable and thirdly that

Box 2.4

Improving health outcomes requires a renewed focus on tackling the social determinants of ill-health and placing health at the centre of all policies through strong stewardship and intersectoral action. Without this, the excessive specialization of health care providers and the narrow focus on disease management programmes that discourages holistic care will continue to predominate (p.10).

adequate information is available to be able to assess the services, which are provided. Finally, those structures are in place whereby patients are empowered to take action. The need for stewardship and citizen engagement is also emphasised as critically important as the following quote demonstrates;

2.4.3   Strategy 3: Reorienting the Model of Care

For Strategy 3, the focus is on reorientation models of care aligning, prioritising primary, and community care services with active engagement of citizens in the co-production of health. From a health care professional and individual citizen perspective, it encompasses the shift from inpatient to ambulatory and outpatient care, and the need for a fully integrated and effective referral system (World Health Organisation 2016, p. 27). The strategic focus for strategy three also includes investment on holistic models of care, which include interventions on health promotion and on ill health prevention supporting health and wellbeing to support social determinants of health. Challenges listed on reorientating models of care include addressing the Hospital "dominance" in terms of service organization and budget allocation. At a hospital organisational level key implications on the service approach of relevance in this text include

1. Ensuring that hospitals form part of a coordinated/integrated health services delivery network that balances budget allocations across all care settings
2. Improved coordination with rest of care providers to ensure continuity of care for patients with increased focus on quality, safety and person-centred care
3. Greater accountability for population health outcomes and clinical results (World Health Organisation 2016, p. 28).

Figure 2.1 provided in the earlier Sect. 2.2.1 demonstrates care plan on how a model of care for a citizen is structured (Mullaney et al. 2016).

2.4.4   Strategy 4: Coordinating Services Within and Across Sectors

Strategy 4 of the WHO PIC framework calls for better care co-ordination as a critical enabler for delivery of this framework drawing on material discussed in Sect. 2.2.1 and other associated strategies listed in the WHO Interim report. Arguing the case that the core purpose of co-ordinating services across sectors is to overcome the fragmentations in care delivery, which undermines the ability of health care service teams and families to provide safe, accessible, high quality and cost-effective care in order to improve care experiences and outcomes for people (World Health Organisation 2016, p. 30). Supporting the aforementioned quadruple aim by Bodenheimer and Sinsky (Bodenheimer and Sinsky 2014), Strategy 4 draws the integration of key public health functions including surveillance, early detection and rapid emergency response capacity into the health service delivery system to address emergencies and potential hazards faced by the contemporary health care systems. From a health care professional perspective, the WHO report recommends moving from the traditional service delivery patterns, which have focused on episodic and vertically oriented interactions between individuals and health care providers. Such approaches fail to respond to the inherent complexity of people's health problems. What is required are co-ordinated systems that are sustainable and capable of evolving to better address patient needs.

2.4.5 Strategy 5: Creating an Enabling Environment

In order to make the four previous strategic plans an operational reality, The WHO framework for patient centreed care advocates the need to create an enabling environment that brings together the different stakeholders to undertake transformational change. Recognising the complexity of this task the following critical enablers are recommended and illustrated in the following Fig. 2.4 which summarises structures required for an enabling environment.

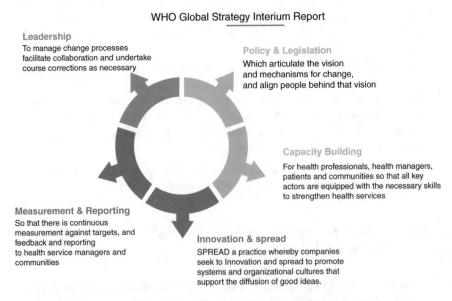

Fig. 2.4 Structures for enabling environment (World Health Organisation 2016)

As is evident from the material presented here to advance universal health care and align the WHO global strategy on people-centred and integrated health services at each system level of development and design, there is extensive work needed to implement the changes required. From a health informatics perspective, interoperability is considered the core foundation stone or building block required to realizing structural functional and behavioural shifts in care delivery to underpin integrated care. This is required across all three system viewpoints the macro mesa and micro. Recognised as difficult to achieve (Benson and Grieve 2016), Interoperability is not solely about sharing data but rather sharing knowledge across a number of different dimensions of the health care domain (Blobel 2019). This chapter therefore includes a brief introductory section on interoperability.

2.5 Interoperability and Risk

Described as difficult to achieve interoperability is at the heart of building next generation models of care at the systems level. Considered as a critical springboard to drive transformation at a global and national level, Interoperability and its clinical counterpart integrated care, form the foundation stone for connecting digital and eHealth services. Both are linked to patient safety, are complex and dynamic to deliver effectively, and require adoption of standards across services for successful deployment (Benson and Grieve 2016). As such an essential topic we believe it is important for nurses to understand some of the theory underpinning interoperability and therefore provide the reader with some finer points on the topic some of which will be expanded upon in Chap. 6.

2.5.1 What Is Interoperability and Why Is It Important

Interoperability is defined in the literature in many different ways. Experts from the European Health Informatics Standards Working Groups (CEN Portal 2020) emphasise the need to consider interoperability as having social, political, and technical dimensions. Indicating that any development initiative relating to interoperability needs to consider all three dimensions concurrently in service requirements design. Alternatively, Palfrey and Glasser suggest interoperability has four layers namely Technology, Data, Human, and Institutional layers which require analysis (Palfrey and Gasser 2012). The most widely used definition adopted is by the IEEE in 1990 which states that

> Interoperability is the ability of two or more systems or components to exchange information and to use information that has been exchanged IEEE 1990 (IEEE 1990).

The core message is that interoperability is a multidimensional dynamic and evolving phenomenon. Different perspectives need careful consideration across the aforementioned system levels, focusing solely on one dimension for deployment in a programme does not fully address the complexity of the topic (Beránková et al. 2010). At the organisational level, for example it is critically important to be cognisant to potential barriers that work against national agendas for sharing and access to data. In large scale deployment of enterprise wide systems project managers must be diligent at the initial procurement stage to ensure vendors conform with national approved standards for interoperability in order to optimise future care co-ordination nationally. In addition, the value proposition and maximising a return on investment for organisations and national bodies needs to be evident. There is much evidence, which demonstrates negative impact towards cost containment on original budget. A core aspect of the procurement process includes avoiding vendor lock in, ensuring privacy concerns are addressed and access by individual patients are realised (Fortune 2020).

Some core principles in procurement to minimise risk and anticipated return on investment include adopting a system wide approach underpinned by focused engagement and consultation during the pre-tender process. Procurement processes should include a competitive procedure, which involves negotiation to cultivate innovative partnerships. Procurement should also use a balanced approach developing procurement in lots ensuring that the appropriate procurement approach is selected. This is achievable by reviewing all procurement options with value based award criteria in order to choose the option that best suits the technology (Davis and Brady 2015).

The 36 billion dollars investment by Obama care is a good case study, which illustrates problems encountered in organisations where a number of issues were identified. Some of major issues relate to interoperability and access of patients to their health records (Fortune 2020). Reporting Fred Schulte and Erika Fry conducted a review of the Obama based programme entitled Meaningful Use, which was published in Fortune Magazine. Summarising the issues identified related to the following; Access to health information across and between hospitals communities and individual patients. Poor integration and closed systems design. Spiralling costs at the local and organisational level Poor interface design accuracy of data and an overall absence of standards conformance. A review of clinical information capture in Electronic Health Records in Ireland published in 2019 identified 21 key issues from the literature from the literature through an advisory group approach. These issues could be defined in three sections.

Firstly in regards to data entry methods, what and how personal health information is stored and used in accordance with data protection and security is important. In additon to considering how health care professionals practice recording health information or use patient information. Otherwise information systems and associated workflow are inefficient and may have unintended consequences leading to workarounds.

Secondly, a broad approach to clinical data types is recommended. The need for unstructured, structured, coded and semi structured data types should be included to accommodate different clinical scenarios and for secondary use of data which is considered important.

Finally data entry by patients should be included and capacity to connect adjunct devices to interface to the Electronic health record in the future should be considered (Fortune 2020; Fennelly 2019b).

Chapter 10 discusses Data Protection and Data Security in detail. Increasingly with new regulations enacted in the·European Union in 2018 organisations are obliged to uphold the the General Data Protection Regulation laws across member states. Failure to adhere to the privacy and security standards regulations leaves organisations open to paying harsh fines. Considered the toughest privacy and security law in the world Europe with this latest regulation adopts a firm stance on data privacy and security. This they argue is warranted at a time when more people are entrusting their personal data with cloud services and breaches are a daily occurrence. The regulation itself is large, and has far-reaching consequences on industry and organisations and we include here a summary of the detail and core concepts defined in the new regulation (GDPR 2018).

- GDPR defines personal data as any information any information that relates to an individual who can be directly or indirectly identified.
- Data processing involves any action performed on data, whether automated or manual. This includes collecting, recording, organizing, structuring, storing of information.
- Data subject is described as the person whose data is processed including site visitors on webpages.
- Data controller is the person who decides why and how personal data will be processed and relates to the owner of an organisation.
- Data processor is a third party that processes personal data on behalf of a data controller. The GDPR has special rules for these individuals and organizations.

There are seven protection and accountability principles, which individuals must comply with, and these are;

- Lawfulness
- Fairness and transparency
- Purpose limitation
- Data minimization (Collect and process only as much data as absolutely necessary for the purposes specified)
- Accuracy
- Storage limitation
- Integrity and confidentiality (Processing must be done in such a way as to ensure appropriate security, integrity, and confidentiality e.g. by using encryption)
- Accountability (The data controller is responsible for being able to demonstrate GDPR compliance with all of these principles) (GDPR 2018).

As individuals increasingly adopt digital in society, the debate on data protection grows more important. Considering GDPR it is important to achieve the optimal balance and level of interoperability particularly for data access and sharing of sensitive health information. As the Vice President-Designate of the European

Commission for a Europe fit for the Digital Age Margarethe Vestager in an EU interview on digital deployment within the EU says, *what we will accept and what we will not accept in society should not be any different in a digital world* (European Commission 2020).

A body of work is required to define the ways systems work together and to consider what data the systems shall and shall not share. This is best achieved by building case studies called Use Case to identify core functionality and structural elements of any planned system. Use Case can then be used to test prototypes and determine how they should interact with each other to support care co-ordination without undue patient risk or comprising patient confidentiality. This approach will be further expanded upon in Chap. 5 of this text.

Today Digital transformation continues to bring unprecedented changes to every aspect of the economy and society, it is important to remember that it brings both new opportunities challenges and risks and these risks need be monitored carefully. From a systems wide perspective the challenges standards and solutions paper published by Blobel to address the interoperability challenge is summarised (Fig. 2.5). This diagram is followed by a short description of the core elements discussed in this paper which need to be considered at both the information and the organisation level (Blobel 2018; Blobel and Oemig 2016).

A number of the core concepts as identified in Fig. 2.5 will be discussed in detail in the proceeding chapters, in this initial chapter on connecting health we provide summary of this structure with some broad examples for clarity.

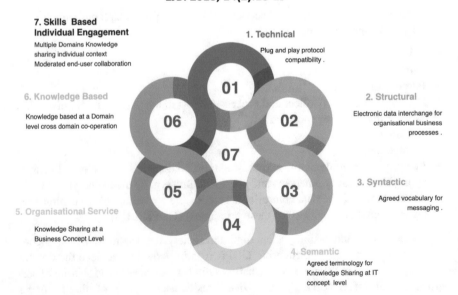

Fig. 2.5 Summary representation of *Blobel Interoperability Levels* (Blobel 2018)

1. The *Technical* challenge is required to address connectivity of systems. Examples of technical solutions for connecting health include protocols for compatibility such The File Transfer Protocol (FTP). As standard FTP is a network protocol used for the transfer of computer files between a client and server on a computer network (Fennelly 2019b).

2. The *Structural* challenge addresses the different levels of data exchange. Examples provided by Blobel include Electronic Data Interchanges (EDI) for exchange of business transaction documents across a network of different service providers.

3. The *Syntactic* challenge deals with structured messages such as clinical documents using an agreed vocabulary. This approach is addressed in health care systems with messaging standards such as HL7 and a set of structured protocols such as IHE profiles, which are expanded upon in detail in Chap. 5.

4. The *Semantic* Challenge is well documented in the evidence base. Here the challenge relates to the creation of detailed coded data sets underpinned by common information models and common terminologies. Much progress has been made in the past 20 years globally on defining detailed semantic platforms to share concepts and terms in health and social care records. The most commonly referenced one being Snomed CT (Fennelly 2019b). This is topic is expanded upon in Chap. 6.

5. The *Organisational* challenge has been discussed above. Core to addressing the issues raised in the organisational challenge is the need for a well defined business case which describes in detail the common business processes from both the functional and behavioural aspects of the system to meet defined business objectives. Here we also include additional earlier references from Blobel (Blobel and Oemig 2016, p. 16). What is also noted in the organisational challenge is the need for correct representation of the domains of knowledge using domain ontologies. For nursing engagement in domain ontologies see (Hussey and McGlinn 2019).

6. The *Knowledge based* challenge is described by Blobel as those domains of discourse which use domain specific terminologies which are underpinned with defined ontologies. They shoud align with business objectives and be defined by domain experts. An example of a domain of discourse could be the family of WHO classifications such as the International Classification for Nursing Practice (ICNP©) (ICN 2020).

7. The need for *Skills Based Individual* Engagement where different domains share knowledge explain and share context and end-user collaboration is moderated is the final challenge to achieve interoperability. Advances in the global diffusion of Open Innovation 2.0 principles aligns well to this agenda. Key aspects of this methodology include defining a platform, participating in ecoystems for focused group discussions on planning for adoption on new models of care. This approach also needs to be underpinned with agile production innovation and engagement with industry to advance data driven agendas. For a case example of how nursing informaticians are engaging in this process see earlier work by the author (Hussey and McGlinn 2019; Curely and Salmeli, 2018).

2.5.2 Immersion of Digital in Connected eHealth

New frontiers with digital are now a reality with global organisations recommending a strong push for public funding investment with AI and robotics, and machine learning. Chapter. 16 discusses new frontiers in a futures chapter. Here we provide a summary of what such technologies involve and consider key factors including the human and ethical implications for the profession. It is only by focusing on the virtues that guide us in our human interactions in society that we can proactively use democratic processes and take control of the frameworks in which we build to make platforms to support our interactions.

Academic publications on translational science in AI report that there is much published in the media about the seemingly limitless power of AI to truly revolutionise patient healthcare. The father of AI Marvin Minsky described AI as simply a machine that is able to do a task, which is considered an intelligent one performed by a human being. Dividing the capacity of AI into two tasks, firstly, as an attempt to reproduce the capabilities of the human mind, and secondly for the creation of tools to carry out tasks which today need a human action. AI can also be understood as a concept presented as an abstract object of thought that enables it to associate the various perceptions that it has of that object (Laï et al. 2020, p. 2). Definitions that are more recent are included in the following Boxes Artificial Intelligence Box 2.5 and Machine Learning Box 2.6.

Durant (AACC 2020) suggests that there are examples of AI and ML increasingly evident in everyday life in society. For example, when on social media, companies provide sites with targeted adverts which are sent to an individual user. This targeting is based on what the user has been searching on the internet perhaps a holiday destination. Other examples include AI tools presenting a viewer with a "best matched" movie selection based on previous choices on television streaming services such as Netflix.

Box 2.5 Definition of Artificial Intelligence (AACC 2020)
AI as the ability of a machine to demonstrate intelligent behavior. It can be further divided into two types of algorithms exhibiting rule based or non-adaptive functions or machine learning adaptive functions (AACC 2020).

Box 2.6 Definition of Machine Learning (AACC 2020)
Machine learning (ML) which can provide adaptive functions is a type of artificial intelligence, which uses mathematical models to automatically map inputs into desired outputs in a way that does not rely on explicit rule based programming (AACC 2020).

There is much discussion on the widespread potential for adoption and integration of machine learning and digital in health and social care (Curley 2018; Laï et al. 2020; AACC 2020; Risling and Low 2020; Healthcare Innovation 2018; Skiba 2018; The Royal College of Nursing 2020). Despite this being the case, a study by Risling and Low (2020), suggests there is very little nursing consultation in relation to the use and potential implications of AI Integration within the profession. Specific areas where implementation of AI relating to nursing occurs include patient decision support particularly in the field of diagnostics and in robotic devices to support the process of care delivery. Results on a literature review conducted in 2020 report only two articles were identified which included discussion on the nursing role or professional view about AI use in healthcare (Risling and Low 2020, p. 38). Qualitative studies, which included professional and public service engagement completed in France, support the need for more focused analysis on impact and use of AI within the health and social care domain. Moving on from innovative research findings on potential benefits there is a need to conduct focused analysis on how AI Tools can meaningfully support service improvements and to identify where best to apply AI tools in practice (Laï et al. 2020). Stressing the need to consider the impact of automation of tasks on human interactions will be important, for example is there potential for loss of competence and skills by humans on tasks that they no longer perform and is there a risk of deskilling of professionals in their roles (Laï et al. 2020; Skiba 2018).

Regulation is required particularly for adoption and use of AI within health care domain, and as the gatekeepers of care both clinician and patient opinion are important in order to decide what is good for practice integration in addition to what is good for patients.

To develop reliable AI tools for predictive modelling and clinical decision making immense amounts of individual health data are essential for testing, training and refining models and this data must be accessed in accordance with the General Data Protection Regulation. Studies suggest that initial integration of AI in health will happen in radiology, but what is key is the translation of research and innovation into tools that focus on utility and service effectiveness (Davis and Brady 2015, p. 6). AI can have a direct impact on organisational of health care systems; there is a need to define responsibilities of AI tools within organisations particularly to avoid error. In the study by Lai et al. findings suggest that radiologists appear to be the least reluctant to integrate AI tools in their practice (Laï et al. 2020).

From an industry perspective,vendors are increasingly introducing machine learning into their electronic health record systems (Healthcare Innovation 2018), however in many instances vendors package machine learning software into clinical decision support blending machine learning with clinical medicine and this can raise concerns as implemented regulation is still under developed in this domain. Knowing where machine learning can be applied and understanding what it is good and not good for in deployment of health and social care is essential to optimise safety and minimise risk. Some institutions have successfully developed and integrated machine learning systems into their laboratory systems and associated workflows, however few have successfully transitioned to clinical practice (AACC 2020; Risling and Low 2020). With a view to the future, and specifically considering the

> **Box 2.7 Skiba Quote on AI and Nursing (Skiba 2018, p. 265)**
> With the intersection of data, devices and AI who will be your health care professional in the future. Will your health care provider partner with you as an invisible AI assistant?
>   Will it be Molly your virtual nurse?
>   Or will it just be the invisible AI wizard on your smartphone?
>   Nurses will not disappear in the future but their roles and responsibilities will change.
>   Skiba (2018, p. 265)

profession of nursing we conclude this section with a quote from Diane Skiba which summarises well the challenges facing the profession in terms of AI going forward.

2.6   Conclusion

In Chap. 2 we have discussed the topic of connecting health using eHealth and digital. We have approached the topic from the perspective of the grand societal challenges which nursing as a profession must meet and actively have a role in addressing. Since the birth of fifth generation computing in 2010 where search engines have been using Artificial Intelligence to mine Internet data on platforms, giant leaps have been realised with a surge of applications to support smart and mobile devices. Health administrators are designing new approaches to data collection, examining data flows and monitoring the transformative nature of how care can be delivered more effectively and efficiently. At a citizen level, Individuals are using smart devices and increasingly embracing digital in their daily routines. They are generating significant data with supporting personalised devices and this provides potential to create new knowledge for understanding health care delivery. This poses the profession with a number of questions

- What role will nursing play in delivery of care?
- Who will design the devices and algorithms that provide silos of data from connected health?
- As regulation of this industry is yet under developed, how can nurses trust the data produced?

The indications are that such questions are currently in debate although early indications are that nursing is not as involved, as it could be. More focused engagement is perhaps now required.

Two key truths are recognising that our existing care models are not sustainable and use of AI and machine learning in society is now inevitable. In the realm of health and social care, citizens need support to be lifelong, self-directed learners who can avail of digital to assist in managing their health. Leadership will be key and nursing today is at a crossroads. The professsion needs to grow digital capabilities and informatics competencies to provide a clear direction for nursing to evolve as a practice based profession. This will be instrumental to understand the evolving roles and responsabilities for the profession that will inevitably come to pass in a digitally enabled and connected health society.

Review Questions
Template One for Group and Individual Assignment Work

1. Consider using template below to formalize your thoughts on what you have read in Chap. 2 on the WHO strategic plans for patient centered integrated care. How you would instigate a project to address a problem based on your current or past work experience, which could bring about a patient centered service initiative?

Template 1 pattern of an information handling activity
Problem: Describe the problem in one or two sentences
Solution: Provide a summary of the solution that you would like to propose
Aim: State the aim to be achieved in the short medium or long term
Objective: Explain what you will have delivered by the end of the module and how it will or could affect the problem
Evaluate: Explain how you would evaluate

2. Consider using template two to formalise your thoughts on what you have read in Chap. 2 and how you could plan a project based on your current or past work experience to implement digital smart or mobiles devices in to your practice?

Template 2 Plan—Do—Study—Act

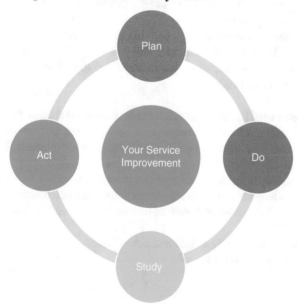

3. *Learning activity* Access the Millenium Development Goal website and view this video https://youtu.be/0XTBYMfZyrM and consider to be completed.

Glossary

Architecture A specific design approach to determine how the information system will work. A variety of architectures exist such as conceptual, operating system, software, etc.

CARE An acronym within nursing informatics initially devised by Hannah and Ball and adapted within this text to refer to Connected health administration research and education

C-HOBIC Canadian Health Outcomes for Better Information and Care

Clinical intelligence The electronic aggregation of accurate, relevant and timely clinical data into meaningful information and actionable knowledge in order to achieve optimal structures, processes, and outcomes" (Harrington 2011, p. 507)

eHealth The use of information and communication technologies (ICT) for healthcare delivery WHO defines it as the transfer of health resources and healthcare by electronic means

EHR Electronic Health Record

Health Informatics Health informatics is the intersection of information science, computer science and health care. Health informatics is the intersection of clinical, IM/IT and management practices to achieve better health Source http://www.imia-medinfo.org/new2/node/66

HRQoL Health-related quality-of-life

IHE IHE is a world-wide initiative created by healthcare professionals and industry to improve the way computer systems in healthcare share information by working together on interoperability use cases. IHE promotes the coordinated use of established standards such as DICOM and HL7 to address specific clinical needs in support of optimal patient care

Information Facts provided or learned about something or someone

Interoperability IEEE in 1990 defined Interoperability is the ability of two or more systems or components to exchange information and to use information that has been exchanged IEEE 1990

IoT Internet of Things

mHealth A collective term used to describe cellular type of mobile technology

Nursing Data Any information element obtained by a nurse during an encounter relating to the assessment of a client's health state, diagnostic of ailments/diseases and/or treatments

Nursing Informatics Nursing Informatics science and practice integrates nursing, its information and knowledge and their management with information and communication technologies to promote the health of people, families and communities world wide" IMIANI.

OECD Organisation of economic co-operation and development

PREMS Patient Reported Experience Measures

PROMS Patient Reported Outcome Measures

SDG Sustainable Development Goals devised by the United Nations

Self Efficacy People's judgements of their capabilities to organise and execute courses of action required to attain designated types of performance. It is concerned not with the skills one has but with the judgements of what one can do with whatever skills one possesses (Bandura 1986, p. 391)

Self Management Support An approach providing education and support to optimize patients' self management and ability to make informed decisions about their health

Theory An abstract generalisation that presents a systematic representation about relationships among phenomena

UN United Nations

Use Case An integration profile used as a guideline for implementation of a specific process called use case. The use case provides precise definitions of how standards can be implemented to meet specific clinical needs for a specific purpose. For example, integration profiles organize and leverage the integration capabilities that can be achieved by coordinated implementation of communication standards, such as DICOM, HL7, W3C and security standards in Digital Health

WHO World Health Organisation

Appendix: Simulation Exercise and Review Questions

1. Review the scenario case study presented in this chapter. Complete this case based exercise which is linked to Box 2.3 and Figs. 2.3a, 2.3b as a role playing simulation and consider the value proposition on the use of connected digital sensors in the home from a patient safety perspective.
2. What are the benefits of implementing digital devices as described in the simulation exercise?
3. What are the potential barriers to implementation and how can they be address?

   Appendix 1 of Chapter 2 Detail is as follows;

Additional Scenarios Case Study

John wakens from a fitful sleep and is conscious he needs to go to the toilet as a matter of urgency. He gets out of bed puts his slippers on and uses his Zimmer frame to go to the toilet.

Day of Week & Time	Location	Activity—Patient	Monitoring/Sensors in Place in Location	Action from Sensor	Nurse/Carer Activity
Saturday Morning 02:30hrs	John's bedroom Bathroom	Sleeping for short periods waking to go to the toilet—urgency to pass urine. Restless Legs	1. Motion sensor—bedroom 2. Plug paired with strip light 3. Fit Bit Watch 4. Sleep Tracking Mat 5. Toilet sensor	Status—monitoring all sensors	Carer in bed
Saturday Morning 02:45hrs	John's bedroom	John sits up in the bed and begins to get out of the bed John places his feet onto the floor and he attempts to put on his slippers and get his Zimmer frame	1. Motion sensor 2. Plug paired with strip light 3. Fit Bit Watch 4. Sleep Tracking Mat Toilet sensor	Status—monitoring 1. Motion sensor activated 2. Light strip activated in bed room	Carer alerted by alarm Carer responds to alarm
Saturday Morning 02:50hrs	John's walks/shuffles from bedside to bathroom using Zimmer frame	John walks to bathroom and puts on light and enters the bathroom with his Zimmer frame. Goes to the toilet after flushing the toilet washes his hands	1. Motion sensor in bathroom activated 2. Toilet Flush sensor activated 3. Fit Bit Watch	Status—monitoring 1. Motion sensor activated 2. Light in bathroom activated 3. Toilet Flush sensor	

Day of Week & Time	Location	Activity—Patient	Monitoring/Sensors in Place in Location	Action from Sensor	Nurse/Carer Activity
Saturday Morning 02:55hrs	Bathroom	After flushing the toilet John washes his hands-water spills on to the floor and he then slips as he turns to reach for the towel which is on the bath (Zimmer frame is occupying circulating space)	1. Motion sensor in bathroom activated 2. Falls alert sensor device		Carer arrives having been alerted to John being out of bed and being on the move at 0245hrs

03:00hrs	Bathroom	John is assessed for injury post fall—no HI or evidence of bony injury. John manages to get himself up off the floor with the assistance of the carer and a chair is brought into the bathroom for him to rest on for a short while.	1. Fit Bit Watch 2. Ambient lighting or SMART lighting		Clinical assessment post fall
03:15hrs	Bedroom	John is escorted back to bed with his Zimmer frame and made comfortable. He is feeling a little shaky following the fall. BP recorded, reassured and drink offered before settling.	1. Motion sensor 2. Plug paired with strip light 3. Fit Bit Watch 4. Sleep Tracking Mat Toilet sensor 5. Digital BP Cuff		Assessment complete. Zimmer frame and slippers are placed by bed appropriately by carer

Physical Props Required for Scenario 2	Actors Required for Scenario 2	Technology IT Props Required for Scenario 2
All sensors active as listed Links to Hub working Curtains/blind closed Slippers Pyjamas Zimmer frame Drink at bedside Towel in bathroom on side of bath Small chair to move into bathroom post fall	John (service user) Carer Observer	• All sensors active as listed • Links to Hub working • Messaging device to alert carer to motion sensor being activated—**mobile phone send text message—Carer located in CeIC Centre**

Evaluation	

Scenario Background 3

At 07:30hrs John begins to get himself out of bed as per his normal routine—his Zimmer frame and slippers are always left beside his bed.

Day of Week & Time	Location	Activity—Patient	Monitoring/Sensors in Place in Location	Action from Sensor	Nurse/Carer Activity
Sunday Morning 07:30hrs	John's bedroom	Awakening-keen to get up and get his breakfast.	1. Motion sensor—bed room 2. Plug paired with strip light 3. Fit Bit Watch 4. Sleep Tracking Mat	Status—monitoring	With other service users in other location
Sunday Morning 07:40hrs	John's bedroom	John sits up in the bed and begins to get out of the bed John places his feet onto the floor and he attempts to put on his slippers and get his Zimmer frame	1. Motion sensor 2. Plug paired with strip light 3. Fit Bit Watch 4. Sleep Tracking Mat	Status—monitoring 1. Motion sensor activated 2. Light strip activated	Carer alerted by alarm Carer responds to alarm

Day of Week & Time	Location	Activity— Patient	Monitoring/Sensors in Place in Location	Action from Sensor	Nurse/Carer Activity
Sunday Morning 07:45hrs	John's walks/ shuffles from bed side to kitchen on his way to the bathroom	John walks/ shuffles to the kitchen and fills kettle with water, puts mug out with tea bag and puts bread in toaster— shuffles to bathroom	1. Motion sensor in bathroom activated 2. Fit Bit Watch	Status— monitoring 1. Motion sensor activated 2. Light strip activated in bathroom	
Sunday Morning 07:55hrs	Bathroom	John walks to bathroom and puts on light and goes to the toilet after flushing the toilet washes his hands and is distracted in the bathroom. Toast burning in the kitchen	1. Motion sensor in bathroom activated 2. Toilet Flush sensor activated 3. Smoke sensor activated in kitchen from toaster		
Sunday Morning 08:00hrs	Kitchen	John returns to kitchen carer arrives and toaster turned off and smoke sensor deactivated	1. Motion sensor in kitchen activated 2. Fit Bit Watch 3. Smoke sensor in kitchen		Carer arrives having been alerted to John being out of bed and being on the move.
	Bedroom	John returns to his bedroom assisted by carer—John uses his Zimmer frame and is complaining of feeling a little light headed.	1. Motion sensor in bedroom activated 2. Fit Bit Watch 3. BP & HR & Temp recorded		

Physical Props Required for Scenario 3	Actors Required for Scenario 3	Technology IT Props Required for Scenario 3
All sensors active as listed—including Smoke Sensor for this scenario Links to Hub working Curtains/blind closed Slippers Pyjamas Zimmer frame Drink at bedside Towel in bathroom on side of bath Toaster, Kettle, Mug Bread/Butter/Jam, Tea Bags, Sugar Plate Knife Milk	John (service user) Carer Observer	• All sensors active as listed • Links to Hub working • Messaging device to alert carer to motion sensor being activated—**mobile phone send text message—Carer located in Reception of Skills Centre** • Sensor data recorded and visualisation accessed through John's profile

Evaluation	

References

AACC. Machine learning and laboratory medicine: now and the road ahead I AACC.org. 2020. https://www.aacc.org/publications/cln/articles/2019/march/machine-learning-and-laboratory-medicine-now-and-the-road-ahead. Cited 30 Jan 2020.

Auraaen AL, Slawomirski NK. (2018) The economics of patient safety in primary and ambulatory care: flying blind. Paris: OECD Publishing. OECD Health Working Papers, No. 106.

Bandura, A. (1986). Social foundations of thought and action: A social cognitive theory. Englewood Cliffs, NJ: Prentice-Hall.

BELLERIN MLS. First EU citizens using ePrescriptions in other EU country thanks to CEF Telecom. Innovation and Networks Executive Agency – European Commission. 2019. https://ec.europa.eu/inea/en/news-events/newsroom/first-eu-citizens-using-eprescriptions-other-eu-country-thanks-to-cef-telecom. Cited 30 Jan 2020.

Benson T, Grieve G. (2016) Principles of health interoperability SNOMED CT, HL7 and FHIR. 3rd ed. London: Springer-Verlag. (Health Information Technology Standards).

Beránková M, Kvasnička R, Houška M. Towards the definition of knowledge interoperability. In 2010 2nd international conference on software technology and engineering. 2010. p. V1-232–6.

Berwick DM, Nolan TW, Whittington J. The triple aim: care, health, and cost. Health Aff. 2008;27(3):759–69. https://www.healthaffairs.org/doi/10.1377/hlthaff.27.3.759. Cited 29 Jan 2020.

Blobel B. Interoperable EHR systems – challenges, standards and solutions. ejbi. 2018;14(2). https://www.ejbi.org/scholarly-articles/interoperable-ehr-systems%2D%2Dchallenges-standards-and-solutions.pdf. Cited 30 Jan 2020.

Blobel B. Challenges and solutions for designing and managing pHealth ecosystems. Front Med. 2019;6:83. https://www.frontiersin.org/article/10.3389/fmed.2019.00083.

Blobel B, Oemig F. Why do we need an architectural approach to interoperability? Interoperability is more than just technology. Eur J Biomed. 2016. https://www.ejbi.org/scholarly-articles/interoperability-is-more-than-just-technology.pdf.

Bodenheimer T, Sinsky C. From triple to quadruple aim: care of the patient requires care of the provider. Ann Fam Med. 2014;12(6):573–6. http://www.annfammed.org/cgi/doi/10.1370/afm.1713. Cited 29 Jan 2020.

CeIC. The Nex Project 1. Centre for eIntegrated Care – Dr Pamela Hussey, DCU CeIC. 2020. https://www.ceic.ie. Cited 30 Jan 2020.

CEN Portal. 2020. https://login.cen.eu/portal/. Cited 20 Jan 2020.

Chen J. Integrated Care Patient reported outcome measures and patient reported experience measures – a rapid scoping review. Australia: University of New South Wales: Simpson Centre for Health Services Research; 2015. p. 116. https://www.aci.health.nsw.gov.au/__data/assets/pdf_file/0009/281979/ACI_Proms_Prems_Report.pdf.

Connecting Europe Facility. Innovation and Networks Executive Agency – European Commission. 2015. https://ec.europa.eu/inea/en/connecting-europe-facility. Cited 30 Jan 2020.

Curley MSB. Open Innovation 2.0. Switzerland: Springer; 2018.

Davis P, Brady O. Are government intentions for the inclusion of innovation and small and medium enterprises participation in public procurement being delivered or ignored? An Irish case study. Innovation. 2015;28(3):324–43. https://doi.org/10.1080/13511610.2014.985192.

Davra. Industrial Internet of Things (IoT) Platform for Enterprise • Davra. 2020. https://davra.com/. Cited 30 Jan 2020.

EU Commission. Digital Europe Programme: a proposed €9.2 Billion of funding for 2021–2027. Digital Single Market – European Commission. 2019. https://ec.europa.eu/digital-single-market/en/news/digital-europe-programme-proposed-eu92-billion-funding-2021-2027. Cited 29 Jan 2020.

EUR-Lex – 52018DC0233 – EN – EUR-Lex. 2020. https://eur-lex.europa.eu/homepage.html. Cited 30 Jan 2020.

European Commission. State aid and a green, digital future. European Commission. 2020. https://ec.europa.eu/commission/commissioners/2019-2024/vestager/announcements/state-aid-and-green-digital-future_en. Cited 31 Jan 2020.

Fennelly O. Factors for success in electronic health record implementation: literature review and key considerations. eHealth Ireland Dublin: insight Centre UCD; 2019a. p. 1–66. https://www.ehealthireland.ie/Strategic-Programmes/Electronic-Health-Record-EHR-/Information-Resources/Factors-for-Success-in-EHR-Implementation-Literature-Review-and-Key-Considerations.pdf.

Fennelly O. Clinical information capture in the electronic health record: literature review and key considerations. Dublin, Ireland: eHealth Ireland; 2019b. p. 30. https://www.ehealthireland.ie/Strategic-Programmes/Electronic-Health-Record-EHR-/Information-Resources/Clinical-Information-Capture-in-the-EHR-Literature-Review-and-Key-Considerations.pdf.

Food and Drug Administration. Guidance for industry – patient-reported outcome measures: use in medical product development to support labelling claims. U.S. Department of Health and Human Services, Food and Drug Administration. 2009.

Fortune. Death by a thousand clicks: where electronic health records went wrong. Fortune. 2020. https://fortune.com/longform/medical-records/. Cited 30 Jan 2020.

GDPR. What is GDPR, the EU's new data protection law?. GDPR.eu. 2018. https://gdpr.eu/what-is-gdpr/. Cited 30 Jan 2020.

Greenhalgh T, Wherton J, Papoutsi C, Lynch J, Hughes G, A'Court C, et al. Beyond adoption: a new framework for theorizing and evaluating nonadoption, abandonment, and challenges to the scale-up, spread, and sustainability of health and care technologies. Eysenbach G, editor. J Med Internet Res. 2017;19(11):e367. http://www.ncbi.nlm.nih.gov/pmc/articles/PMC5688245/.

Harrington L. Clinical intelligence. J Nurs Adm. 2011 Dec;41(12):507–9. https://doi.org/10.1097/NNA.0b013e318237eca0. PMID: 22094613.

Health Service Executive. Self management support for chronic conditions. HSE.ie. 2020. https://www.hse.ie/eng/health/hl/selfmanagement/self-management.html. Cited 30 Jan 2020.

Healthcare Innovation. Why analytics is at the foundation of healthcare transformation. Healthcare Innovation. 2018. https://www.hcinnovationgroup.com/home/article/13011305/why-analytics-is-at-the-foundation-of-healthcare-transformation. Cited 30 Jan 2020.

Hussey P, McGlinn K. The role of academia in reorientation models of care—insights on eHealth. Informatics. 2019;6(3):37. https://www.mdpi.com/2227-9709/6/3/37. Cited 31 Jan 2020.

ICN. International Classification for Nursing Practice about ICNP. ICN – International Council of Nurses. 2020. https://www.icn.ch/what-we-do/projects/ehealth-icnp/about-icnp. Cited 31 Jan 2020.

IEEE. IEEE standard computer dictionary compilation of IEEE standard computer glossaries. The Institute of Electrical and Electronics Engineers, Inc. 1990.

IPPOSI – The Irish Platform for Patient Organisations, Science and Industry. IPPOSI. 2020. https://www.ipposi.ie/. Cited 29 Jan 2020.

Kerr J. Legacy: 15 lessons in leadership: what the All Blacks can teach us about the business of life. 2013.

Laï M-C, Brian M, Mamzer M-F. Perceptions of artificial intelligence in healthcare: findings from a qualitative survey study among actors in France. J Transl Med. 2020;18(1):14. https://doi.org/10.1186/s12967-019-02204-y. Cited 30 Jan 2020.

Maier CB, Aiken LH, Busse R. Nurses in advanced roles in primary care: policy levers for implementation. 2017. https://www.oecd-ilibrary.org/social-issues-migration-health/nurses-in-advanced-roles-in-primary-care_a8756593-en. Cited 30 Jan 2020.

McEvoy P. Chronic disease management: a new paradigm for care. Boca Raton, FL: CRC Press; 2014.

Mullaney C, O'Reilly O, Quinn G. Development of a national self management support framework for Ireland, for patients with cardiovascular disease, COPD, asthma and diabetes. Int J Integr Care. 2016;16(6):176. https://www.ijic.org/article/10.5334/ijic.2724/. Cited 29 Jan 2020.

O'Connell S, Palmer R, Withers K, Saha N, Puntoni S, Carolan Rees G. Requirements for the collection of electronic PROMS either "in clinic" or "at home" as part of the PROMs, PREMs and effectiveness Programme (PPEP) in Wales: a feasibility study using a generic PROM tool. BioMedicalCentral. 2018. https://pilotfeasibilitystudies.biomedcentral.com/articles/10.1186/s40814-018-0282-8.

OECD. OECD Going Digital Toolkit. 2019. https://goingdigital.oecd.org/en/themes/. Cited 29 Jan 2020.

OECD. Measuring the digital transformation – a roadmap for the future – en – OECD. 2020a. https://www.oecd.org/publications/measuring-the-digital-transformation-9789264311992-en.htm. Cited 30 Jan 2020.

OECD. Measuring the digital transformation: a roadmap for the future. 2020b. https://www.oecd-ilibrary.org/science-and-technology/measuring-the-digital-transformation_9789264311992-en. Cited 30 Jan 2020.

Organizational Change | | Bill Hogg. 2020. https://www.billhogg.ca/tag/organizational-change/. Cited 30 Jan 2020.

Palfrey JG, Gasser U. Interop: the promise and perils of highly interconnected systems. New York: Basic Books; 2012. p. 296.

Regional Office of the Americas World Health Organisation. Pan American Health Organisation. PAHO eHealth. 2020. https://www.paho.org/ict4health/index.php?lang=en.

Risling T, Low C. Advocating for safe, quality and just care: what nursing leaders need to know about artificial intelligence in healthcare delivery. Nurs Leadersh (Tor Ont). 2020;32(2):31–45. https://www.longwoods.com/content/25963. Cited 30 Jan 2020.

Skiba D. The invisible health care professional: exploring the intersection of data, devices, and artificial intelligence. Nurs Educ Perspect. 2018;39(4):264–5.

Stenberg K, Hanssen O, Edejer TT-T, Bertram M, Brindley C, Meshreky A, et al. Financing transformative health systems towards achievement of the health Sustainable Development

Goals: a model for projected resource needs in 67 low-income and middle-income countries. Lancet Glob Health. 2017;5(9):e875–e887. https://www.thelancet.com/journals/langlo/article/PIIS2214-109X(17)30263-2/abstract. Cited 30 Jan 2020.

The Royal College of Nursing. eHealth | Clinical | Royal College of Nursing. The Royal College of Nursing. 2020. /clinical-topics/ehealth. Cited 30 Jan 2020.

Thompson C, Sansoni J, Morris D, Capell J, Williams K. Patient-reported outcome measures an environmental scan of the Australian healthcare sector. Wollongong Australia: Centre for Health Service Development, Australian Health Services Research Institute; 2016. https://www.safetyandquality.gov.au/sites/default/files/migrated/PROMs-Environmental-Scan-December-2016.pdf.

Topol E. The patient will see you now: the future of medicine is in your hands. Boulder: Basic Books; 2016. http://public.ebookcentral.proquest.com/choice/publicfullrecord.aspx?p=4786012. Cited 30 Jan 2020.

Tutorialspoint. Computer—fifth generation—Tutorialspoint. 2020. https://www.tutorialspoint.com/computer_fundamentals/computer_fifth_generation.html. Cited 30 Jan 2020.

United Nations D of E and SA. Division for Sustainable Development Goals. Sustainable Development Goals Knowledge Platform. 2019. sustainabledevelopment.un.org.

United Nations Economic and Social Council. E/2019/68 – E – E/2019/68. Special edition: progress towards the Sustainable Development Goals Report of the Secretary-General. 2019. https://undocs.org/E/2019/68. Cited 30 Jan 2020.

World Health Organisation. Ottowa Charter for Health Promotion. 1986. https://www.who.int/healthpromotion/conferences/previous/ottawa/en/.

World Health Organisation. National eHealth toolkit. eHealth. 2012. https://www.who.int/ehealth/publications/overview.pdf. Cited 29 Jan 2020.

World Health Organisation. Framework for people centred integrated care services. 2016. http://www.who.int/servicedeliverysafety/areas/people-centred-care/en/.

World Health Organisation. Classification of Digital Health Interventions v1.0. Geneva: WHO; 2018. p. 20. (Health Research Impact). Report No.: WHO/RHR/18.06. https://apps.who.int/iris/bitstream/handle/10665/260480/WHO-RHR-18.06-eng.pdf?sequence=1&ua=1. Cited 30 Jan 2020.

WHO | eHealth at WHO [Internet]. WHO. 2020. http://www.who.int/ehealth/about/en/. Cited 30 Jan 2020.

Chapter 3
Nursing Informatics: A Core Competency for the Profession

Pamela Hussey and Kathryn J. Hannah

Abstract This chapter provides the reader with a summary of nursing informatics, considering how it has evolved over a 50-year timeframe to become a core competency for the profession of nursing in twenty-first century healthcare. In this chapter we describe the background and context of nursing informatics and why it is a critical enabler for the advancement of the profession. Drawing on nursing theory and historical milestones on development of informatics within health and social care service delivery. This chapter uses an adaptation of the CARE acronym with four core concepts namely Connected health, Administration, Research, and Education to present the evidence and provide insights on key influences shaping the development and advancement of digital within the profession. Specifically this chapter focuses on introducing the reader to critical factors are which driving the practice of nursing informatics in order to impact upon patient outcomes, and deliver a quality orientated global health and social care service over time. This chapter therefore acts as a primer for chapters which follow in this fifth edition, and presents the fundamental concepts of nursing informatics in context. It provides an introductory and summative chapter for those who do not have a background in this topic and who wish to understand how nursing informatics is emerging as a core competency for the profession.

Keywords Health informatics · Nursing informatics · eHealth · Connected health
Nursing role · Digital health

Electronic Supplementary Material The online version of this chapter (https://doi.org/10.1007/978-3-030-58740-6_3) contains supplementary material, which is available to authorized users.

P. Hussey (✉)
School of Nursing Psychotherapy and Community Health, Dublin City University,
Dublin, Ireland
e-mail: pamela.hussey@dcu.ie

P. K. Hannah
Professor (Adjunct), School of Nursing, University of Victoria,
Victoria, BC, Canada

Key Concepts
Health Informatics
Nursing Informatics
Nursing Role

Learning Objectives for the Chapter
1. Understand how nursing information can be used efficiently and responsibly to make nursing care evident in documentation of patient care through the use of digital data.
2. Understand the importance of nursing informatics competencies and digital literacy in professional practice of nursing.
3. Gain a deeper understanding of historical roots of nursing informatics and its association with nursing theory over the lifecycle of electronic health care delivery.
4. Appreciate the Impact of digital transformation on the profession of nursing especially in regards to connected health.

In Chap. 2, we explained the seismic shift in care design transitioning to new models of care underpinned by digital health. We considered how global leaders are looking to information and communications technology (ICT) as an enabler to support health care professionals and assist individuals to age well in place. In this chapter, we focus on the changing landscape of healthcare and consider what it means for the profession of nursing. The increasing use of digital and technology integration in the domain of health means that nursing leaders must adopt a proactive approach on the digital transformation within both health and social care. Specifically we argue the case that nursing informatics specialists can provide a much-needed scaffold for the profession to build stronger evidence based infrastructure and guidance supporting nursing education, research, and practice. We demonstrate how nursing informatics is a core nursing competency and critical to the practice of the profession in the delivery of twenty-first century health care. Projected figures on the need for nursing leadership to engage with informatics specialists to advance eHealth and digital health are noteworthy. The American Medical Informatics Association estimates that as many as 70,000 nursing informatics specialists or analysts will be needed in the next 5 years (Spring 2020, p. 12). Focused nursing informatics activities and associated deliverables are influencing patient outcomes. This is a core message that needs to be amplified so that a wider audience can understand it. The scope and influence of clinicians with advanced informatics knowledge and analytics expertise is poorly understood, not only in the profession, but also in the wider context of care delivery (Peltonen et al. 2019). As a means of background and context, this chapter provides an overview of the journey of informatics theory. Using the CARE acronym as outlined in Chap. 1, we use this CARE acronym (see Fig. 1.1) to discuss key concepts, which underpin the material presented in this chapter. In this edition, CARE is presented as an acronym for Connected Health, Administration, Research and Education.

Key definitions of nursing informatics are included in addition to insights from the evidence base on the nursing contribution to and role of informatics within practice. This chapter is structured in three sections. Firstly, this introduction, then Sect. 3.1 provides an historical view of informatics and its origins. This section also includes the nursing contribution within informatics and how the nature of nursing influences and informs the field of informatics over the past 50 years. Section 3.2 reviews the CARE acronym in the context of Nursing Informatics considering Connected Health, Administration and Research and Education from the perspective of related evidence to inform nursing agendas. The chapter concludes with a final discussion on critical factors that situate nursing informatics as a core competency for the profession.

3.1 Historical Overview of Informatics

Francois Gremy of France is widely credited with coining the term informatique medical, which was translated into English as medical informatics. Early on, the term medical informatics was used to describe "those collected informational technologies which concern themselves with the patient care, medical decision making process") (Greenburg 1975). Another early definition, in the first issue of the Journal of Medical Informatics, proposed that medical informatics was "the complex processing of data by a computer to produce new kinds of information"(Anderson 1976). As our understanding of this discipline developed, Greens and Shortliffe (Greens and Shortliffe 1990) redefined medical informatics as "the field that concerns itself with the cognitive, information processing and communication tasks of medical practice, education, and research, including the information science and the technology to support these tasks. An intrinsically interdisciplinary field … [with] an applied focus, … [addressing] a number of fundamental research problems as well as planning and policy issues." Shortliffe et al. (2001) also defined medical informatics as "the scientific field that deals with biomedical information, data, and knowledge—their storage, retrieval and optimal use for problem-solving and decision-making."

One question consistently arose: "Does the word medical refer only to physicians, or does it refer to all healthcare professions?" In the first edition of this book, the premise was that medical referred to all healthcare professions and that a parallel definition of medical informatics might be "those collected informational technologies that concern themselves with the patient care decision-making process performed by healthcare practitioners." Thus, because nurses are healthcare practitioners who are involved in the patient care and the decision-making process that uses information captured by and extracted from the information technologies, there clearly was a place for nursing in medical informatics. Increasingly, as research was conducted and medical informatics evolved, nurses realized there was a discrete body of knowledge related to nursing and the use of informatics. During the early 1990s, other health professions began to explore the use of informatics in their disciplines. Mandil (1989) coined the phrase "health informatics," which he defined as the use of information technology (including both hardware and software) in combination with information management concepts and methods to support the delivery of healthcare. Thus, health informatics has become the umbrella term encompassing medical, nursing, dental, and pharmacy informatics among others. Health informatics focuses attention on the recipient of care rather than on the discipline of the caregiver. The evolution of technology supporting health and professional nursing practice can be illustrated in Fig. 3.1, which demonstrates the steady progression of innovation with technology. From the 1970s onwards, there is an acceleration of technology to support practice and improve patient outcomes across the context of health care, including how the use of ICT for distance activities related to health. One example being the introduction of telehealth facilities for remote access to diagnostic and therapeutic support resources to enhance quality of care. Telehealth services provided scope to reduce geographical limits and accommodate access to population and mobile health services. Core over this time line is the integration of computers and technology originally as two separate entities they have today become one. This is well articulated by Time Magazine brief history of the computer (Time Magazine 2020) and the Computer History Museum Timeline of Computer History (CHM 2020).

Within healthcare, the progressive deployment of electronic health records (EHR) evolved. Hospital administrators became more aware of the possibilities of

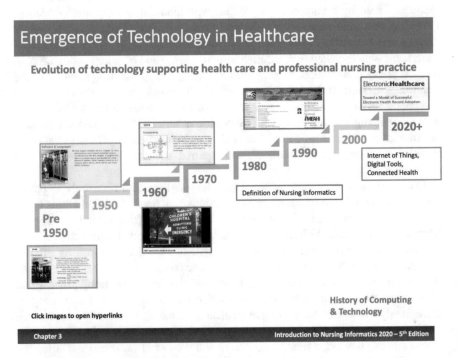

Fig. 3.1 Emergence of technology in healthcare

automating health care activities beyond business office procedures. Health care professionals began to develop patient care applications and vendors began to realise the potential of the market in healthcare. The stages of EHR cycle in terms of capability and integration over time are illustrated in Fig. 3.2 which is adapted from Nagle and Catford (2008).

Originally published in 2008, Fig. 3.2 presented above depicts the various stages of electronic health record cycles over time is still very much relevant in 2020. Sensmeier (2017) describes health care as one of the most data rich industries driven by digital health image capture and widespread EHR adoption. Between the various EHRs in existence, the average person will leave a trail of more than one million gigabytes of health related data in their lifetime.

On review of the early literature on nursing and informatics. The nurse's early role in medical informatics was that of a consumer. The literature clearly shows the contributions of medical informatics to the practice of nursing and patient care. Early developments in medical informatics and their advantages to nursing have been thoroughly documented by Hannah (1976). These initial developments were fragmented and generally restricted to automating existing functions or activities such as automated charting of nurses' notes, automated nursing care plans, automated patient monitoring, automated personnel time assignment, and the gathering of epidemiological and administrative statistics. Subsequently, an integrated approach to medical informatics resulted in the development and marketing of sophisticated hospital information systems that included nursing applications or modules. Pioneers from this time include Maureen Scholes from the United Kingdom who was involved in the London Hospital Real Time Computer Project in 1967, and Harriet Werley from the USA who from the 1960s worked with the American Nurses Association on communication and decision making in nursing.

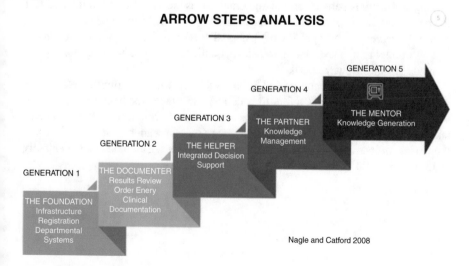

Fig. 3.2 EHR lifecycle adapted from Nagle and Catford (2008)

Box 3.1 Definitions of Nursing Informatics (Harrington 2015; Newbold 2016)

Nursing informatics (NI) is the specialty that integrates nursing science with multiple information and analytical sciences to identify, define, manage and communicate data, information, knowledge and wisdom in nursing practice. ANA 2015 (Harrington 2015).

Nursing Informatics science and practice integrates nursing, its information, knowledge, and their management with information and communication technologies to promote the health of people, families and communities worldwide. IMIA NI SIG 2009 (Newbold 2016).

Harriet Werley was also involved in the 1980s in the development of Nursing Minimum Dataset with Norma Lang (Scholes et al. 2000).

Dr. Marion Ball introduced the term nursing informatics (NI) initially at the 1983 International Medical Informatics Association (IMIA) Conference in Amsterdam. Nursing informatics as then originally defined by Hannah, in 1984, (Ball et al. 2000, p. 181), referred to the use of information technologies in relation to those functions within the purview of nursing carried out by nurses when performing their duties. We include here two additional definitions of nursing informatics from the American Nursing Association and the International Medical Informatics Association Special Interest Group for Nursing in Box 3.1.

Today, we see there is a further evolution of related definitions that encompasses core concepts relating to informatics, Digital Health and Connected Health under an umbrella of Digitally Connected Health. Both of these terms are briefly described here and will be expanded upon further in Sects. 3.2 and 3.3.

Digital Health is patient centred and emphasizes the use of information and ICT to enable people to better track, manage, and improve their own and their family's health. (Adapted from Topol (2016).) Digital Health is the use of patient centred ICT solutions "to improve health, transform quality and reduce health system costs" (Canada Health Infoway 2020).

Connected Health encompasses terms such as wireless, digital, electronic, mobile and tele-health and refers to a conceptual model for health management where devices, services or interventions are designed around the patient's needs, and health related data is shared in such a way that the patient can receive care in the most proactive and efficient manner possible (Caulfield and Donnelly 2013, p. 704).

3.2 Nursing Informatics CARE

3.2.1 Connected Health

Considering the impact of digital transformation in connected health, it is evident from the literature that almost every country claims to have a digital transformation initiative in progress. Digitally Connected Health is the broadest term and encompasses the use of information and ICT that will empower nurses and assist healthcare systems in achieving a Primary Health Care focus. Evolving from the convergence of the digital and genomic revolutions with health and wellness, healthcare, living, and society. Digitally Connected Health includes Social Networking, Information and Communication Technology, Interoperability (both functional and semantic), Infrastructure and Processes, Solutions and Applications. Digitally Connected Health also includes the use of best practice guidelines/pathways, electronic order sets, smartphone apps (e.g., drug manuals, calculators), point of care documentation tools (e.g., bar-code readers), and access to internet resources which can all faciliate and support evidence-informed practice as well as patient generated data such as exercise, diet, vital signs.

The International Telecommunication Union (ITU) suggest at its core digital transformation in connected health is about creating a vision. Putting an emphasis on how digital services and connected health applications will change and "transform" citizen's experience and how improvement in quality of life and wellbeing and the attainment of Sustainable Development Goals can be achieved. Sustainable Development Goals (SDG) were discussed in detail in Chap. 2, often described as global goals, they were adopted by all United Nations Member States in 2015 as a universal call to action to end poverty, protect the planet and ensure that all people enjoy peace and prosperity by 2030 (Saha 2019; Sustainable Development 2020). https://www.undp.org/content/undp/en/home/sustainable-development-goals.html.

A thematic report published on digital transformation in 2019 by the ITU offers some principle insights relating to connected health (Saha 2019). ITU in this report identify six fundamental attributes of services that classify a transformation as digital. For example digital services need to be personalised, paperless, cashless, presence less, integrated and consent based to be transformational. Three of these attributes are of interest to connected health and nursing related activity and are therefore listed for consideration.

- Personalised services are designed and delivered to suit the specific requirements of those who consume them. Personalisation is generally achieved by way of giving citizens a great experience that meets their needs and expectations.
- Paperless services are automated by adopting widespread automation. Paperless services are a consequence of extensive business process reengineering and significant fundamental rethinking.

- Consent-based services refer to security and data privacy, two imperatives that have to be focused on with utmost priority. In the digital era, people share huge amounts of information, citizen consent has a hugely significant impact on the effectiveness of digital services. People must know what data is being collected, who is collecting it, and for what purposes is it going to be used.

Nowadays, countries and organizations need to develop specific capabilities to be able to deliver connected health digital services for effective transformation. ITU describe this as the value chain and propose organisations consider some key questions incrementally over the life course of any transformational programme. They suggest organisations follow a high-level process and address some core issues iteratively throughout the programme of change. These issues are illustrated as questions in Fig. 3.3.

Considering Fig. 3.3 from a clinical perspective, digitally connected health offers potential for a value chain in the area of integrated care. Effective transitioning of care delivery mechanisms across services i.e. from a primary to secondary care, and then back to primary care in a coordinated fashion underpins the vision and ambition for integrated care. To achieve integrated care effectively access to quality data is needed. Quality data is considered as information that are relevant, accurate and reliable. Key features relating to quality data are presented in Fig. 3.4 that describes core components of a data quality framework.

Underpinning a quality data framework is the need to use agreed and shared vocabularies. From a nursing informatics perspective, agreed vocabularies for patient assessment tools need to be embedded in electronic health records and digital devices linked to performance indicators for monitoring of interventions and

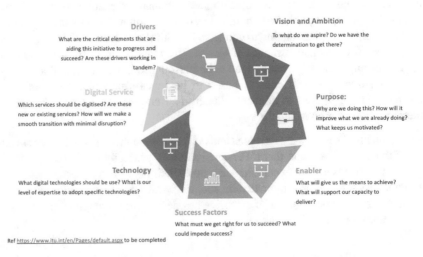

Fig. 3.3 ITU report adapted (Saha 2019)

Data quality framework

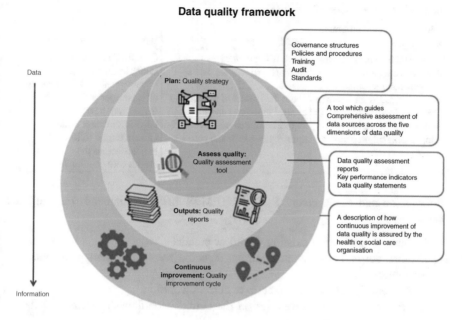

Fig. 3.4 HIQA key components for a data quality framework (Flynn 2018)

symptom management. This is a core requirement discussed in Chaps. 2, 5 and 6 from a computer science and standards perspective. Here, however we provide some examples of systems interfaces and processes that can assist with advancing data quality from connected health and integrated care initiatives.

A large-scale programme entitled C-HOBIC full title being the Canadian Health Outcomes for Better Information and Care. This dataset introduces a common, structured terminology for use in patient assessment and in electronic health record (EHR) documentation in acute care, complex continuing care, long-term care and home care. This data set includes terminology in the following areas:

- Functional status and continence
- Symptoms: pain, nausea, fatigue, labored breathing
- Safety outcomes: falls, pressure ulcers
- Readiness for discharge

This dataset is now entering its third phase of deployment in Canada and is integrated into the core National Nursing Data Standards (NNDS) with the goal of optimising the nursing contribution to care delivery (White 2020).

Table 3.1 provides a summary of the process of workflow engagement for C Hobic in health care services and describes how the impact of nursing is made evident in client or patient outcomes across different points in service delivery.

Integrating programmes such as C-HOBIC requires detailed workflow to be completed as outlined in Table 3.1 to optimise workflow mapping the Healthcare

Table 3.1 C-HOBIC CIHI (White 2020)

Direct health care programs and services	Health research	Health care system
C-HOBIC data informs and evaluates operational decisions and resource allocation, helps set industry benchmarks and provides real-time information to support clinical practice	C-HOBIC provides standardized clinical data to answer research questions about the impact of practice on clinical outcomes and to support research on new approaches to clinical practice	C-HOBIC empowers Better health system Management decision making, offers deeper Insight into how Facilities manage clinical Outcomes and follows Patients across the Health care continuum

Information and Management Systems (HIMSS 2019) recommend some initial key steps;

- Conduct an analysis of existing workflow practices
- Explore the end user input regarding specific roles in current paper record workflows
- Review and finalise documentation of current workflow
- Identify waste and opportunities on the current workflow diagrams, and then redesign workflow practices.
- Identify and implement the electronic health record system and the new agreed workflow process in practice
- Analyse new electronic health records workflow and refine the process as needed (HIMSS 2019) (Fennelly 2019, p. 21)

Workflow is critical to ensure that there is good alignment between the existing systems of paper workflows and the new automated workflows using technology for data entry of health records. Poor alignment from "as is" infrastructure to the "to be" planned new workflow can have a number of negative outcomes. Reports from the United States provide examples such as issues with technology-induced errors that impact on patient safety and nursing practice. Technology-induced errors is a new category of errors identified with the introduction of electronic health records in the United States. These errors occur at the interaction between the information technology interface and the health care providers during clinical use. As a consequence focused interventions are now in place across the US to develop pre-emptive activities involving new workflow processes to detect such technology errors in EHR before they occur (Spring 2020).

Figure 3.5 provides an illustrative workflow completed by nursing informaticians on bed management and referral of a patient to facilitate integrated care delivery.

As the largest stakeholder group in health care delivery, nursing can provide insights on patient safety in regards to technology induced errors. Defining detailed workflow on medication management processes and patient safety checks for example can assist in minimising negative impacts on transition from paper to electronic prescribing systems. In the following section, we provide some screen shots of

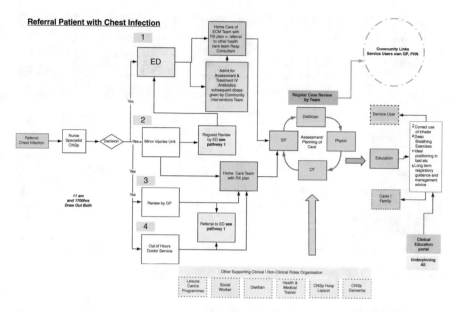

Fig. 3.5 Workflow of care transition for patient with chest infection

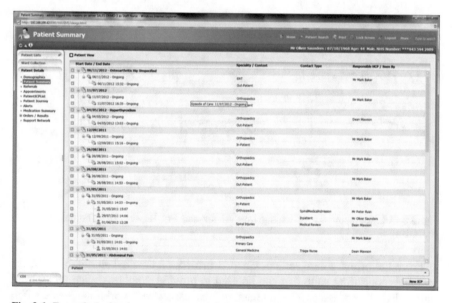

Fig. 3.6 Example 1 of patient summary module in electronic record system

electronic health records from secondary care services that offer examples of care planning and patient summary record systems. Such systems are routinely now used by nurses and implemented across Europe and Canada (Figs. 3.6 and 3.7).

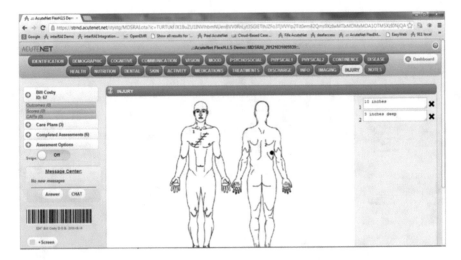

Fig. 3.7 Example 2 of patient summary module in electronic record system

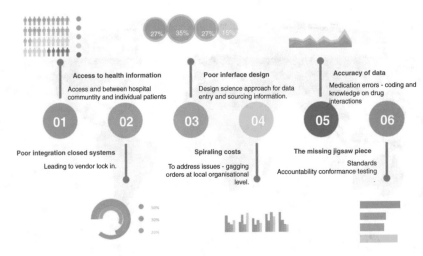

Fig. 3.8 Adapted summary of finding from Shultz and Fry Report 2019 (Fortune FS Erika Fry 2019)

From the primary care setting, Chap. 2 provides a detailed summary of Davra personal monitoring suite that can be used to provide supporting data on assisted care delivery processes. The interaction and associated workflow issues often encountered between the information technology, transitional care and the associated system interface of data access is highlighted in 2019 Report by Shultz and Fry in the Fortune Report Case Studies. These issues are illustrated in Figure 3.8 and summarised Box 3.2.

Box 3.2 Case Study Detail on Transitional Care

Reports of progress on connected health of electronic health records and integrated care are variable. In the United States, for example the Health Information Technology for Economic and Clinical Health Act (HITECH) was signed into law in 2009 to deliver meaningful use for interoperable electronic health care records. Ten years after this initiative was signed into law, Obama Care and the Meaningful Use programme has been implemented nationally, a controversial report by Schulte and Fry published in Fortune magazine indicate the results are often lacking in terms of anticipated benefits. Costing over 36 billion dollars a wide review of the impact of deployment of Meaningful Use described at the flagship programme to deploy electronic health records across the United States provides concerning results. Rather than an electronic ecosystem of information, the authors suggest that the nation's thousands of EHRs largely remain fragmented and in a number of initiatives disconnected. The authors of this specific report spoke with more than 100 physicians, patients, IT experts and administrators, health policy leaders, attorneys, top government officials and representatives at more than a half-dozen EHR vendors, including the CEOs of two of the companies. Describing the interviews in this report the authors maintain that they reveal a tragic and missed opportunity (Fortune FS Erika Fry 2019), key findings suggest six core factors, which are impeding anticipated benefits. They include,

1. Poor integration of health systems and use of closed rather than open systems. The benefits of open systems are provided in Chap. 5 integrating the Health Care Enterprise.
2. Access to health records across and between health services and to individual patients.
3. Poor interface design, the strategic fit between the systems deployed and the needs of the user of this system to complete their role-increased time to do routine tasks using the technology and systems deployed than previous operation of routine tasks.
4. Spiraling costs the authors indicated that in interviews users of the systems and the service administrator had gagging orders enforced upon them.

   EHR vendors often impose contractual "gag clauses" that discourage buyers from speaking out about safety issues and disastrous software installations—though some customers have taken to the courts to air their grievances (Fortune FS Erika Fry 2019).
5. Accuracy and quality of data was noted as a concern, the report indicated that the process of linking the correct medical record to the correct patient, even when made by the same EHR vendor, often failed. This finding is also evident in other reports. For example the Kaiser Foundation tracking poll reports nearly half of those with EHRs have concerns about errors in their records (40% of total), one in five overall (21%) say that they or a family

member have noticed an error in their EHR. The most-reported errors are incorrect medical history (9%); fewer report incorrect personal information (5%), incorrect lab or test results (3%), incorrect medication or prescription information (3%), and billing issues (less than 1%) (Muñana 2019).

6. The missing jigsaw piece described by an interviewee as an inability for systems to connect across and between services. This is cited in the article, as follows "we didn't think about how all these systems connecting with one another. That was the real missing piece." (Fortune FS Erika Fry 2019) Figure 3.8 provides a summary illustration on this report by Schulte and Fry.

Anecdotal discussions with scholars from the US who have drafted Chap. 14 suggest that incremental improvements are emerging in different care service providers. Enhancements include revisions of existing systems and provide changes on how care is being provided to advance integrated care. For example, the patient portal is impacting on citizen access to their records in a positive way. https://www.dmc.org/portal (TH Medical 2016–2020). The implications of this comprehensive report by Fortune Magazine however suggest that the nursing informatics contribution for large-scale deployment is clearly warranted. Nursing has a core role to play particularly in designing and addressing patient safety and participating in detailed workflow mapping to optimise quality of care in transitioning to electronic health records. Examples where nursing engagement influences direct and indirect patient care increasingly will include the use of digital in the domain of connected health and supporting activated patients to manage their own care.

3.2.2 Administration and Research

In Chap. 9, the authors provide a comprehensive overview of administration systems and their increasing use in nursing and research. Here in Sect. 3.2.2, we provide some introductory background on the topic of nature of nursing and practice based evidence that contributes to progress nursing as a profession over time.

Research by Matney et al. (2011) recognises nurses as knowledge workers who translate data to information, information to knowledge and knowledge to wisdom. While nursing has a rich history of theoretical thinkers, who explore the knowledge of nursing, with advances in artificial intelligence and machine learning there are increased opportunities to advance nursing knowledge accelerating the research of practice theory. This is often articulated as a quest for a theoretical basis for the practice of the profession, and will be expanded upon further in the Chaps. 12–14 of this text (McQueen and Kickbush 2007; Saba and McCormack 1986).

It is not only the concept of practice theory that is important to consider to advance informatics, seminal work on the nature of nursing is also important. Virginia Henderson has in 1964 for example explored the Nature of Nursing and argued the case that an occupation especially a profession such as nursing that affects human life must clearly define its function (Flynn 2018). Today this notion is translated into terms such as evidence based practice and nursing scholarship as described by AACN published in 2018.

Nursing scholarship is the generation, synthesis, translation, application and dissemination of knowledge that aims to improve health hand transform health care. Scholarship is the communication of knowledge generated through multiple forms of inquiry that inform clinical practice nursing education policy and healthcare delivery (American Association of Colleges of Nursing (AACN) 1999, p. 2).

Schlodfeldt and Cody (1989) described the two criteria for a profession as a social mission and a calling for examiners to assist in knowledge generation to support advancement of practice. In the context of twenty-first century, health care Nursing's social mission is as important today as it has ever been. Nursing theory continues to evolve at an accelerated rate with the proliferation of digital data in society and access to such large volumes of data will challenge the boundaries of conventional thinking not only in the profession of nursing but at the interface of inter-professional working relationships.

Inter-professional clinical models are important and models such as Bonnie Wesorick Clinical Practice Model (CPM) are useful to reference in this context. The CPM framework is designed to assist practitioners to focus on practice priorities, evidence based clinical decision support, and practice expertise to ensure improved patient outcomes, compliance with national patient safety standards, and inter-professional staff collaboration satisfaction is achieved. This CPM framework also includes a health informatics model with evidence based clinical practice guidelines to support professional scope of practice and care processes (Troseth et al. 2017). Underpinned by core beliefs, principles, and theories and clinical practice models, the CPM Framework includes the following concepts: Health and healing care, Partnership and culture, Interdisciplinary integration, International consortiums, Health informatics, Applied evidence based practice, and central to the framework, the patient family and community care giver. Further information on the CPM framework is available from the following website https://www.elsevier.com/solutions/care-planning/professional-practice-services (Professional Practice Services 2020), that is to appraise and assist human beings in their quest to optimize their health status, health assets, and health potential" (Schlodfeldt and Cody 1989, p. 17).

In 2010, the International Council of Nursing defined nursing as:

Nursing encompasses autonomous and collaborative care of individuals of all ages, families, groups and communities, sick or well and in all settings. Nursing includes the promotion of health, prevention of illness, and the care of ill, disabled and dying people. Advocacy, promotion of a safe environment, research, participation in shaping health policy and in patient and health systems management, and education are also key nursing roles (International Council of Nurses (ICN) 2020).

More recent publications from Royal College of Nursing provide eight key principles relating to nursing practice describing what citizens can expect from the profession of nursing. These eight principles are

1. Principle A: Nurses and nursing staff treat everyone in their care with dignity and humanity; they understand their individual needs, show compassion and sensitivity, and provide care in a way that respects all people equally.
2. Principle B: Nurses and nursing staff take responsibility for the care they provide and answer for their own judgments and actions—they carry out these actions in a way that is agreed with their patients, and the families and carers of their patients, and in a way, that meets the requirements of their professional bodies and the law.
3. Principle C: Nurses and nursing staff manage risk, are vigilant about risk, and help to keep everyone safe in the places they receive healthcare.
4. Principle D: Nurses and nursing staff provide and promote care that puts people at the centre, involves patients, service users, their families and their carers in decisions and helps them make informed choices about their treatment and care.
5. Principle E: Nurses and nursing staff are at the heart of the communication process: they assess, record and report on treatment and care, handle information sensitively and confidentially, deal with complaints effectively, and are conscientious in reporting the things they are concerned about.
6. Principle F: Nurses and nursing staff have up-to-date knowledge and skills, and use these with intelligence, insight and understanding in line with the needs of each individual in their care.
7. Principle G: Nurses and nursing staff work closely with their own team and with other professionals, making sure patients' care and treatment is coordinated, is of a high standard and has the best possible outcome.
8. Principle H: Nurses and nursing staff lead by example, develop themselves and other staff, and influence the way care is given in a manner that is open and responds to individual needs (Royal College of Nursing 2019).

Each of the eight principles identified by RCN and listed above can be linked with nursing informatics knowledge skills and competencies. Principle B recommends nursing taking responsibility for care provision in accordance with patient's families and the law or Principle D recommends promoting patient centered care designed to aid decision making across the continuum of care. Principle E, F G and H include concepts such as communications, confidentiality, acquired knowledge and skills and provision of coordinated care for all.

The implications on the above definitions and principles of nursing practice on the specialty of informatics are increasingly evident. It is important to stress that nursing functions include both delegated tasks as illustrated in the CPM inter professional framework in addition to autonomous nursing activities, all of which have a direct bearing on the design and use of information systems for integrated care in practice. By nursing performing a dual role, the focus for nursing activity can be identified both as an independent practitioner and as part of an inter-professional team. As nursing is one of the largest stakeholder groups in most countries engaged in direct and indirect patient care, their voice within the specialty of Health informatics needs to be a strong one.

The ever-expanding impact of informatics on clinical nursing practice is therefore inevitable. It is therefore not surprising that institutions such as the National Academy of Medicine have consequently developed a dedicated committee to address technology roles in nursing, providing a series of focused sessions to inform practice and advance equity for use of digital. As technology increases in daily nursing practice, they consider nurses wellbeing and the impact of technology on patients and caregivers important factors to take into consideration (Spring 2020; Troseth et al. 2017). In the United Kingdom the Royal College of Nursing in 2019 launched its programme entitled Every Nurse an eNurse (Royal College of Nursing 2019).

The first report on this initiative is entitled Improving Digital Literacy (RCN NHS Health Education 2017) and the executive summary stresses that nursing is in the *midst of a technological revolution and digitalisation is developing at an incredible speed. It will continue to impact on many aspects of our lives and has the potential to transform the art and science of healthcare creating many opportunities for the population and those who care for them* (RCN NHS Health Education 2017, p. 3).

This report stresses the need to rethink the nurse patient and nurse citizen relationship and provides key definition for digital literacy as

Definition: Digital literacies are the capabilities, which fit someone for living, learning, and working, participating and thriving in a digital society.

To become a digitally-literate person the report suggests involving and developing specific functional skills, plus attitudes, values and behaviors' that can be categorised under the following domains:

- Digital identity, wellbeing, safety and security
- Communication, collaboration and participation
- Teaching, learning and personal/professional development
- Technical proficiency
- Information, data and media literacies
- Creation, innovation and scholarship. (RCN NHS Health Education 2017)

Jo and Ha (2019) sought to develop and validate an instrument to measure nursing information literacy competency. Reviewing information theoretical conceptual competency frameworks for education by RCN, ACRL Nurse and Tiger (Royal College of Nursing 2011; Phelps 2013; O'Connor et al. 2017). Through conducting a quantitative study using factor analysis 27 items in total were agreed for selection in the final scale. The authors suggest the results provide a basic direction for developing a nursing information literacy programme. The items are summarised as follows;

1. Competency for identifying a problem for example selecting key concepts or topics to find the information needed to solve the nursing care problem.
2. Competency for potential sources for information for example selection of the most appropriate information source to solve the nursing problem.

3. Competency for searching fine information for example checking of clinical information systems nursing records or test results in order to solve the nursing problem.
4. Competency for evaluating information for example identifying whether the retrieved information is valid reliable accurate and current.
5. Competency for acquiescing and managing of information for example extracting the core content needed to sort the nursing problem from various sources of data and information material.
6. Competency for using the information ethically for example the collected information is legally available to use and if required transfer, there has been no abuse of use of information access use of password or ID in an electronic health record.
7. Competency for integrating new information for example the main content of the collected information to use as a basis to resolve the nursing problem is appropriate Ref. Jo and Ha (2019, p. 32).

This section provides some initial detail on how to use data to develop a plan of care, we suggest there is a need to expand further the use of data through the nursing process and use digital compentencies for patient assessment intervention and evaluation for a one to one action and the use of data for population health.

The ubiquitous nature of smart and mobile devices in the twenty-first century provides new opportunities for nursing informatics, particularly to enhance professional influence and empower the profession to tackle health challenges. Examples of global initiatives, which situate nursing at the core of global policy, include the Nursing Now campaign. This initiative focuses on raising the profile and status of nursing (ICN 2020). It seeks to disseminate to wider audiences the triple impact of nursing which includes better health, greater gender equality and stronger economies. Reports from the Nursing Now campaign unpack core elements of the value of the nursing contribution. Examples include intimate hands on care, professional knowledge and person centered humanitarian values (Crisp et al. 2018, p. 4).

Nursing Now as a campaign, has created five programme areas to enable the profession to achieve campaign goal of improving global health by raising the profile and status of nursing worldwide. Briefly, we expand on the programmes in Table 3.2 and further information and resources are available from the Nursing Now Website (ICN 2020) https://www.nursingnow.org/join-the-campaign/.

It is evident from the literature and policy reviewed that the profession of nursing globally is at a crossroads and nursing informatics is critical in preparing the profession to practice in a digitally enabled society. Some of our existing models of care are evolving. There is a growing need for nursing as a profession to engage with community based interventions that support home and integrated care service. Underpinning such services are systems that can provide disease prevention, health promotion and self-management support interventions. Skiba et al. (2016) reports that deployment of Meaningful use and adoption of EHRs presents a fundamental change in how nurses plan, deliver, document, and review clinical care. For the academic community it suggests a change is needed in how we educate and train

Table 3.2 Nursing now progamme areas

Programme areas	Description
Universal Health Coverage	Programmes that provide access to essential health services to achieve universal health coverage require investment in nursing WHO can engage with communities and provide leadership on health promotion and prevention in partnership with community health workers. Recommendation call on WHO and world bank to invest in nursing as champions of universal health coverage
Evidence of impact	Increase of nursing capacity to build evidence on the nursing's contribution to health, economic development and gender equity. Recommendation initiate new studies where there are significant gaps in available research; work with partners to improve and disseminate evidence; promote the role of research to strengthen the impact of nursing; and develop global collaborations between researchers
Leadership and development	Appointment of a new Chief Nursing Officer by the World Health Organisation Recommendation—Instigate senior roles and provide support and training for senior nurse leaders in both policy and practice agendas globally
Sharing effective practice	Through focused dissemination and publishing of the best examples of innovation and effective practice. The nursing now campaign will work with the World Health Organization, International Council of Nurses and others to develop better ways of disseminating and improving access to existing collections of effective practice
The Year of the Nurse 2020	The Year of the Nurse in 2020 instigates a number of focused initiatives including inspiring 1000 employers worldwide to enable 20,000 young nurses and midwives to build their skills as advocates and influential leaders in healthcare. This is possible through initiatives such as the nightingale challenge

next generation nurses Chap. 15 by Prof Diane Skiba will discuss technology enabled learning in nursing, the final section on education in this chapter uses a framework from Skiba et al. (2016) to illustrate critical factors for digitally connected care. This final section explores core concepts to underpin educational and training requirements for practicing nurses.

3.2.3 Education

As illustrated earlier in this chapter, nursing and global policy recommends that nursing as a profession is expected to use a variety of technological tools and complex information management systems. This will require skills in analysis and synthesis of information to improve the quality and effectiveness of care delivery. Skiba et al. (2016) in a paper discusses preparation for next generation nursing on connected care. Identifying critical factors where nursing influences can align to achieve optimal results for care delivery. Under the theme of education, the concepts on this Framework for Nursing Informatics and Digitally Connected Care are adapted to present the evidence on next generation nursing informatics in context (Skiba et al. 2016) (Fig. 3.9).

Fig. 3.9 Skiba et al. (2016) framework for nursing informatics and digitally connected care adapted

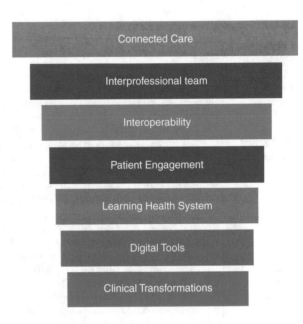

Table 3.3 Key factors for successful EHR Implementation (Fennelly 2019)

Organisational factors	Human factors	Technological factors
Governance leadership and culture	Skills and characteristics	Usability
End user involvement	Perceived benefits and incentives	Interoperability
Training	Perceived changes to the health ecosystem	Infrastructure
Support		Regulation standards and policies
Resourcing		Adaptability
Workflows		Testing

An Inter-Professional Team

For inter-professional team engagement, nurses globally are working across disciplinary fields providing leadership and insights on deployment of electronic health systems. Recent reports from Ireland that provide nursing leadership in inter professional team engagement and report on what the profession considers as key factors for successful deployment in electronic health records. Working as part of a inter disciplinary group team three core strands and themes are identified relating to organisational factors human factors and technological factors for successful electronic health care record deployment nationally.

These factors are listed below in Table 3.3.

Examples of educational inter-professional team programmes on digital transformation in eHealth have been introduced in Ireland. For example in January 2020, a new interdisciplinary programme on digital health transformation was introduced with a number of different academic institutions across the country. This innovative programme is working collaboratively to fully operationalise the concept of inter-professional collaboration in practice the goal of this innovative programme is preparation of leaders to implement large-scale change involving digital health technologies, to accelerate active participation where all disciplines are working in a harmonised and connected health fashion to advance innovations based on citizens needs (McElligot 2019). In the United States, the advanced practice nursing roles are expanding through certified nurse practitioner programmes to deliver primary care health services by 2025. Focusing on ability to attain skills, which support the healthcare organization to deliver clinical, leadership, and informatics skills across the care continuum. These initiatives will be discussed further in Chap. 16.

Interoperability

The theory underpinning Interoperability and investigating why interoperability is an important priority to grow capacity on with health care professionals is discussed in detail Chaps. 2, 5 and 6 of this text. It will therefore not be expanded upon further in this chapter other than to say that interoperability is increasingly described as the missing jigsaw piece in delivery of integrated care services (Blobel and Giacomini 2019; Blobel and Interoperable 2018; Blobel 2019). It is critically important therefore that nursing informatics education include related theory and evidence underpinning this important topic into educational syllabus. In this fifth edition the adoption and wide use of standards is discussed from different viewpoints with examples by authors across a number of chapters. As it is considered a critically important topic for nurses to understand and promote in their associated practice. Chapter. 2 that discusses new models of care as defined by global leaders emphasizes the need to connect systems and devices as a priority to address the fragmentation of care. Without the integration of standards within large scale national programmes of eHealth and digital, there is little chance of achieving the anticipated benefits of accessing quality information across and between systems. Indirectly this also can have an impact on patient safety and outcomes. Further information on standards for integrated care is available in Chap. 5 and a full chapter introducing standards is available as Chap. 6.

Patient Engagement

The third trend that requires focused attention in nursing informatics education is the rise of patient engagement and their uptake and use of digitals tools. The engagement of patients, families, caregivers and consumer in their health care is an important component of the transformation of health care. Leonard Kish refers to Patient Engagement "as the blockbuster drug of the century (Skiba et al. 2016).

If as already indicated in Sect. 3.2, the profession of nursing's mission is to appraise and assist human beings in their quest to optimize their health status, health assets, and health potential. The nurse patient relationship is at the heart of our professional scope of practice. As new inter professional working roles emerge, and some of traditional models of care delivery are revised, the people patient involvement agenda (PPI) becomes a critical driver to include in nursing informatics education. Understanding what the benefits for patients are with digital, the notion of empowerment and choice of services are just some of the key instigators within connected health. Underpinning this is the need to recognise the importance of design science and the fit of systems for their specific purpose to address patient need. This is best achieved by placing patients at the heart of health innovation within informatics. Ensuring patients are the driving force, informed through co-participatory methods of engagement in order to translate their needs into planned service delivery using digital and connected health (IPPOSI 2020).

Learning Health System

A Learning Healthcare System is defined, by the Institute of Medicine in 2015 (IoM)), as a system in which, "science, informatics, incentives, and culture are aligned for continuous improvement and innovation, with best practices seamlessly embedded in the delivery process and new knowledge captured as an integral by-product of the delivery experience" (McLachlan et al. 2019).

Learning health systems (LHS) were developed as a vehicle to advance clinical safety and health research and improve patient-centered care. Learning systems are closely aligned with the progression of Electronic Health Records (EHR) and share similar barriers and facilitators with implementation of EHR particularly from a human factors perspective. Learning health systems are possible by advancements in integrating patient data in to care, knowledge management, data analytics and documentation practices underpinned with legal ethical and data privacy agendas. Core to the adoption of a learning health system is the constant generation and use of new clinical knowledge and evidence based practice collated from digital data streams informing public policy. Such data presents new opportunities to provide benefits in care delivery efficiencies and inform quality and safety and patient outcomes (Friedman et al. 2015). Addressed in the future chapters critical questions that may be addressed by a learning health system may include how can the financial and emotional costs of care to patients be reduced? Alternatively, what is the impact of dashboards on nursing clinical decision making on patient outcomes?

For access to health, systems in progress see the following link, http://www.learninghealthcareproject.org/section/background/learning-healthcare-system (Foley 2020).

Digital Tools

The advancement and uptake of digital tools is increasingly mainstream in society today, In the United States for example, over 80% of citizen's use a smart phone or tablet to access social media, the use of email and text is now the preferred choice of communication rather than face-to-face communications. In the text The Patient Will See You Now published in 2015, Topol argues the case that individuals are increasingly expecting more from technology and less from each other (Topol 2016, p. 43). At the time of drafting, this chapter there is 3.50 billion smart phones in the world. Statistics reviewed in February 2020, including both smart and feature phones, the current number of mobile phone users is 4.78 billion, which makes 61.62% of people in the world a cell phone owner. Feature phones are the basic cell phones without apps and complex OS systems, are more prominent in developing countries. (Source: statista 2019.) We therefore are conditioned to engage with digital tools and Artificial Intelligence in our daily social and professional lives. For example, we use the Internet of Things (IoT); assistive devices such as the Amazon Alexa in the home to check weather listen to music or schedule our diaries. We see AI integrated in the clinical practice setting with devices such as infusion pumps. Such devices are underpinned with algorithms that include sequential instructions to complete a task in a sequenced order. Such algorithms provide assistance in managing the patient safety agenda, they are underpinned by a set of well-constructed rules for conformances such as checking an infusion rate is correct or setting a warning, that it has exceeded the pre-programmed limits. Driven by the global workforce decline of nurses, robotics has experienced a steady growth in the use of nursing particularly in aging population and in countries like Japan (Maalouf et al. 2018, p. 590). They define the use of robotics in nursing as into two distinct types assistive to support physical care including service and monitoring tasks and social assistive focused on the cognitive and emotional well-being of patients in need of companionship (Glauser 2017).

Spring identifies three key levels in which digital and technology is integrated into nursing practice

1. Use of digital device system and products including ICT used in daily routine working practices.
2. The act of using the technology for example pushing a button to turn on a device.
3. Technology as a service or purpose using the device and systems to deliver a function. For example, decrease in medication errors by using a bar coded medication administration system. (Spring 2020, p. 11).

It is essential to understand that such digital tools do not in any way replace nursing judgements and as required health care professionals can overwrite such tools as necessary (Spring 2020, p. 10). Stressing the importance of considering the legal and ethical dimension in the uptake and use of digital in practice setting, Jo and Ha (2019) deliberate on what impact the ever-increasing volume of accumulated data is on the practice of the profession.

The scale of digital information across healthcare organisations is ever increasing. It is therefore necessary to understand nursing information literacy from the perspective of nurses' ability to focus on what key information they need. This is achievable by fully understanding a nursing related problem in context, searching for the necessary information to address the identified problem. Having the ability to evaluate selected information and to use the accurate information to address the identified problem (Fortune FS Erika Fry 2019; Jo and Ha 2019). Other authors stress the need for educationalists to ensure that the skills associated with nursing informatics competencies are aligned with different roles and contexts within nursing and across different levels of health system delivery. This is best achieved by allocating better supports for the development of NI education, practice and research globally (Peltonen et al. 2019).

Clinical Transformation

Publications on clinical transformation and adoption of a comprehensive electronic health record EHR are associated with more positive usability ratings and higher quality of care within the profession. For example, in recent studies by Kutney-Lee et al. (2019) findings suggest that at the EHR adoption level, the hospital work environment plays a significant role in how nurses evaluate EHR usability and whether EHRs have their intended effects on improving quality and safety of care. Evaluation studies completed in Taiwan on the Implementation of a Mobile Nursing Information System (MNIS) found that the domain relationship of registered nurses years and managers' support for the use of the MNIS were positively related. Listing quality of care and user satisfaction as the most powerful predictor in both behavioral intention and actual use of the MNIS, this study also reported upon Managers' support as having a significant impact on implementation of digital systems in clinical setting (Cheng et al. 2019).

A core reason for user satisfaction being unmet relates to human factors and the fit of the system in to organisations.

Managing clinical transformation presents nursing with a number of challenges, all of which require important change management and implementation processes.

For clinical transformation change, literature suggests that altering practice involves two key implementation process firstly change processes and secondly transition processes. (McLean 2011). Both of these concepts can be distinguished as follows; change can be described as observable things that happen or are done differently usually involving alteration of structural processes on work practice routines. While transition processes relate more to the emotional aspects around what people feel, experience, or consider important in their practice. Early recognition that both concepts are required for successful implementation of national eHealth programmes is important (Hewitt-Taylor 2013). Failure to address change management processes can be a costly business and it therefore important to include the topic in nursing informatics educational programmes.

Change management theory emphasise the importance of establishing both frameworks and models to facilitate sharing and collaborating on the transition process in order to ensure a smooth translation from paper based records to electronic records is achieved. Bridging the gap between what we know and what we do in order to maximise the translation of evidence into practice requires effective and focused communication (Thompson et al. 2013, p. 20). The importance and complexity of communication within the change management/transition process is well illustrated in the following quote:

> eHealth program is best conceptualised not as a blue print and implementation plan for a state of the art technical system but as a series of overlapping, conflicting, and mutually misunderstood language games that combine to produce a situation of ambiguity, paradox, incompleteness and confusion. (Greenhalgh et al. 2011, p. 534)

Identifying the need for change with practitioners and devising strong leadership with clear aims and objectives are critical levers for success (Hewitt-Taylor 2013). Other key requisites for change include realisation and communicating a vision (Kotter 1995; Alonso 2013). Change management programmes need to be rooted in practitioner's wisdom (Greenhalgh et al. 2011, p. 7). Advancing clinical transformation and eHealth agendas therefore requires change management programmes, not only to succeed in single organisations structures, but at the wider cross-institutional boundaries to facilitate patient centered connected care. The consequences of such innovations affect health care professionals working practices and organisation need to invest significant effort on acquiring new skills on security measures, training on routine documenting and referral practices whilst concurrently managing patient care to avoid adverse outcomes. Clarity on realisable benefits or incentives not just for the organisation but for the individual practitioners involved by identifying why they should make such a time investment needs to clearly articulated (Peppard et al. 2007).

3.3 Conclusion

This chapter has summarised nursing informatics in the context of contemporary health and social care, considering how it has evolved over the past 50 years. Chapter 3 highlights, that the field of informatics is increasingly considered a core professional competency for nursing. Using an adaptation of the CARE acronym namely connected health, administration, research, and education Chap. 3 has sought to present the evidence and provide the reader with insights on the critical factors which are driving the practice of informatics within the profession. Programme initiatives such as the Nursing Now campaign are critical to migrate key values from the nature and scope of nursing activities in twenty-first century health and social care. As the needs of our patients change so too does the clinical specialist and advanced practice roles within nursing. Effectively communicating the value of nursing informatics to a wider audience in health and social care policy is essential, and we would argue critical for the profession at this time. The need for robust and rigoursly designed nursing informatics infrastructure to enhance the use of ICT and digital across the different levels of care delivery to support nursing workforce and patient outcomes has never been greater. A poorly designed and implemented Electronic health record can make nursing practice harder to deliver, and in the longer term potentially compromise patient care and outcomes. This explains why we consider that different informatics roles are needed across the care environment ensuring that nursing informaticians are involved from the outset on any planned digital transformation. Specifically nursing engagement in procurement, selection of technologies, enhanced equipment deployment and software design. At the time of writing this chapter, the world is in the midst of fighting a global pandemic Covid-19. Nurses globally are practicing 24 h a day 7 days a week on the front line to care for citizens, many of whom will not survive. Never before has there been such as need to accelerate innovation and advance knowledge skills and competencies in the field of nursing and health informatics to assist in care delivery.

Clinical Pearls
Nursing informatics skills are now considered a critical competency in delivery of health and social care and global policy agendas for new models of care.

The nursing contribution in the development of eHealth and digital is critical to optimise the value proposition specifically in regards to efficiency effectiveness and sustainability of electronic health records in the future.

The expanding and new roles within the profession are underpinned with connected digital health solutions, attaining digital competencies are therefore increasingly considered a priority skill set for nurses.

3.4   Review Questions

3.4.1   Questions

1. Having reviewed this chapter, list what you consider are the critical factors that require careful consideration in the context of your own health care context to advance connected digital health.
2. Access the website and publications on the Nursing Now campaign from the following link (ICN 2020) https://www.nursingnow.org/join-the-campaign/
3. One of the nursing now initiatives is the Nightingale Challenge established for the Year of the Nurse 2020. A total of 27,295 nurses and midwives from 719 employers in 71 countries have accepted the Nightingale Challenge. Review the associated links and select an example of one initiative which uses nursing informatics to demonstrate empowerment of nurses and midwives as leaders, practitioners and advocates in health.

3.4.2   Answers

1. The response to question one should include reference to Sect. 3.2.3 specifically material relating to Interoperability, Patient Engagement, Learning Health System, Digital tools and Clinical Transformation. The response should demonstrate contextual material from the participants professional practice context or experiences.
2. The response to question two should reference publications from the Nursing Now Resources homepage and specifically the Toolkit which has structured resources on social media, advocacy materials and Nursing Now guidelines and slides.
3. The response to question three should provide a selected example and list detail of how this example incorporates nursing informatics as detailed in this chapter.

Glossary

Careflow A mapping activity of the healthcare encounter or service delivery process between health care professionals and patients, which describes the health and social care service activity through one to many service and data flow points

C-HOBIC Canadian Health Outcomes for Better Information and Care

CIHI Canadian Institute for Health Information

Cloud computing A term used to describe a new form computing, "cloud" computing relates to remote based computing, instead of storing and processing all of your information locally, all computation and storage is done remotely on the "cloud" which is an external server or network of servers

Co-production Co-production is about care that is delivered in an equal and reciprocal relationship between clinical and non-clinical professionals and the individuals using care services, their families, carers and communities. Co-production therefore goes beyond models of engagement, since it implies a long-term relationship between people, providers and health systems where information, decision-making and service delivery become shared

CPM Clinical Practice Model

CPOE Computerised provider order entry system

DHC Digital Health Canada

Digital Health Digital Health is used as an umbrella term for areas including eHealth, telehealth, mHealth and more. Digital Health is the integration of all information and knowledge sources involved in the delivery of healthcare via information technology (IT)-based systems. This includes information created by caregivers, often within electronic health record systems at a hospital or GP practice, and information created by patients using apps, monitoring devices and wearable sensors. Digital health information also includes management and administrative information needed to co-ordinate and manage activities within the healthcare system

eHealth eHealth is the use of information and communication technologies (ICT) for health (WHO 2005)

Empowerment Empowerment is about supporting people and communities to take control of their own health needs resulting, for example, in the uptake of healthier behaviours, the ability of people to self-manage their own illnesses and changes in people's living environments

EMR Electronic medical system

Engagement Engagement is about people and communities being involved in the design, planning and delivery of health services, enabling them to make choices about care and treatment options or to participate in strategic decision-making on how, where and on what health resources should be spent. Engagement is also related to the community's capacity to self-organize and generate changes in their living environments

FHIR Fast Healthcare Interoperability Resources Specification is a set of standards that guides how systems code, transmit, and receive data using smart and mobile devices

Health Health as a state of complete physical, mental and social wellbeing, and not merely the absence of disease and infirmity (WHO 1948)

Interoperability Interoperability is the ability of two or more systems or components to exchange information and to use information that has been exchanged

ITU International Telecommunication Union

mHealth A term for medical and public health practice supported by mobile devices such as mobile phones, patient monitoring devices , and other wireless devices

NNDS National Nursing Data Standards

PAHO Pan American Health Organisation

Personalization Services designed specifically for individuals and their unique healthcare needs

Telehealth The delivery of healthservices using ICTs, specifically where distance is a barrier to health care

Workarounds A strategy for working around a software misfit in order to solve the problems that the poorly designed software fails to address

Workflow Depiction of actual sequence of the operations or actions taken in a process Ref Systems of Concepts for Continuity of Care ISO 13940

References

Alonso I. Navigating triage to meet targets for waiting times. Emerg Nurse. 2013;21(3):20–6.

American Association of Colleges of Nursing (AACN). Defining scholarship for the profession of nursing. American Association of Colleges of Nursing Position Statement. 1999. https://www.aacnnursing.org/News-Information/Positions-White-Papers/www.aacnnursing.org/News-Information/Position-Statements-White-Papers/Defining-Scholarship. Cited 30 Mar 2020.

Anderson J. Medical informatics. J Med Inform. 1976;1:1.

Ball MJ, Hannah KJ, Newbold SK, Douglas JV. Nursing informatics: where caring and technology meet. 3rd ed. New York: Springer; 2000.

Blobel B. Challenges and solutions for designing and managing pHealth ecosystems. Front Med. 2019;6:83.

Blobel B, Giacomini M. Phealth 2019: Proceedings of the 16th international conference on wearable micro and nano technologies for personalized health, 10–12 June 2019, Genoa, Italy. Amsterdam/Washington, DC: IOS Press; 2019. p326. (Studies in health technology and informatics).

Blobel B, Interoperable EHR. Systems – challenges, standards and solutions. EJBI. 2018;14(2). https://www.ejbi.org/scholarly-articles/interoperable-ehr-systems%2D%2Dchallenges-standards-and-solutions.pdf. Cited 31 Mar 2020.

Canada Health Infoway. What is digital health. 2020. https://infoway-inforoute.ca/en/what-we-do/benefits-of-digital-health/what-is-digital-health. Cited 30 Mar 2020.

Caulfield BM, Donnelly SC. What is connected health and why will it change your practice? QJM. 2013;106(8):703–7.

Cheng C-C, Chan RC-L, Chen PL, Guo SH-M, et al. Evaluation of the implementation of a mobile nursing information system. 2019. https://www.himss.org/resources-evaluation-implementation-mobile-nursing-information-system. Cited 31 Mar 2020.

CHM. History of computing. Computer History Museum. 2020. https://computerhistory.org/. Cited 30 Mar 2020.

Crisp N, Brownie S, Refsum C. Nursing and midwifder the key to rapid and cost effective exapanisin of high quality universal health coverage. Qatar: ICN Nursing Now Campaign; 2018. p. 34. (Word Imnnovation Summit for Health). https://www.wish.org.qa/wp-content/uploads/2018/11/IMPJ6078-WISH-2018-Nursing-181026.pdf.

Fennelly O. Factors for success in electronic health record implementation: literature review and key considerations. Dublin; 2019, 64. https://www.ehealthireland.ie/Strategic-Programmes/Electronic-Health-Record-EHR-/Information-Resources/Factors-for-Success-in-EHR-Implementation-Literature-Review-and-Key-Considerations.pdf.

Flynn R. Guidance for a data quality framework. Dublin, Ireland: Health and Informatin Quality Authority; 2018. p. 64. https://www.hiqa.ie/sites/default/files/2018-10/Guidance-for-a-data-quality-framework.pdf.

Foley T. The learning health care project. Institute of Health and Society, Newcastle University. 2020. http://www.learninghealthcareproject.org/section/background/learning-healthcare-system. Cited 31 Mar 2020.

Fortune FS Erika Fry. Death by 1,000 clicks: where electronic health records went wrong. Kaiser Health News. 2019. https://khn.org/news/death-by-a-thousand-clicks/. Cited 30 Mar 2020.

Friedman C, Rubin J, Brown J, Buntin M, Corn M, Etheredge L, et al. Toward a science of learning systems: a research agenda for the high-functioning learning health system. J Am Med Inform Assoc. 2015;22(1):43–50.

Glauser W. Artificial Intelligence automation and the future of nursing. Canadian Nurse. 2017. https://www.canadian-nurse.com/.

Greenburg AB. Medical informatics: science or science fiction. Unpublished. 1975.

Greenhalgh T, Russell J, Ashcroft RE, Parsons W. Why national eHealth programs need dead philosophers: Wittgensteinian reflections on policymakers' reluctance to learn from history: why national eHealth programs need dead philosophers. Milbank Q. 2011;89(4):533–63.

Greens R, Shortliffe EH. Medical informatics: an emerging academic discipline and institutional priority. J Am Med Assoc. 1990;263(8):1114–20.

Hannah KJ. The computer and nursing practice. Nurs Outlook. 1976;24(9):555–8.

Harrington L. American Nurses Association releases new scope and standards of nursing informatics practice. AACN Adv Crit Care. 2015;26(2):93–6.

Henderson V. The Nature of Nursing. Am J Nurs. 1964;64(8):62.

Hewitt-Taylor J. Planning successful change incorporating processes and people. Nurs Stand. 2013;27(38):35–40.

HIMSS. About the workflows and capabilities. 2019. https://www.himss.org/about-workflows-and-capabilities. Cited 30 Mar 2020.

ICN. Nursing now. Nursing Now Campaign. 2020. https://www.nursingnow.org/join-the-campaign/.

International Council of Nurses (ICN). ICN – International Council of Nurses. https://www.icn.ch/homepage. Cited 30 Mar 2020.

IPPOSI. Irish Platform for Patient Organisations, Science & Industry. IPPOSI. https://www.ipposi.ie/. Cited 31 Mar 2020.

Jo M, Ha Y. Development and validation of an instrument to measure nursing information literacy competency. J Korean Acad Community Health Nurs. 2019;30(1):25.

Kotter J. Leading change: why transformation efforts fail. Harvard Business Review. 1995. http://lighthouseconsultants.co.uk/wp-content/uploads/2010/08/Kotter-Leading-Change-Why-transformation-efforts-fail.pdf.

Kutney-Lee A, Sloane DM, Bowles KH, Burns LR, Aiken LH. Electronic health record adoption and nurse reports of usability and quality of care: the role of work environment. Appl Clin Inform. 2019;10(01):129–39.

Maalouf N, Sidaoui A, Elhajj IH, Asmar D. Robotics in nursing: a scoping review. J Nurs Scholarsh. 2018;50(6):590–600.

Mandil S. Health informatics: New solutions to old challenges. World Health. 1989;2:5.

Matney S, Brewster PJ, Sward KA, Cloyes KG, Staggers N. Philosophical approaches to the nursing informatics data-information-knowledge-wisdom framework. Adv Nurs Sci. 2011;34(1):6–18.

McElligot A. University of Limerick. MSc Digital Health Transformation. 2019. http://www.digitalhealthtransformation.ie.

McLachlan S, Dube K, Johnson O, Buchanan D, Potts HWW, Gallagher T, et al. A framework for analysing learning health systems: are we removing the most impactful barriers? Learn Health Syst. 2019;3(4). https://onlinelibrary.wiley.com/doi/abs/10.1002/lrh2.10189. Cited 31 Mar 2020.

McLean C. Change and transition: what is the difference? Br J Sch Nurs. 2011;6(2):78–81.

McQueen DV, Kickbush I. Critical issues in theory for health promotion. In: Health and modernity the role of theory in health promotion. New York: Springer; 2007. p. 21–42.

Muñana C. Data note: public's experiences with electronic health records. The Henry J. Kaiser Family Foundation. 2019. https://www.kff.org/other/poll-finding/data-note-publics-experiences-with-electronic-health-records/. Cited 30 Mar 2020.

Nagle LM, Catford P. Toward a model of successful electronic health record adoption. Health Q. 2008;11(3):84–91.

Newbold S. IMIA NI SIG. IMIA. 2016. https://imia-medinfo.org/wp/sig-ni-nursing-informatics/. Cited 30 Mar 2020.

O'Connor S, Hubner U, Shaw T, Blake R, Ball M. Time for TIGER to ROAR! Technology informatics guiding education reform. Nurs Educ Today. 2017;58:78–81.

Peltonen LM, Nibber R, Lewis A, Block L, Pruinelli L, Topaz M, et al. Emerging professionals' observations of opportunities and challenges in nursing informatics. Nurs Leadersh (Tor Ont). 2019;32(2):8–18.

Peppard J, Ward J, Daniel E. Managing the realisation of business benefits from IT investments. MIS Q Exec. 2007;6:1–11.

Phelps SF. Designing the information literacy competency standards for nursing. Med Ref Serv Q. 2013;32(1):111–8.

Professional Practice Services. Elsevier. 2020. https://www.elsevier.com/solutions/care-planning/professional-practice-services. Cited 30 Mar 2020.

RCN NHS Health Education. Improving digital literacy. England: NHS; 2017. p. 11. Report No.: RCN publication code: 006 129. https://www.rcn.org.uk/-/media/royal-college-of-nursing/documents/publications/2017/july/pub-006129.pdf?la=en.

Royal College of Nursing. Royal College of Nursing RCN Competencies: finding , using and managing information [Internet]. RCN Competencies. 2011. https://www.rcn.org.uk/-/media/royal-college-of-nursing/documents/publications/2018/april/pdf-006854.pdf?la=en.

Royal College of Nursing. Every nurse is an eNurse. eHealth Digital Capabilities for 21st Century. 2019. https://www.rcn.org.uk/clinical-topics/ehealth/every-nurse-an-e-nurse.

Saba VK, McCormack KA. Essentials of computers for nurses. Philadelphia: Lippincott; 1986.

Saha P. Digital transformation and the role of enterprise architecture. International Telecommunications Union; 2019. p. 18. Report No.: 978-92-61-29021-4 (EPUB version). https://www.itu.int/dms_pub/itu-d/opb/str/D-STR-DIG_TRANSF-2019-PDF-E.pdf.

Schlodfeldt R, Cody W. Structuring nursing knowledge: a priority for creating nursing's future. Philosophical and theoretical perspectives for advancing nursing practice. 5th ed. Burlington, MA: Jones and Bartlett; 1989. p. 15–21.

Scholes M, Tallberg M, Pluyter-Wenting E. International nursing informatics: a history of the first forty years 1960–2000. British Computer Society. 2000; BCS Swinford.

Sensmeier J. Harnessing the power of artificial intelligence. Nurs Manag. 2017;25(2):18–20.

Shortliffe EH, Perreault LE, Weiderhold G, Fagan LM. Medical informatics: computer applications in healthcare and biomedicine. 2nd ed. New York: Springer -Verlag; 2001. p. 21.

Skiba DJ, Barton AJ, Estes K, Gilliam E, Knapfel S, Lee C, et al. Preparing the next generation of advanced practice nurses for connected care. Stud Health Technol Inform. 2016;225:307–13.

Spring B. Nursing 2.0: Care in the age of technology. Ohio Nurses Association; 2020. https://www.ce4nurses.org/nursing-2-0-care-in-the-age-of-technology-2/.

statista. Mobile internet usage worldwide. 2019. www.statista.com. Cited 31 Mar 2020. https://www.statista.com/topics/779/mobile-internet/.

Sustainable Development. Sustainable Development Goals. Sustainable Development Knowledge Platform. 2020. https://sustainabledevelopment.un.org/?menu=1300.

TH Medical. I'm A patient | My Health Rec, our patient portal. DMC Hospital. https://yourhealth.tenethealth.com/corporate-content-blocks/corporate-content/i-m-a-patient. Cited 30 Mar 2020.

Thompson L, Schneider J, Wright N. Developing communities of practice to support the implementation of research into clinical practice. Leadersh Health Serv. 2013;26(1):20–3.

Time Magazine, editor. A brief history of computing. Time Magazine. 2020. https://time.com/search/?q=history+of+computing+. Cited 30 Mar 2020.

Topol EJ. The patient will see you now: the future of medicine is in your hands. New York: Basic Books; 2016. p. 374.

Troseth M, Mayo D, Nieves R, Lambrecht S. Case study 12.1: Clinical practice model (CPM) framework approach to achieve clinical practice interoperability and big data comparative analysis. In: Big data –enabled nursing education, research and practice. Cham Switzerland: Springer International Publishing; 2017.

White P. CHobic. CIHI 2020. https://www.cihi.ca/en/c-hobic-infosheet_en.pdf.

WHO | eHealth at WHO. 2005. WHO. Retrieved October 13, 2020, from http://www.who.int/ehealth/about/en/.

Chapter 4
The Mechanics of Technology and Digital

Christopher Henry

Abstract In this short chapter an overview of technology currently in use in health care is discussed. Both hardware and software are explained offering the reader a high level summary of critical components used in conventional computing. Comparisons between computer functionality and human activity such as riding a bike or driving on a motorway are described. Cloud computing is introduced and the example of how mobile technology applications on health and wellbeing can be used is discussed.

Keywords Hardware · Software · ICT · Cloud computing · Architecture · Digital

Key Concepts
Hardware
Software
ICT
Cloud Computing
Mobile Applications
Digital

Learning Objectives for the Chapter
1. Understand foundation concepts relating to hardware and how hardware is used in delivery of computer programmes.
2. Acquire a foundational understanding of software and its relationship to emerging developments in computer science such as cloud computing.
3. Determine how software applications are acquired and how mobile applications are sourced.

Electronic Supplementary Material The online version of this chapter (https://doi.org/10.1007/978-3-030-58740-6_4) contains supplementary material, which is available to authorized users.

C. Henry (✉)
FINEOS, Dublin, Ireland

© Springer Nature Switzerland AG 2021
P. Hussey, M. A. Kennedy (eds.), *Introduction to Nursing Informatics*, Health Informatics, https://doi.org/10.1007/978-3-030-58740-6_4

We don't know where we get our ideas from. What we do know is that we do not get them from our laptops .....

—John Cleese

4.1 Introduction

Society is increasingly technologically knowledgeable and yet increasingly dependent. Rather than relying on information committed to memory, our brains "outsource" information to repositories accessed through smart phones and computers. Consider how many phone numbers people memorize compared to a number of years ago? The availability and power of technology impacts our behavior; it influences how we socially communicate, how we write, read, and what we choose to remember. As a healthcare professional, it is crucial to have an appreciation of the latest advances with digital technologies and a basic understanding of how they operate. This understanding is needed as technological breakthroughs with Artificial Intelligence and Machine Learning are constantly being uncovered in the pursuit of improved patient outcomes, and to improve the care delivery process for clinicians. These topics are discussed in detail in Chaps. 2 and 16 (AACC 2020).

This chapter presents an overview of technology that is in use today and provides a brief explanation as to how they operate in society both in communities and in our health care organisations. It also offers some insight into the emerging paradigm in communications technology mTechnology and offers one example of how mobile applications can be used in healthcare.

This chapter will focus on the fundamentals of computing technologies. It will also explore some of the more recent technologies and explain how they can support eHealth solutions to assist health care professionals and individual patients in their daily practice and lives.

4.2 What Is a "Computer"

The vast array of twenty-first century technological advances have made it difficult to use the term "computer" to convey the conventional desktop or laptop models. Today, computers exist in almost every part of day-to-day life, from the fuel management system in a car, the program selection unit in a washing machine, the digital temperature control gauge in a refrigerator, to a Smartphone. In this sense, technology and computers are considered ubiquitous, since they are a part of everyday life activities, and so common that most people no longer consider them to be out of the ordinary, their uptake and use in society is inevitable.

Despite the many different appearances and occurrences of computers, they are all composed of two elements—hardware and software. The hardware of a computer can be defined as being the physical components that create the computer and the software can be defined as being the stored set of instructions that allow computers to do what they do. While the overall complexity of computers today may initially seem daunting, it is important to remember that every computer is based on Boolean logic. The term Boolean relates to mathematical algebra and can be associated with variable values. Simply stated Boolean values offer a true and false variable often denoted as either 1 or 0 (on or off) in the field of computer science. This simple true/false or on/off logic forms the platform upon which all computer functionality is built. In order to achieve this Boolean functionality, computer manufacturers use electronic components called Transistors.

A transistor can be described as a semi-conductor device, which essentially amplifies and switches electronic signals and power. Transistors build upon the differentiation between off and on Boolean logic to create complex processes that integrate together to achieve the final communications and processing tool, that is the end-user's computer.

4.2.1 Hardware

Hardware consists of the physical elements of a computer. Essentially, hardware can be defined as being the physical computer itself. A conventional computer model's hardware would consist of a Central Processing Unit (CPU), a monitor, a mouse and a keyboard. These components are the "seen" elements of a computer. The term hardware also covers the unseen or internal elements of a computer such as the computer's motherboard, ram, graphics card, hard drive. Table 4.1 lists some hardware components and briefly explains their function.

Table 4.1 Components of computer hardware

Component	Description
Monitor	Computers screen, used for viewing output from a computer
Mouse	Input device used to obtain motion-based input from the user
Trackpad	Similar to a mouse but obtains data directly from user's touch
Keyboard	Input device used to obtain static predefined symbol input
CPU (Central Processing Unit)	Processes tasks given to it by the computers operating system (explained later)
RAM (Random Access Memory)	RAM is used as temporary storage space for task data that is being processed
ROM (Read Only Memory)	ROM is a type of computer memory used mainly to store core computing software
Hard Drive	Is used to store data that will persist after the computer has powered off
Graphics Card	Used to compute the image values to be displayed on a graphical output
Bus	A network architecture in which a set of clients are connected via a shared communications structure in the single cable called a bus
Cache	A collection of data duplicating original values stored elsewhere on a computer
Persistent data	Information that continues to be stored even after power is no longer applied to it

Random Access Memory (RAM)

The term, memory, in computing has a lot of confusion surrounding it. People often automatically equate memory with storage, which although technically correct, uses the word memory out of context. Memory, as part of a computer's specifications, does not relate solely to the amount of storage capacity a computer has. Memory on a computer is not about how many movies, songs or photos it can hold.

Computers require a minimum amount of "memory" or working capacity in order to process information and execute the various programs in use. Thus, the term memory relates both to how much storage memory (See section on ROM below) and also how much random access memory (RAM) a computer has available to engage in processing information.

RAM can be thought of as the platform on which tasks are processed by the machine's processor. The processing unit runs the programme by fetching the instructions from RAM evaluating the programmes in sequence and executing them. In a way, it can be compared to a bridge on a highway where cars are tasks, the motorway's speed limit is the processor's speed and the lanes on the motorway are the processor's speed capability. When traffic converges onto the bridge, if the bridge doesn't have enough lanes or capacity to deal with the number of cars (tasks) that the highway is capable of processing then there is going to be a traffic jam. This process is demonstrated in Figs. 4.1 and 4.2.

Adding another lane (RAM memory bank) to the bridge will significantly increase the amount of traffic crossing the river. The processor speed still has a major contribution to the overall processing of tasks. There is no point in having a four-lane bridge on a small highway that has a speed limit of 30 km/h as most of these lanes would be left idle.

Fig. 4.1 RAM Functionality 1

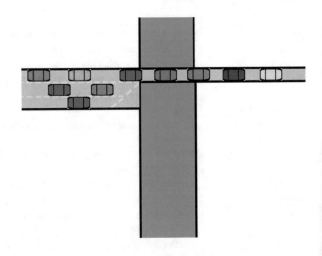

Fig. 4.2 RAM
Functionality 2

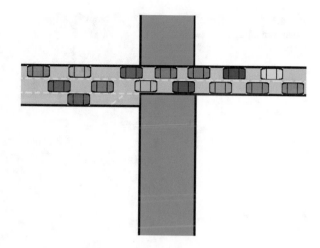

ROM (Read Only Memory)

When discussing RAM, we considered real-time processing of tasks and how RAM integrates into a computer. The downfall of RAM is that its memory is not persistent through a cut-off of power. As RAM is only capable of storing memory when power is supplied to it, another type of memory is also needed to create a conventional computer. As it would be very inefficient to constantly apply power to the computer to store information that is infrequently accessed and not likely to be modified. Persistent data is needed in computing to store the start-up instructions of a computer, i.e. "boot "the computer. ROM differs from RAM in that its stored data persists even after power is no longer applied to it. Thus, ROM is ideal for use as the computer's booting memory. ROM is also the type of memory used in hard drives to store data such as movies, music and documents. The higher the ROM capacity, the greater is the storage capability available in a computer.

Operating Systems (OS)

The computer's operating system is the fundamental set of instructions that drives the operation of the computer. It manages all the computer's hardware and ties it to the computer's software. Technically speaking, the computer's operating system is software, but it is the main software that interprets all other software.

There are predominantly two types of Personal Computer (PC) operating systems. These are Win and Unix systems. These types of systems are the basis for the Windows and Macintosh (Mac) operating systems, with the Windows operating system being developed by Microsoft and the Mac operating system being developed by Apple.

Fig. 4.3 An overview of
basic computing
architecture

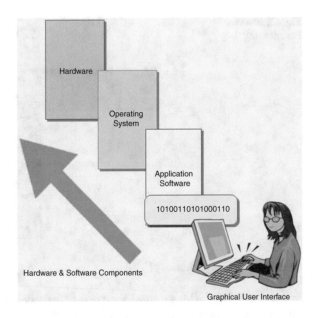

As illustrated in the diagram below, the operating system for a computer can be interpreted as sitting between the hardware and application software for a computer (Fig. 4.3).

The Apple or "Mac" the overall layout, functionality and file structure is different to that of a conventional windows (Microsoft) personal computer. This is not because of the hardware that is used in producing the different machines; it is because of the operating system that they are using.

The operating system in an Apple "Mac" uses different system architecture than a traditional windows machine and therefore, has different capabilities and ways of doing things. In order to get a better understanding of a computer's hardware specification, Table 4.2 outlines some perspective, relative to computing technology in 2013.

Networks

The topic of networks is a broad and comprehensive subject that has changed dramatically over the past 30 years. Briefly, a network is comprised of two or more nodes that can transfer data between each other. These nodes can be classified as any entity capable of interpreting the data that it receives. In computing terms, the node will mainly refer to some form of computational device. The computational device can refer to a large spectrum of entities. On a large scale, it can refer to a server but if we reduce our spectrum, we can technically define a computer itself as being a network.

Table 4.2 Computer components specification

Specification detail	Low	Medium	High
Processor	1 GHz	2.0 GHz	3 GHz
Memory	2 GB	8 GB	32 GB
Hard Drive	128 GB	750 GB	2 TB
Graphics Video Card	Graphics cards vary depending make and model. In order to get a better understanding of a particular model, searching through reviews will provide some great insight		
Sound Card	Sound card quality tends to be consistent through computer manufacturers. Like graphics cards, it would be best to find reviews online		
Disk Drive	Disk Drive specifications on average are very similar for most computers. The only distinction between most would be different capabilities such as the ability to burn DVD's		
Screen	Screen specifications have a lot of different contributing factors. These include screen size, resolution capabilities and display technology i.e. LCD, HD		

LCD liquid-crystal-display, *HD* high definition, *GB* gigabyte, *TB* terabyte, *GHz* gigahertz, *MB* megabyte, *DVD* digital video disk

Computers are comprised of multiple pieces of hardware communicating with each other through internal networks managed by the computer's operating system. This concept of sharing data between small components to create a computer can be expanded to sharing data between computers to create a larger network such as an in-office emailing system or chat network. This concept of communication gave rise to what we know today as the Internet. The Internet isn't a physical entity, it's a term used to describe the global exchange of data between computers and servers worldwide. This exchange of data is most commonly facilitated by a network protocol known as Hyper Text Transfer Protocol (http). Additional detail relating to networks can be sourced from the www3Schools resource and a related paper on machine learning from the perspective of clinical laboratory (AACC 2020; WWW3 Schools 2020).

4.2.2   Software

Computer software can be defined as the stored procedures that control the internal workings of a computer. The role of software can be illustrated in the example of riding a bicycle (Fig. 4.4). In order for a person to ride a bike, their brain has a set of instructions to make the overall process possible. The rider's brain has a stored set of instructions to keep their legs peddling while maintaining balance with their overall body positioning and movement. This is exactly what software is,—in order to run a program (a game for example) on a computer, the computer has a stored set of instructions to display images on the screen and to compute the physics required to make the game realistic.

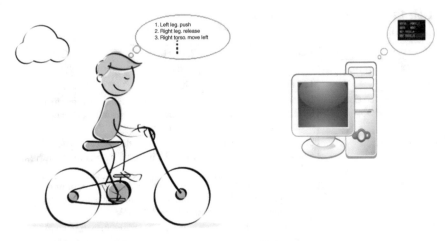

Fig. 4.4 Computer functionality

4.3   Emerging Technologies for eHealth Solutions

As computing advances in fifth generation computing, services such as cloud computing and services orientated architecture come to the forefront. Here we briefly outline some of the addtional elements that are required to deliver the fifth generation computing paradigm.

4.3.1   Service Orientated Architecture (SOA) and Web Services

Service oriented architecture can be described as a dynamic framework, which establishes a set of protocols to deliver integrated services across different health care providers.

The framework comprises of a set of methods for specifying and standardizing services and includes a dynamic model for detailing interactions between and among these services. SOA emerged from the progression of delivering web-based services to advance integration and access of health data across and between service providers. Briefly, web services can glue together applications running on different messaging platforms and enable information from one application to be used by others. Web services software has grown to include a rich set of specifications and standards to facilitate interoperability across and between services. These include the ability to describe, compose, package, and transport messages and ensure that security in service access is accomplished. In the domain of healthcare a state of the art application used for message transfer is entitled Fast Healthcare Interoperability Resources. This specification is developed by Health Level Seven International (commonly known as HL7), and it supports interoperability specification for the exchange of healthcare information electronically. This specification is described in detail in Chap. 5 (Health Level 7 2020).

Clinicians will see SOA in action when clinical records using information from diverse sources (laboratory, radiology, primary care providers, hospital information systems, etc. can be viewed with a single sign on an integrated record of health information.

Despite the rapid progression of web services within the business and financial industry, its growth within the healthcare industry has been slower than in other service industries. A key reason for this directly relates to the limited uptake of health informatics standards in the healthcare industry. Although there is potential for this to advance now with the introduction of a web services such as Fast Healthcare Interoperability Resources Specification FHIR (Health Level 7 2020) In addition, healthcare information is considered to be sensitive data, therefore for successful implementation of shared or integrated records a robust security and data privacy platform from which healthcare service professionals can access and transfer patient records is essential. The topic of standards in healthcare is discussed in Chap. 6 and patient safety and confidentiality will be discussed in detail in Chap. 10.

4.3.2 Cloud Computing

Demand for persistent and accessible data storage has contributed to the genesis of virtual storage platforms. The technologies which focus on the delivery of a virtual system, such as cloud computing aim to facilitate access to large amounts of computing power by aggregating resources and offering a single system view to the user often referred to as a portal or platform. This view is however usually at a cost and is based on a business model for the "on demand" delivery of computing power or in recent developments, can be pre-purchased based on expected usage.

The utility service for cloud computing includes the processing of information, the storage of information and the associated data and software resource requirements (Foster 2003). As a relatively new phenomenon several definitions exist on what cloud computing is. Additional information relating to the deliverables of cloud computing eHealth and digital is available to view in Chap. 2.

4.3.3 Wireless Technologies and the Mobile Internet

Wireless technologies are a means of transferring data from one entity to another without the use of a cable or wire. This means of communication typically relies on radio waves with specific frequencies (Marshall and Wilson 2020). The mobile internet is a term used to describe internet access using Smartphones or other mobile technologies. The most common type of this communication today is known as mobile broadband, which relies on encrypted radio waves resonating at high frequencies. The progression of fifth generation technologies in society is having a direct impact on not only how we communicate, but also how we observe the physical space in which we live. By combining the power of cloud computing, search engines, and databases, individuals will have immediate access to information using mobile technology anytime and anywhere (Raychaudhuri and Gerla 2011, p. 10).

Within the domain of healthcare, mobile technology and sensors are considered significant tools for future healthcare provision, enabling remote monitoring and improved access to health information for both clinicians and consumers. Chapters. 2 and 3 describe case examples of how these technologies are being used in healthcare. Due to the low cost of deployment associated with wireless devices, wireless networks will continue to be an attractive option for connecting to the Internet of the future. Such new perspectives also present several challenges.

As wireless networks become more integrated into the design of future eHealth systems, questions arise as to how secure the network infrastructures can or will be used most effectively and ethically particularly from a patient centered perspective. Traditional healthcare systems that functioned in isolation will not be able to provide wider access for mobile and eHealth resources and new security protocols are progressing (Trappe et al. 2011). This topic is explored further from a health care perspective in Chaps. 5 and 10.

4.4 A Mobile Application within Health Care

One simple example of technology use in contemporary society is in the case of individuals managing their health and wellbeing. This is particularly relevant for individuals who wish to manage chronic disease and monitor their symptoms thus recognizing early any deterioration of their health. In addition, push notification through alerts can assist individuals to actively engage in health seeking behaviors such as a planned exercise regime and or healthy eating. An example of a smartphone WHO application that supports active health and wellbeing is featured through Digital Health article (Downey 2019) and additional access to World Health Organisation Digital Health Atlas is available from this link https://digitalhealthatlas.org/en/(World Health Organisation 2020). Further information on smart digital app to enhance health and wellbeing of individuals is included in Chap. 15.

4.5 Conclusion

This chapter presented the basic components of computers for traditional and current computing, while exploring some of the emerging technologies of fifth generation computing. (Segars 2019). We have considered how technology is changing our behaviour. The pace of development in ICT over the past 30 years has been rapid and as we currently exist in a digital world, it is difficult to estimate just how mTechnology will impact on future healthcare provision. Current mTechnology such as android phones offer a resource for outsourcing information and designing new ways to communicate, read and write. This chapter concludes with revisiting the opening quote from Mr. John Cleese which suggests that: We don't know where we get our ideas from. What we do know is that we do not get them from our laptops …. John Cleese (2010). Outsourcing some of our memory to smart phones and laptops should leave time for reflection; create a space for creativity, and the development of some smart ideas to enhance individual care. In many instances this is not the case. A core function of nursing informatics may then be to create time to consider just how technologies can be harnessed through design science to offer additional time to enhance direct care. This theme will be revisited in the proceeding chapters of this edition.

Glossary

API Application Programmable Interface—Essentially documentation around the capabilities of a certain technology

ASCII American Standard Code for Information Interchange, common form character encoding

Asynchronous Non-synchronized usually applies to network communication where communication is event based rather than time based

Bit Digital Unit, one bit can either be represented by a 1 or a 0

Browser Used to visually/audibly interpret data received either locally or via a form of transfer protocol

Byte Digital Unit, one Byte is a representation of 8 bits and can store a value of up to 2^8 or 256

Cache Usually applies to the storage of retrieved data, most networks have a cache to prevent the need to request the same information multiple times from the same source

Clinical decision support Clinical decision support—Tools used in clinical practice for enhancing health-related decisions and actions with pertinent, organized clinical knowledge and patient information to improve health and healthcare delivery

Cloud A term used to describe a new form computing, "cloud" computing relates to remote based computing, instead of storing and processing all of your information locally, all computation and storage is done remotely on the "cloud" which is an external server or network of servers

CPU Central Processing Unit—the primary mechanism of processing driving the core operations of a computer

Database Database Most common form of persistent data storage

Encryption Mathematical operation to change the original format of data

Ethernet Form of computer networking technology, commonly used for Local Area Networks (LAN)

External hard drive A data storage device

GUI Graphical User Interface, where icons are used to identify programs, files, and other processing options

Interface Multiple meanings, in oop programming an interface is a blue print for a class, can be used as another term for GUI as well

Interoperability The ability of disparate and diverse organisations to interact towards mutually beneficial and agreed common goals, involving the sharing of information and knowledge between the organisations, through the business processes they support, by means of the exchange of data between their respective ICT systems. Source EIF Report http://bookshop.europa.eu/is-bin/INTERSHOP. enfinity/WFS/EU-Bookshop-Site/en_GB/-/EUR/ViewPublication-Start?Publica tionKey=KK0113147

Interoperability Framework An interoperability framework is an agreed approach to interoperability for organisations that wish to work together towards the joint delivery of public services. Within its scope of applicability, it specifies a set of common elements such as vocabulary, concepts, principles, policies, guidelines, recommendations, standards, specifications and practices

LAN Local Area Network

Modem Physical device used to transmit digital data through analogue communication

PDA Personal Digital Assistant, can be used to describe a range of digital devices

Protocol In ICT a set of invisible computer rules that govern how an internet document gets transmitted to your screen

RAM Random Access Memory

ROM Read Only Memory

Secure Sockets Layer Most commonly used as an encryption layer for Hyper Text Transfer Protocol (HTTP)

Semantic interoperability Semantic interoperability refers to the ability of computer systems to transmit data with unambiguous, shared meaning

Synchronous Usually applies to network communication where both ends of the network are synchronized to expect communication at particular time

USB Universal Serial Bus—form of data transfer

Use case Specific scenarios designed to illustrate and provide context for testing a specific digital task or functionality

VPN A virtual private network which extends a private network across a public network such as the Internet

VOIP Voice Over Internet Protocol

Wide Area Network Wide Area Network

WLAN Wireless Local Area Network

References

AACC. Machine learning and laboratory medicine: now and the road ahead I AACC.org. 2020. https://www.aacc.org/publications/cln/articles/2019/march/machine-learning-and-laboratory-medicine-now-and-the-road-ahead. Cited Jan 30 2020.

Downey A. World Health Organisation launches app to improve care for the elderly digital news. 2019. https://www.digitalhealth.net/2019/10/world-health-organisation-elderly-care-app/. Accessed 25 Apr 2020.

John Cleese on creativity. Dr Shock. 8 Sept 2010. http://www.shockmd.com/2010/09/08/john-cleese-on-creativity/. Accessed 24 Apr 2020.

Foster. The grid: computing without bounds. Sci Am. 2003;288(4):78–85.

Health Level 7 Fast Healthcare Interoperability Resources (FHIR). 2020. https://www.hl7.org/fhir/overview.html. Accessed 25 Apr 2020.

Marshall B, Wilson TV. How WIFI works. 2020. http://computer.howstuffworks.com/wireless-network1.htm. Accessed 24 Apr 2020.

Raychaudhuri D, Gerla M. Emerging wireless technologies and the future of mobile internet. Los Angeles, USA: Cambridge University Press; 2011. p. 1.

Segars S. The fifth wave of computing is built on AI, 5G and a secure IoT. 17 Apr 2019. https://www.arm.com/blogs/blueprint/the-fifth-wave-of-computing-ai-5g-iot. Accessed 28 Apr 2020.

Trappe W, Baliga A, Poovendran R. Opening up the last frontiers for securing the future wireless internet in Raychaudhuri and Gerla, emerging wireless technologies and the future mobile internet, vol. 9. New York: Cambridge University Press; 2011. p. 242–79.

World Health Organisation. World Health Atlas. 2020. https://digitalhealthatlas.org/en/. Accessed 24 Apr 2020.

WWW3 Schools. 2020. http://www.w3schools.com/. Accessed 24 Apr 2020.

Chapter 5
Health Information Exchange: The Overarching Role of Integrating the Healthcare Enterprise (IHE)

Karima Bourquard and Alexander Berler

Abstract Innovative solutions are needed in Healthcare to deliver interoperable and secure digital services. Big data and Artificial Intelligence (AI), Personalized medicine, are considered as the main priorities by the European Commission for the coming years. As such, topics are placing high demands on medical data to ensure that they are consistent, relevant, and structured. In order to achieve this degree of consistency data that is to be exchanged, needs to be underpinned with protocols and standards which need to be clearly understood by those charged with implementation. To increase data quality, integration guidelines called profiles allow a harmonious combination of standards for answering specific clinical needs and workflows. Alignment and conformity of the IT systems to the requirements is the preferred approach to build trusted healthcare IT ecosystem. The chapter describes a comprehensive process that allows reaching the goal of developing Digital Health Space. Based on two concrete examples, firstly, the Integration Healthcare Enterprise (IHE) is a profiling organization that proposes a use case driven methodology for successfully deploying interoperable systems that are tested during events called Connectathons. Secondly, The Conformity Assessment Scheme for Europe (CASforEU) designed in the European project EURO-CAS completes the process by proposing a rigorous evaluation of the conformity of products and solutions for better confidence of the interoperability implementation. This chapter initially introduces the concept of interoperability and then describes in detail how to implement the process in healthcare setting, It also provides some concrete examples of

Electronic Supplementary Material The online version of this chapter (https://doi.org/10.1007/978-3-030-58740-6_5) contains supplementary material, which is available to authorized users.

K. Bourquard (✉)
IN-SYSTEM, IHE-Europe, Brussels, Belgium
e-mail: Karima.bourquard@ihe-europe.net, Karima.bourquard@in-system.eu

A. Berler
IHE-Europe, Brussels, Belgium
e-mail: Alexander.berler@ihe-europe.net

deployment projects, and introduces the concept and process of the conformity assessment scheme for healthcare IT products and solutions.

Keywords Digital health · Interoperability · Health information exchange Concept · Use case · Interoperability framework · Testing tools · Conformity assessment Scheme · Certification · Projectathon · Connectathon

Learning Objectives for the Chapter

Many countries in Europe and beyond are developing interoperability frameworks at the national or regional levels in order to serve their programs and objectives that include

1. Secure Access for citizens to their health data.
2. Increase interoperability among systems for sharing electronic health data.
3. Increase the quality of electronic health data.

This chapter will focus mostly on the interoperability understanding, one of the key challenges of the Digital Transformation processes of Health and Care in the Digital Single Market (Health and care in the digital single market - ICPerMed 2020). The main objectives are the following:

- Provide a common understanding of the concept of interoperability including the difference between standards and integration in eHealth;
- Introduce IHE as an international organization that collects use cases from healthcare professionals, defines IHE profiles, tests the conformance and interoperability during the Connectathon and deploys the profiles within national/regional programs;
- Provide the reader with some concrete examples of the use of IHE methodology;
- Provide insights to the reader on the data quality and how IHE impacts on better use of data in big data analysis and artificial intelligence by promoting the conformity assessment for interoperability in eHealth;
- Introduce the reader to general considerations on the use of certification and conformity assessment in digital health.

The official website of the office of the national coordinator for health information technology[1] in USA reports, the *"Electronic health information exchange (HIE) allows doctors, nurses, pharmacists, other health care providers and patients to appropriately access and securely share a patient's vital medical information electronically—improving the speed, quality, safety and cost of patient care"* (What is HIE?|HealthIT.gov 2020). Even nowadays, despite the widespread existence of secure information transfer technologies, most citizens' healthcare information is still stored on paper in hospitals, primary care settings and in patients' homes. When that set of information is shared between providers, it happens by

---

[1] https://www.healthit.gov/topic/.

hand, mail, fax and usually by patients themselves, who have to carry their records from one point of care to another. While electronic health information exchange cannot replace patient-provider necessary physical communication, it can surely enhance the completeness of patient's medical records, as patient summaries, structured discharge letters, lab results, current medications and other information are needed during visits. Proper and well-timed sharing of vital patient information can better inform decision making at the point of care and facilitates providers to

- Avoid unnecessary readmissions;
- Avoid prescription errors adverse drug reactions;
- Improve the quality of medical diagnoses;
- Decrease or eradicate duplicate tests.

To reach the aforementioned goals listed above, it is expected that interoperable systems need to share structured (or even unstructured) information, by applying commonly accepted and used terminologies, and standards. The role of Standardization Development Organizations (SDOs) such as DICOM, HL7 Inc. and others is of critical importance. Their role is discussed in detail in Chap. 6. In addition, the role of profiling organizations such as Integrating the Healthcare Enterprise (IHE) is also of overarching importance because it introduces the terms of integration profiles and provides much needed detail for testing infrastructure to support same.

With interoperable systems, data can be exchanged and stored automatically rather than re-typed into the different point of care systems each time. Data is unfortunately today not always available in a usable format, thus hindering the integration of data from various sources in use cases for secondary use of medical information. As a solution to create widely used and accepted data format, the integration profiles process has been proposed as a way to enable end-to-end interoperability by sharing structured (and unstructured data) between the point of care systems (Hoerbst and Ammenwerth 2010). An integration profile is a guideline for implementation of a specific process called use case. The use case provides precise definitions of how standards can be implemented to meet specific clinical needs for a specific purpose. For example, integration profiles organize and leverage the integration capabilities that can be achieved by coordinated implementation of communication standards, such as DICOM, HL7, W3C and security standards in Digital Health. Recently, the European Commission, in relation to the Article 292 of the EU (Commission implementing regulation (EU 2018) (the GDPR regulation on the lawful processing of personal data and the ability of citizens and healthcare providers to securely access and share electronic healthcare records), released the important Commission Recommendation of 6.2.2019 on a European electronic health record exchange format (EHRxF) (Transformation of health and care in the digital single market 2019; Commission recommendation on a European Electronic Health Record exchange format 2019) which set the grounds for a secure, standardized and proper set of exchange formats. These recommendations should form the basis of any future developments in the domain of lawful and legitimate reuse of clinical data for research and Big Data analytics within the so-called Health Data Space (Digital health progressing towards more interoperability for the digital cross border exchange of health data in Europe 2020).

The achievement of Interoperability in Digital Health will facilitate the adoption of innovation when many countries are today heavily involved, by developing the medicine of the future using Artificial Intelligence and big data analysis. Interoperability is also the vehicle to ensure seamless exchanges or shared data among systems when they are distributed among public and private healthcare organizations or within healthcare providers, for example by involving a broad range of ICT systems that include medical devices (EHR, radiology Information system, modalities, laboratory information System, pump infusion) applications (appointment system), mobile applications and many other types of applications of concern.

Traditionally, ICT systems in healthcare providers have been working as standalone systems with no connection to other systems across the continuum of healthcare settings. Systems and applications were operated as silos. This is increasingly no longer the case. Health care providers and the systems they deploy from applications in silos, the systems are now more and more connected and exchange data in order to support the care processes that can involve multiple actors, healthcare professionals and patient. Behind the complexity of the health care world, the interoperability is not a simple concept but covers multiple dimensions that will be analyzed in this chapter. Implementation of interoperability cannot be a success without taking into account the end-users who will use in their daily work the systems that support their activities and tasks (Bourquard et al. 2014). This is why IHE[2] has been developing for many years a methodology that allows deployment of care systems in organizations. This methodology is presented and is followed by some concrete examples. Finally, quality of the health data is the main goal to be achieved: even if standards and integration profiles specifications are essentials (Witting 2015), vendors developing their systems have not always the same interpretation of the specifications or customize them to fit to their developments. Therefore, many countries are developing certification schema or conformity assessment in eHealth interoperability and a European project called EURO-CAS has created a Conformity Assessment Scheme for Europe which is now presented in this chapter.

In conclusion, because Interoperability is one of the key challenges in the coming years, the next section will provide oversight on the Interoperability and related concepts to better understand this challenge: Interoperability is a complex concept that impacts upon all levels of the societal health organization. It will be followed by a section on how to implement the interoperability infrastructure using IHE and its methodology with examples of deployment in various countries to complete this section. The quality of medical data will be highlighted in the last section where the conformity assessment in Europe for interoperability digital health is described based on the European project EURO-CAS and based on existing testing environment.

---

[2] Integration the Healthcare Interoperablity (www.ihe.net).

5.1   Interoperability and Concepts

Interoperability is a characteristic of a product or system, whose interfaces are completely understood, to work with other products or systems, at present or in the future, in either implementation or access, without any restrictions (Definition of interoperability 2020). While the term was initially established for information technology or systems engineering services, a broader definition considers social, political, and organizational factors that impact on system to system design performance (Slater 2012). Interoperability implies the use of Open standards by definition.

Open standards are publicly available and follow some principles as established by the joint meeting of several organization and standard development bodies (IEEE, ISOC, IETF, IAB[3]):

1. Cooperation between members;
2. Acceptance of the following principles:

    (a) A clear process where decisions are developed with equity and respect among members;
    (b) Broad consensus;
    (c) Transparency;
    (d) Balance: no domination by one of the groups of interest, company or person;
    (e) Openness: open to all interested parties;

3. Collective empowerment commitment;
4. Availability: standards shall be FRAND;[4]
5. Voluntary adoption of standards.

The new European Interoperability Framework promotes seamless services and data flows for European public administrations (New European Interoperability Framework 2017). This framework defines the principles and makes recommendations for interoperability by defining the minimal characteristics for a specification for open standards.

When a vendor is forced to adapt its system to a dominant system that is not based on Open standards, it is not interoperable e.g. able to exchange data with any other systems only those systems which are compatible. As a result, interoperability can be seen as an opportunity to safeguard the potential of open free markets societies.

Open standards rely on a broadly consultative and inclusive group of individuals including representatives from vendors, academics and others holding a stake in the development process which discusses and debates the technical and economic merits, demerits and feasibility of a proposed common protocol. After focused discussion, the doubts and reservations of all members are addressed, the resulting

---

[3] See Glossary.

[4] FRAND: FAIR, Reasonable and Non-Discriminatory.

common document is endorsed as a common standard. Then anybody is entitled to use the standard to achieve interoperability in a specific context.

In the healthcare sector, HIMSS[5] provided the best current definition of healthcare interoperability as

> "the ability of different information systems, devices and applications ('systems') to access, exchange, integrate and cooperatively use data in a coordinated manner, within and across organizational, regional and national boundaries, to provide timely and seamless portability of information and optimize the health of individuals and populations globally".

Health data exchange architectures, application interfaces and standards enable data to be accessed and shared appropriately and securely across the complete spectrum of care, within all applicable settings and with relevant stakeholders, including by the individuals.

HIMSS defined four layers of interoperability (What is interoperability in Healthcare? 2013):

- Foundational (Level 1)—establishes the inter-connectivity requirements needed for one system or application to securely communicate data to and receive data from another;
- Structural (Level 2)—defines the format, syntax, and organization of data exchange including at the data field level for interpretation;
- Semantic (Level 3)—provides for common underlying models and codification of the data including the use of data elements with standardized definitions from publicly available value sets and coding vocabularies, providing shared understanding and meaning to the user;
- Organizational (Level 4)—includes governance, policy, social, legal and organizational considerations to facilitate the secure, seamless and timely communication and use of data both within and between organizations, entities and individuals. These components enable shared consent, trust and integrated end-user processes and workflows.

This definition is also in line with what has been proposed in Europe by the ISA[2] program—Interoperability solutions for public administrations, businesses and citizens, managed by the European Commission. The European position on interoperability is stated in (European Interoperability Framework for pan-European eGovernment Services 2004), communication from the commission to the European, parliament, the council, the European economic and social, committee and the committee of the regions, European Interoperability Framework—Implementation Strategy document as:

---

[5]The Health Information and Management Systems Society (https://www.himss.org).

Interoperability is a key factor in making a digital transformation possible. It allows administrative entities to electronically exchange, amongst themselves and with citizens and businesses, meaningful information in ways that are understood by all parties. It addresses all layers that impact the delivery of digital public services in the EU, including: legal issues, e.g. by ensuring that legislation does not impose unjustified barriers to the reuse of data in different policy areas; organizational aspects, e.g. by requesting formal agreements on the conditions applicable to cross-organizational interactions; data/semantic concerns, e.g. by ensuring the use of common descriptions of exchanged data; technical challenges, e.g. by setting up the necessary information systems environment to allow an uninterrupted flow of bits and bytes.

Those four layers of interoperability are the foundation of the European Interoperability Framework (EIF) which is part of the reference: Communication (2017) from the European Commission adopted on 23 March 2017. The framework gives specific guidance on how to set up interoperable digital public services. It offers public administrations 47 concrete recommendations on how to improve governance of their interoperability activities, establish cross-organizational relationships, streamline processes supporting end-to-end digital services, and ensure that both existing and new legislation do not compromise interoperability efforts. The new EIF is undertaken in the context of the Commission priority to create a Digital Single Market in Europe. The public sector, which accounts for over a quarter of total employment and represents approximately a fifth of the EU's GDP through public procurement, plays a key role in the Digital Single Market as a regulator, services provider and employer. The successful implementation of the EIF will improve the quality of European public services and will create an environment where public administrations can collaborate digitally.

Standards and specifications are fundamental to interoperability. The European Interoperability Framework (EIF) distinguishes **six steps** to managing standards and specifications appropriately:

- **Identifying** candidate standards and specifications based upon specific needs and requirements;
- **Assessing** candidate standards and specifications using standardised, transparent, fair and non-discriminatory methods;
- **Implementing** the standards and specifications according to plans and practical guidelines;
- **Monitoring** compliance with the standards and specifications;
- **Managing change** with appropriate procedures;
- **Documenting** standards and specifications, in open catalogues, using a standardised description.

The European Interoperability Framework (EIF) also includes a conceptual model as presented in Fig. 5.1 for integrated public services. The model is modular and comprises loosely coupled service components interconnected through shared infrastructure.

The conceptual model promotes the idea of interoperability by design. It means that for European public services to be interoperable, they should be designed in accordance with the proposed model and with certain interoperability and

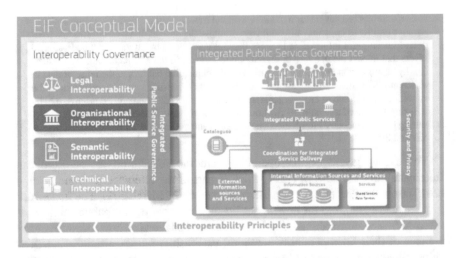

Fig. 5.1 EIF conceptual model. From ISA

reusability requirements in mind. The interoperability maturity model (IMM) developed in the context of the ISA programme can be used to assess a service's readiness for interoperability. The model promotes reusability as a driver for interoperability, recognising that the European public services should reuse information and services that already exist and may be available from various sources inside or beyond the organisational boundaries of public administrations. Information and services should be retrievable and be made available in interoperable formats. This in line with current profiling solutions for the healthcare sector as depicted in ISO/TR 28380[6,7,8] technical report.

For the Healthcare domain the European Commission adopted the Refined eHealth Interoperability Framework. The ReEIF was adopted and endorsed by the eHealth Network[9] in November 2015.

While the EIF 2017 has four layers, the ReEIF describes the organizational and technical layer. This is important because it provides details which results in six layers and takes into account security, privacy, governance principles and agreements:

---

[6] ISO/TR 28380-1:2014 Health informatics—IHE global standards adoption—Part 1: Process, https://www.iso.org/standard/63383.html.

[7] ISO/TR 28380-2:2014 Health informatics—IHE global standards adoption—Part 2: Integration and content profiles, https://www.iso.org/standard/46207.html.

[8] ISO/TR 28380-3:2014 Health informatics—IHE global standards adoption—Part 3: Deployment, https://www.iso.org/standard/61471.html.

[9] The eHealth Network is a network gathering European countries and Norway and created by the directive on the application of patient rights in cross border healthcare in March, 9th 2011 (https://eur-lex.europa.eu/LexUriServ/LexUriServ.do?uri=OJ:L:2011:088:0045:0065:EN:PDF). One of the objective is to develop cooperation among countries.

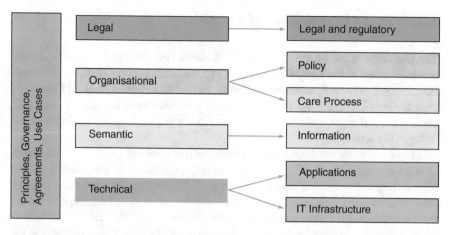

Fig. 5.2 From EIF to ReEIF with the vertical layer Principles, Governance, Agreements, Use Cases. (From Antilope project)

- Legal and regulatory level describes the legal context and constraints;
- Policy level is related to the collaboration agreements as for example healthcare network where healthcare professionals exchange medical data for given patients;
- The care process level identifies and specifies care process among healthcare professionals for alignment and development of a common vision of the processes;
- Information level describes the data and their semantic based on coding systems that are exchanges among Healthcare Professionals;
- Application level identifies the actors, structured messages and standards that will support the medical exchanges as described by the levels above;
- IT infrastructures describes the communication protocols.

These layers are completed by vertical layers for the global governance, security and patient policies and other necessary items necessary for a successful deployment (certification, interoperability framework, etc). An illustration of the EIF to ReEIF is presented in Fig. 5.2.[10]

5.2   Digital Health Strategy Efforts

As a result, the implementation of Healthcare Information Exchange network (HIE) implies a substantial policy and consensus building effort is required. Many such efforts and Digital Health strategies are globally under development. It is important to focus on some examples that have a rather important impact at the global scale. They are briefly expanded upon in this section.

---

[10] eHealth Standards and Profiles in Action for Europe and Beyond Deliverable 4.2r1 Interoperability Guideline for eHealth Deployment Projects, Release 1, 13-03-2017.

5.2.1 In the United States of America

The first effort is led by the Office of the National Coordinator for health information technology in the United States (ONC) (2020–2025 Federal Health IT Strategic Plan 2020) that recently released their draft 2020–2025 Federal Health IT Strategic Plan for public comments. This plan, which was developed in collaboration with over 25 federal organizations, is intended to guide federal health information technology (IT) activities.

The plan's goals are deliberately outcomes-driven, with objectives and strategies focused on using health IT as a catalyst to empower patients, lower costs, deliver high-quality care, and improve health for individuals, families, and communities. ONC and its federal partners have taken and will continue to take steps to ensure that stakeholders in the healthcare sector benefit from the electronic access, exchange, and use of the health information. Specifically, this plan explains how the federal government intends to use health IT to impact on individuals in the following manner:

- Promote Health and Wellness;
- Enhance the Delivery and Experience of Care;
- Build a Secure, Data-Driven Culture to Accelerate Research and Innovation; and
- Connect Healthcare and Health Data through an Interoperable Health IT Infrastructure.

5.2.2 In Europe

The second effort is led by the European Commission that is working to provide its citizens access to safe and top-quality digital services in health and care. For this, the European commission has published a Communication on Digital Transformation of Health and Care in the Digital Single Market, empowering citizens and building a healthier society (Communication on enabling the digital transformation of health and care in the Digital Single Market; empowering citizens and building a healthier society 2020).

The Communication on Digital Transformation of Health and Care in the Digital Single Market identifies three priorities:

- "Citizens' secure access to their health data, this includes across borders enabling citizens to access their health data across the EU;
- Personalised medicine through shared European data infrastructure allowing researchers and other professionals to pool resources (data, expertise, computing processing and storage capacities) across the EU;
- Citizen empowerment with digital tools for user feedback and person-centred care using digital tools to empower people to look after their health, stimulate prevention and enable feedback and interaction between users and healthcare providers."

5.3   IHE (Integrating the Healthcare Enterprise) and IHE Methodology

IHE is a world-wide initiative created by healthcare professionals and industry to improve the way computer systems in healthcare share information by working together on interoperability use cases. IHE promotes the coordinated use of established standards such as DICOM and HL7 to address specific clinical needs in support of optimal patient care.

IHE has been defined a successful process for more than 20 years that identifies four steps (IHE Process 2020):

1. Healthcare Professionals, clinical and technical experts define critical interoperability use cases for information sharing;
2. Technical experts generally originated from Industry identifies and selects established and robust standards and develop detailed integration specifications called IHE profiles for communication among systems to address these specific use cases;
3. Industry implements these IHE Profiles in their systems;
4. Vendors' systems are tested by neutral monitors at carefully planned, controlled and supervised events called Connectathons.

Figure 5.3 provides a visual overview of the IHE process activity.

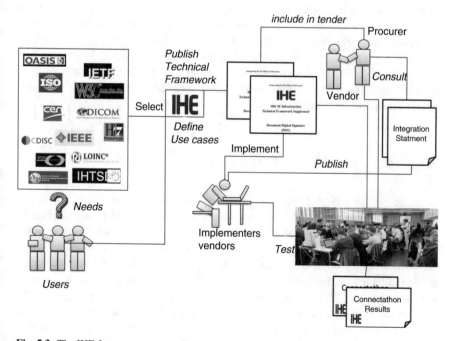

Fig. 5.3 The IHE four steps process. (From IHE)

Beginning in the Radiology Domain back in 1999, IHE has expanded into multiple domains and today 13 medical domains are covered such as Cardiology, Endoscopy, Pathology and Laboratory Medicine, Eye Care, Patient Coordination Care, ITI infrastructure, Pharmacy, Quality research and Public Health and Radiation Oncology, thereby ensuring system interoperability between suppliers and their systems on a very big scale and on an even larger world stage. Various national entities (called National Deployment Committees under IHE's governance model) were established to provide testing, education and support implementation of projects over the world, including IHE USA, IHE Europe, IHE Japan, IHE China, IHE Korea, IHE Australia and many others. They vary widely in composition, size and scope of activities.

IHE also organizes demonstrations of IHE-compliant systems working in real-world at meetings and other venues and conferences over the world. These demonstrations give a sense to the audience on how IT systems interact between them when clinical use cases are working inside hospitals or between healthcare organizations or with the shared EHR/PHR deployed at the regional or national levels or cross countries.

IHE invites clinical practitioners and technical domain experts to become leaders in this work by participating in IHE domain committees and using the IHE methodology, by identifying use cases, selecting operational and robust standards and specifying integration profiles or reviewing the documents they publish at the international level for public comments once the documents are ready. After integrating the comments received worldwide, IHE publish the specifications as supplements in trial implementation for being implementing by vendors in their systems and testing at the Connectathons. When the specifications become stable e.g. with no change proposals that impact the content, the IHE profiles are published in final text and are included in the technical framework of the domain. More than 175 organizations (IHE Member Organizations 2020) from professional societies, government agencies, provider organizations, HIT companies and others- have joined the IHE initiative worldwide.

5.3.1   Benefits of the IHE Approach

Some of Europe's largest countries are made up of autonomous regions with full authority over healthcare decisions and the information systems to support healthcare delivery. For example, Spain is made up of nine autonomous health regions, while in Italy there are 21 independent regions, and Germany is a confederation of 16 federal states. Even large nations with a single national structure, such as France or United Kingdom, have seen the development of diverse health information systems over the past 20 years built around regional university hospitals. This patchwork of regional development of IT for healthcare in Europe has created different, sometimes stand-alone systems for healthcare. Even within regions, documents created by clinical systems for patient care may not interface with administrative systems that determine payment or citizen entitlements for healthcare. The same complexity can be seen in other countries at a global scale.

Healthcare providers, institutions like hospitals organizations or individual doctors and nurses, are working with an increasing number of information systems, all containing relevant data on the patients. Typically, these systems behave like "islands", not sharing patient-related data between systems. This leads to broken work processes, the need for repetitive data entry (with risk of mistakes) and an incomplete view on the patient's record. The same is true when caring for patients coming from abroad.

At the global scale, people are more and more highly mobile, traveling freely, whether for work or vacation, between countries. In the course of one single day, a European citizen for example, might pass through several nations. And each European citizen carries health insurance provided by his or her country of residence. In the case of an accident or a health crisis, a citizen may be treated in a foreign country by nurses and doctors speaking a different language. How can the foreign doctor determine the medications being taken by this patient, or any allergies to medications? What is the medical history of this patient? And, of course, who is paying for the often-expensive emergency medical intervention?

Europe's and other governments, both national and regional, have worked with different suppliers from the private sector to develop equipment or software for stand-alone systems. While this has resulted in a robust base of expertise and solutions for health IT in Europe, an innovative system or successful solution developed by a company often cannot be exported without significant changes to meet variations in standards and requirements in a neighboring country.

Much is at stake for national governments who spend hundreds of billions of euros/dollars each year as the primary insurer of its citizens' healthcare. As discussed in Chap. 2, there is an urgency around the globe which has a rapidly ageing population that soon countries will require greater health expenditure on, while the base for the model for health funding, for the younger working population, is shrinking. These governments see a solution in health information systems that can deliver greater efficiency and productivity, as well as supporting alternative delivery of health services for the chronically ill through community-based clinics and in-home care.

An integrated information system, with proper flow of information from one system to the other, puts the right information in front of the right doctor at the right moment to assure the right treatment.

It's that simple and applies to supporting both local and foreign patients. Adoption of common protocols and standards that are specified within IHE profiles will create a more uniform market for health IT equipment, software and services enabling manufacturers to market their products at the European and even global level with only minor variations. In addition to helping to assure compatibility between systems, a harmonized market will also lower the costs of acquiring best practices solutions for governments and citizens. Greater adoption of IHE Technical Frameworks will also enable the IT industry based in Europe to compete internationally, thereby increasing employment and sustaining the development of this sector of activity in the Global and European economies.

5.3.2 Integration Profiles: A Framework for Interoperability

IHE Profiles provide standards-based specifications for sharing information within care settings and across healthcare networks. They address critical interoperability issues related to information access for care providers and patients, clinical workflow, security, administration and information infrastructure. Each profile identifies the system actors that are involved in the workflow (for example, the Order Filler requesting a prescription of medication), specifies the transactions where messages are described in detail using referencing standards (for example HL7 messages) with the information artefacts. The semantical information is carefully identified and selected in order to address the clinical use case by referencing appropriate terminologies.

The integration profiles that are developed by specialties and are gathered on the Technical Framework contain a number of specific volumes (IHE Domains 2020):

- The Volume 1 describes the use cases, interaction between actors by using transactions;
- The volume 2 specifies each identified transaction in detail that uses messages based on international standards;
- The volume 3 describes the content and semantic details;
- The volume 4 describes the national extensions if any.

All the technical frameworks are freely available on the IHE international website (see reference above).

5.3.3 Connectathons®: Testing Interoperability and Conformance

IHE has been testing the interoperability of Healthcare Information Technology (HIT) systems for more than a decade. At IHE Connectathons held regularly in several locations internationally, trained technical experts supervise testing of vendor systems, making use of advanced testing software developed by IHE and several partner organizations. More than 250 vendors worldwide have implemented and tested products with IHE capabilities. The IHE Product Registry (IHE Product Registry 2020) provides essential information for IT administrators and executives responsible for purchasing and integrating systems at healthcare sites and health information exchanges (IHE User handbooks 2020). Detailed results of testing at IHE Connectathons® over the past several years in Europe, North America and Asia

Fig. 5.4 IHE testing at a Connectathon®

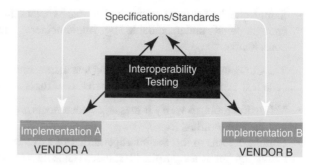

are made available in this easy-to-use online database. In Europe, Connectathons has been organized for more 20 years. Each year IHE-Europe, the European deployment committee, selects a national initiative from one of the European countries for setting up the next yearly Connectathon (comparable but at its size, the selection of the city for the Olympics game!).

The main objective of the Connectathon is to test systems' conformity to IHE Profiles by using validators and the interoperability between systems or simulators in a controlled and neutral environment. Clinical workflow is guidance for testing. The Connectathon allow testing in a controlled and neutral environment. Figure 5.4 distinguishes the interoperability testing from the conformity testing:

- Conformity will be checked using validator tools where the messages that are sent/received by a system are conformed to the required standard specifications.
- Interoperability checking will show that the message sent by one system is received and treated adequately by the receiver.

It is not because a system is conformed to a specific standard that it is interoperable and vice versa. This is mainly true for a specific use case or health care context, for example when the IHE profile is applied to this use case.

The Connectathon is also called Connectivity Test Marathon and can be described as following:

- It allows week-long (5 days) face-to-face testing of the participating products' interoperability developed by industry and implementers;
- Participants implements profiles and standards in their solutions and test them with open source test tools and test plans provided in advance by IHE;
- Vendors, large and small companies, are encouraged to work closely together to solve interoperability issues for the benefit of the healthcare community;
- Participants are allowed to correct their solutions (products or prototypes) non-conformities during the event;
- Thousands of transactions are verified using both test tools and peer tests: they are recorded and the outcomes are checked and validated by neutral Monitors (subject expert matters or knowledgeable testers);
- At the end of the event, successful vendors are registered in the Connectathon Results Matrix published publicly on the IHE website;

- Sanity checks are also performed to see whether the IHE Profiles are clear enough, well understandable by implementers and can be implemented consistently.

The Connectathon test platform using test management software system is called Gazelle test bed. Essentially, several varieties of tools are used:

- Validation tools, to verify if messages/documents are in conformity with specifications and profiles;
- Simulator tools to test the interoperability of a system, not as a reference implementation but as a controlled test cases (Gazelle simulators 2020).

The Gazelle test bed provides Connectathon® participants, Monitors and the management with the tooling to run the event. The process is described in Fig. 5.5:

- Participants share configurations (1), samples and identify test partners through the Gazelle test management tool;
- The tool provides them with a list of tests to be performed and enables them to log evidences of the tests performed (2). Participants are free to run the test at their own environment following the test plan they received;
- Monitors, who are subject-matter experts, verify each test (3) using the Gazelle test management platform;
- As for the participants, they have the ability to check the conformance of the exchanged messages that are most critical, using validation services (4);
- The Management Team is provided with indicators that allow them to monitor the testing progress and grade the participants progress.

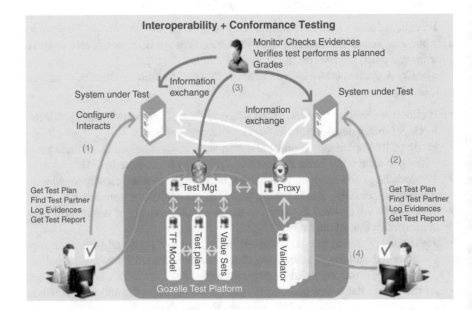

Fig. 5.5 Testing in practice

5.3.4   Conformity Assessment Scheme

The interoperability of healthcare information systems is one of the most important challenges facing both users and suppliers of healthcare solutions.

The accurate, timely and secure exchange of medical records requires unique technical expertise and competencies often beyond the experience of individual vendor or user deployment teams. Medical information details often provide crucial facts needed for optimal healthcare, whether within a hospital, across regional health IT projects, within national networks, or from a hospital to the patient at home. It is critical that vendors and users work together, along with regulatory authorities and standards bodies, to ensure that products, systems and solutions interoperate together to bring quality solutions to the market that perform as they should and result in the best quality patient care. To reduce costs, delays and other risks of incorrect, inappropriate and inadequate product purchases of many products, users have come to depend on trusted, independent third-party testing, which is often called "Conformity Assessment".

To meet these challenges, IHE International is introducing the IHE Conformity Assessment Program (IHE Conformity Assessment Scheme 2014).

The IHE Conformity Assessment testing is based on an ISO/IEC 17025 quality system in accordance with the IHE Conformity Assessment Scheme published by IHE. A specific set of IHE Profiles used for sharing health records is available for testing in accordance with requests from projects users and the industry.

Products submitted must be either market-released products or expected to be released within 6 months after the Conformity Assessment test session. Figure 5.6 describes the process to be engaged in the Conformity Assessment testing:

- The vendor must have passed the IHE Connectathon tests within the prior 2 years for the appropriate IHE Profiles targeted for Conformity Assessment;
- The accredited testing laboratory, authorized by IHE International, will deliver the Conformity Assessment Report (IHE Conformity Reports 2020): it will give more trust on the results when tested by a neutral, competent and recognized testing laboratory;
- The Conformity Assessment Report is published on the IHE International website after successful completion of testing which gives transparency and an overview of qualified products to the end users.

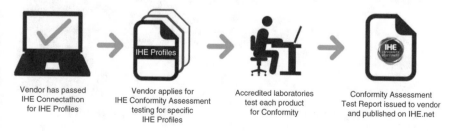

Fig. 5.6 Conformity assessment scheme. (From IHE)

From this, several benefits are identified for Users as well as for industry:

- Users:
  - Large eHealth projects reduce their testing and integration efforts by specifying and procuring products that have been conformity-assessed;
  - It gives confidence that a current/potential supplier has independent proof of the interoperability of their products;
  - It relies on an accredited testing laboratory to validate products before they are installed in an organization or facility, reducing risks and deployment costs;
  - It Improves patient outcome through better and more consistent product quality.

- Suppliers:
  - Interoperability readiness for systems and solutions;
  - Global market credibility by distinguishing the company and its products. For a listing of companies and products, recognized internationally and accepted for "shortlisting" (i.e. pre-qualified for purchasing programs) by being engaged in the quality process governed by the IHE Conformity Assessment Program.
  - Wealth of IHE Profiles and increase an organization's capabilities.

Currently IHE International has today 16 IHE integration profiles included in the IHE CAS program (see Fig. 5.7) that covers the most important identified needs in hospitals, at the regional and national Health Information exchanges and at cross-border. New profiles will be added in the future depending of the user demand. Procurers have to request qualified products in their tenders in order to develop this activity which is considered more and more as mandatory by various healthcare stakeholders.

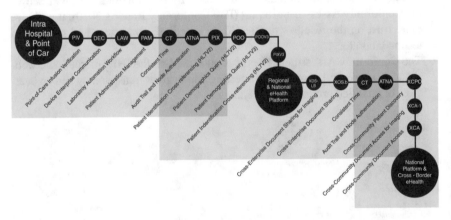

Fig. 5.7 Integration profiles of the IHE Conformity assessment scheme. (From IHE)

5.3.5 Gazelle Test Bed and IHE Services

IHE-Services provides the IHE competency for eHealth consultancy, training services. It organises interoperability test sessions and develops interoperability test tools, leveraging more than 10 years of experience in these domains and a community of hundreds of implementers around the world.

Developed for the annual IHE European Connectathon, these services allow specific projects to complement the product testing performed at the IHE Connectathon and include:

- The IHE Gazelle management software that supervises and coordinates testing activities;
- Unique interoperability test engines for DICOM, XML, HL7, OASIS, IETF and IHE integration profiles;
- Simulators for online, or virtual testing;
- Technical project management and results reporting services to organize and manage special-purpose interoperability testing events.

This Gazelle platform is developed under the ISO/IEC 17025 quality system (same level of quality as ISO 9001) and is composed of the main blocks below:

- Administrative, management and statistics;
- Test plan repositories and management;
- Management of test sessions;
- Management of validation tools (External Validation Service—EVS tool) and specification compliance (assertion manager);
- A portfolio of test tools: validators, simulators, objects Checker, test data sets, etc., some developed by IHE Services while many others from contributors from around the world.

This test management platform is also used remotely to realize the tests directly from the product development sites. Developed under the Apache 2.0 license, this platform can therefore be easily installed for end-users, both companies creating eHealth solutions for health projects and healthcare facilities. It supports a number of regional or national ehealth projects (Belgium, France, Finland, Luxembourg, Veneto Region, Saudi Arabia, Korea, Australia, Japan and North American Connectathons). Figure 5.8 shows that the same IHE Gazelle test platform can be used in many ways that finally provides a continuum of testing aligned with the concept of interoperability:

- At first, the IHE Gazelle test platform is used at the IHE Connectathon supporting implementers in their development of prototypes and products. The Connectathon is also a network of implementers and provides training, support and expertise from the monitors and experts to the product implementers;
- The step forward is the conformity assessment that increases the quality of products and uses also the IHE Gazelle test platform. The conformity assessment

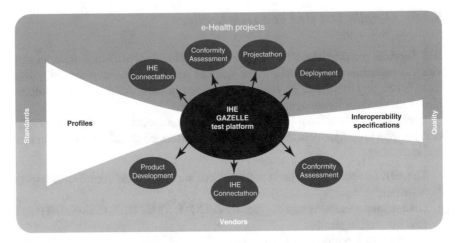

Fig. 5.8 IHE Gazelle test platform. (From IHE)

specifies a more rigorous test plan in a more controlled environment performed by an accredited testing laboratory;

- Finally, when deploying IHE profiles at the project level, the IHE Gazelle test platform is used at the Projectathon which is a type of Connectathon but dedicated to the specifications-based profiles of the eHealth project. The Projectathon has the same role as the Connectathon: it provides support, training and expertise to vendors that are selected for the project deployment.
- The ehealth project and vendors have also their own test environment (pre-production and production) that can be based on the same test bed.

Using a common IHE Gazelle test platform at different stages of development and deployment will reduce effort to build such an environment, reduce the learning phases while promoting robustness and increasing interoperability quality for medical data for their use.

5.4 Examples of Deployment

Carefully implemented interoperability standards are the foundation of the electronic Health records (EHRs), Personal Health Records (PHRs) and Health Information Exchanges (HIE) being established around the world. IHE has developed a foundational set of profiles for secure exchanges of patient information across enterprises. IHE profiles support health information networks in Canada and the U.S.A, as well as several Asian and European countries, and have been accepted as requirements by the U.S. Secretary of Health and Human Services for federal procurement of healthcare IT systems.

IHE case studies describe projects that use IHE profiles to improve systems interoperability and information access for patients and providers within and across care sites. They highlight the advantages of using IHE to improve:

- Operational efficiency in implementing and upgrading systems;
- Productivity and workflow efficiency;
- Communication among care providers and patients and access to vital medical information;
- Patient safety and quality of care.

5.4.1   French Electronic Health Record Program

The French Electronic Health Record (DMP system-Dossier Médical Partagé) developed, implemented and rolled out by the ASIP Santé (National eHealth Agency that is now renamed on ANS (National Digital Health Agency) and the CNAM/TS, the national French health insurance.

The electronic health record (in French, "Dossier Médical Partagé": DMP) system was developed based on a mandate from the French national legislature. DMP is a free service aimed to improve the coordination of healthcare in France that is supported by healthcare professionals and has become part of patient expectations for care. It makes information required for patient care available more easily and quickly and facilitates communication between healthcare professionals and patients. Launched in January 2011, the DMP is being gradually rolled out across the French territories through voluntary adoption by patients and healthcare professionals. It will form the infrastructural and technical base for numerous e-health services, whether proposed by public authorities or private sector.

DMP core specifications have been derived from IHE profiles, especially IHE XDS (Cross-Reference Document Sharing profile).

5.4.2   Hôpitaux Universitaires de Genève, Medical Imaging Facilities

Les Hôpitaux Universitaires de Genève (HUG) is the aggregation of all hospital facilities in the canton de Genève from 1856 until today. HUG is comprised of 2187 beds and a staff of more than 7865 people. HUG provides consultation services for all the Geneva region and handles more than 550,000 patients annually. The imaging workflow utilizes PACS solutions and modalities with digital capabilities.

The workflow at HUG is as follows: Images are routed to the clinical evaluation stations and the image active episode of care services for the Electronic Patient Record (EPR) upon arrival at the Image Manager/Archive. They are then queried and displayed by the Image Display workstation. Preliminary reading by residents doctors and clinical round preparation with senior residents occurs within the Radiology Department.

5.4.3 Geneva, Switzerland: Shared Medication Treatment Plan

The Canton of Geneva Switzerland has built an Electronic Patient Record system aiming at regrouping all important documents for the patient's care. Documents are provided by all stakeholders. The patient is the owner of the patient record (patient centered). An added-value service exists for 3 years now enabling care providers to manage the medication treatment plan. The goal is to have a complete view of all medications taken by the patient. The ongoing project is to link stakeholders' applications (prescription systems, dispensing systems, home care systems) directly with the core system in order to avoid any duplication of data entry and to have a true integration of all primary systems with the central shared medication treatment plan tool. The primary goal of implementing the Shared Medication Treatment Plan (Rosemberg et al. 2015; Spahni et al. 2013), is to achieve a real-time, global view of the past, current and planned medications taken by all patients. Creating this comprehensive picture of patients' medication history will create more complete and up-to-date medical histories that can be accessed anywhere that patient goes to receive care. This project uses IHE pharmacy content profiles.

In conclusion, IHE Profiles specifically implemented to this project include a set of IHE Pharmacy profiles that define the content and format of structured pharmacy documents used in planning, prescribing and dispensing of patient medications:

- Medication Treatment Plan (MTP) describes a medication document generated when a health care professional adds a medication to a patient treatment plan;
- Pharmacy Prescription (PRE) describes a prescription document generated when a health care professional decides that the patient needs a medication;
- Pharmacy Dispense (DIS) describes a dispense document generated when a health care professional dispenses a medication to a patient;
- Pharmacy Pharmaceutical Advice (PADV) describes a pharmaceutical advice document generated when a health care professional validates a prescription item against pharmaceutical knowledge and regulations or manages a medication treatment plan or a dispensation;
- Pharmacy Medication List (PML) describes a medication list document generated when a health care professional requests this information, for example when prescribing.

5.4.4 HEALTH OPTIMUM Project, Veneto Research Center for eHealth Innovation, Veneto, Italy

HEALTHcare delivery OPTIMisation through teleMedicine (HEALTH OPTIMUM) connects today all 34 hospitals in Veneto, one of the 21 Regions of Italy, to 7 specialty centers for neurosurgery., This system manages more than 2300 teleconsultations requests each year and allows 75% of patients to be treated at home medical center.

The Health Optimum network established an interoperability framework as a first common language, as an essential step first step. This framework adopted several IHE profiles such as XDS.b, XDS-I, etc. In order to accomplish information exchanges a common interoperability platform based on IHE XCA gateway (Cross Community Access profile) specifications allowed all hospitals to be linked across the region of Veneto.

HEALTH OPTIMUM applied a layered strategy where specialized hospitals in neurosurgery acted as the hub, and the peripheral hospitals extended the network out into the local communities and primary care settings. This infrastructure was implemented in seven hubs all connected so that all hubs can receive input from the peripheral hospitals, creating a safe network across the region. As a consequence, any physician in any clinic makes available to the expert neurosurgeon at the hub hospital a digitally signed teleconsultation request (HL7 CDA2 document with LOINC Codes) and a set of CT Images (based on DICOM Manifest). The neurosurgeon can then decide if a patient transfer is needed, providing the answer in a reply form. When such a decision is needed, the surgeon automatically begins preparations for therapeutic or surgical intervention while the patient is transferred from the peripheral hospital to the neurosurgeon hub, saving precious time for the patient, and increasing successful treatment and good outcome of care.

The IHE-driven interoperability of the central platform enables an infrastructure lending itself to multiple uses. Additional services have been easily added, such as teleconsultation for ischemic stroke. Extensions of the platform are expected to include laboratory and medical report sharing, e-prescription, and e-referral services for general practitioners and pediatricians (Table 5.1).

5.4.5 Keystone Health Information Exchange, Northeast Pennsylvania, USA

Keystone Health Information Exchange (KeyHIE®) is a network of healthcare providers in more than 31 counties of northeast and central Pennsylvania that serve three million patients yearly, where many of them in medically underserved areas. KeyHIE designed its Health Information Exchange (HIE) to roll out in phases, growing the system's value and capabilities and overall adoption over time. Geisinger Health System is an innovative integrated delivery network based on healthcare IT-supported care coordination, is one of the major and active participants in KeyHIE. Currently, KeyHIE interconnects already Geisinger with five other regional hospitals—Evangelical Community Hospital, Community Medical Center, Mid-Valley Hospital, Shamokin Area Community Hospital, and Moses Taylor Hospital—for a total of seven facilities. Geisinger received a $2.3 million grant from the Agency for Healthcare Research and Quality (AHRQ) to extend and innovate the KeyHIE-connected community by adding additional regional hospitals, home health organizations, long-term care facilities, and physician practices. In addition to attracting more stakeholders, this 5-year AHRQ grant helped to make

Table 5.1 Health Optimum IHE profiles used

Integration profile	System/vendor	IHE actor	IHE transaction
Cross-Enterprise Document Sharing	Solinfo, Exprivia, EbitAET, Intema (Gruppo Dedalus), A-thon	Document Source	Provide And Register Document Set—b (ITI-41) Patient Identity Feed (ITI-8)
	Solinfo, Exprivia, EbitAET, Intema (Gruppo Dedalus), A-thon	Document Consumer	Registry Stored Query (ITI-18) Retrieve document set (ITI-43)
	Solinfo, Exprivia, EbitAET, Indema (Gruppo Dedalus). A-thon	Imaging Document Source	Provide and Register Imaging Document Set (RAD-54) WADO Retrieve (RAD-55)
	Solinfo, Exprivia, EbitAET, A-thon	Imaging Document Consumer	WADO Retrieve (RAD-55)
	Solinfo, Exprivia, A-thon, InsielMercato	Document Registry	Register Document Set (ITI-42) Registry Stored Query (ITI-18) Patient Identity Feed (ITI-8)
	Solinfo, Exprivia, A-thon, InsialMarcato, Intema (Gruppo Dedalus)	Document Repository	Provide and Register Imaging document Set (RAD-54) Register Document Set (ITI-42) Retrieve Document Set (ITI-43)
Notification of Document Availability	Solinfo, Exprivia. A-thon, Ebit-AET, Intema (Gruppo Dedalus)	NAV Sender NAV Receiver	Sand Notification (ITI-25) Receive Notification (ITI-26) Send Acknowledgement (ITI-27) Receive Acknowledgement (ITI-28)
Audit Trail and Node Authentication	All vendors involved	All actors	Record Audit Event
Cross Cummunity Access	Solinfo, Exprivia, A-thon, InsielMercato, Telemedicina Rizzoli	Initialing Gateway	Cross Gateway Query (ITI-38) Cross-Gateway Retrieve (ITI-39) (RAD-55)
Cross-Community Access	Solinfo, Exprivia, A-thon, InsielMercato, Telemedicina Rizzoli	Responding Gateway	(ITI-38) (ITI-39) (RAD-55)

new innovative clinical applications and create new document types to be used within the HIE.

Leveraging KeyHIE's infrastructure is an important element in this Geisinger's $16 million projects, which aims to extend the Health information technology-driven coordinated care models to more constituents and patients. New roles such as case managers can access KeyHIE for patient information and, as a result, reduce substantially the time they spend collecting important and critical patient information locked in different systems. This new online communication is a major enhancement from their current mode of communication, which occurred via fax, email, voicemail, and regular postal service.

KeyHIE's initial phase scope was to provide rapidly critical patient information to all Emergency Department (ED) teams at the point of care—providing the right information at the right time and place. The ED is usually the place where the least information is available about a patient due to the situation of the patients, and speed is a key factor in providing the best treatment in the shortest time possible. Faced with disparate EMR systems that existed in the participating hospitals' emergency departments, it was clear that point-to-point integrations were not the proper technical solution for clinical data transparency and sharing.

KeyHIE selected a large vendor to power their community Health Information Exchange. Today, KeyHIE has successfully incorporated nearly three million patients in the Master Patient Index (MPI) across all seven active hospitals. Using the new solution, KeyHIE adhered to IHE standards, which are thoroughly tested in North American Connect-a-thons.

The use of IHE helped healthcare professionals to resolve interoperability challenges and barriers. The ability to properly and securely access and exchange patient-related health data have for long, been a substantial issue to deal with. The addition of new incentives such as demonstrating compliance to "Meaningful Use' rules and regulations in the United States, and similar regulatory mandates elsewhere in the world, IHE provides a proven and practical solution to resolve health IT interoperability problems based upon the proper reuse of international standards and terminologies. The use of IHE integration profiles creates a stable collaborative environment between healthcare providers and industry leaders to improve the secure and effective exchange of patient-related health information.

5.5   Conformity Assessment Scheme: The EURO-CAS Case

The conformity Assessment Scheme for Europe (CASforEU) is a key deliverable of the European project called EURO-CAS[11] as a mean to demonstrate that ICT systems are conformed to standards and integration profiles, thus ensuring interoperability in countries and across borders.

---

[11] https://www.euro-cas.eu.

5.5.1   Introduction

With the finding of the lack of interoperability that introduces discrepancies among ICT systems that uses the data that are exchanging or shared, it will directly impact of the data quality and their use by the healthcare professionals. For example, a woman coming in hospital gives the married name and the maiden name for patient identification at the entrance. The demographic data are sent to the Electronic Medical Record (EMR) where the medical record is identified by the maiden name. During the workflow exchange, because the developer misinterprets the standard used for such exchanges and the names were reversed in the structured message. When the message is treated by the EMR, a new medical record is created for the women. To avoid errors, testing the conformity is the key to enhance data quality in healthcare.

Based on recommendations from the Antilope project[12] and the state of the art in interoperability testing in eHealth, CASforEU puts in place an operational Conformity Assessment Scheme (CAS) based on ISO/IEC 17067[13] and requires laboratories to be accredited to ISO/IEC 17025.[14] This enables CASforEU to demonstrate product conformance to requirements of European eHealth projects as well as national and regional eHealth programs and provides an EU-wide platform for procurers and vendors of digital health technologies to test their products or solutions.

CASforEU is defined as a sustainable conformity assessment scheme (Fig. 5.9) that consists on a consistent and uniform policy and procedures thereof are a cornerstone for such a scheme. It gives a comprehensive vision of an organization enable to run testing session for products and ICT solutions in order to provide a trusting and confident assessment report for the evaluation of the conformity.

CASforEU specifies

- The governance based on the creation of a non-profit mutual benefit organization called ECO (EURO-CAS organization) characterized by its article of incorporation, corporate bylaws, IPR policy etc. EURO-CAS is composed by members from different constituencies gathering European organization, member states and regions, Industry and accredited test laboratories.
- The mission of the organization;
- The organization that includes the General Assembly, the steering board and technical committees;
- The process of development and maintenance of the scheme;
- The execution process that involves test laboratories, vendors and their products together executing the tests as described in the CASforEU test plan;

---

[12] https://www.antilope-project.eu/front/index.html.

[13] ISO/IEC 17067 Conformity Assessment—Fundamentals of products certification and guidelines for product certification schemes.

[14] ISO/IEC 17025 General requirements for the competence of testing and calibration laboratories.

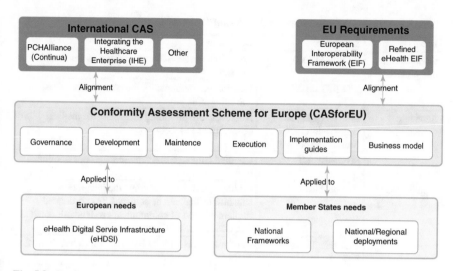

Fig. 5.9 Conformity Assessment Scheme for Europe. (From CASforEU)

- The EURO-CAS test plan that content the set of use cases, the profiles and standards and the test methodology to test product.

In addition, the implementation guidelines provide guidance for the ecosystem that allow stakeholders to implement and to be part of the conformity assessment ecosystem, for example, implementation entities (organization wanted to launch a conformity assessment for their own eHealth program or project, vendors, test laboratory, etc). The business model provides scenarios for sustaining the Euro-CAS Organisation (ECO) at the European level starting by the adoption of CASforEU by European countries (the main goal of the year 2019).

5.5.2 The Content

The CASforEU developed under the supervision of the EURO-CAS organization, is compliant with the deliveries of the international standard bodies (SDOs), which develop and specify standards in eHealth and other domains such as HL7 international,[15] DICOM,[16] IEEE,[17] W3C,[18] ISO,[19] etc) as well as international profile organizations (IHE, PCHAlliance[20]) which develop implementation guidelines. By

---

[15] http://www.hl7.org.

[16] Digital Imaging and Communication in Medicine: https://www.dicomstandard.org.

[17] https://www.ieee.org.

[18] https://www.w3.org.

[19] International Standard organization: https://www.iso.org/fr/home.html.

[20] Personal Connected Health Alliance: https://www.pchalliance.org.

Table 5.2 Examples of standards used for CASforEU

Level	Standards	Description
Organization and process	ISO/IEC 17065	Requirements for bodies certifying products and services
	ISO/IEC 17025	General requirements for the competence of testing and calibration laboratories
Semantic	LOINC ((Logical Observation Identifiers Names and codes)	Nomenclature providing identifiers for medical observations in laboratory
	SNOMED/CT	Codified language that represents groups of clinical terms
Application	IHE profiles	Profile organize and leverage the integration capabilities that can be achieved by coordinated implementation of communication standards, such as DICOM, HL7, W3C and security standards
	HL7 (Health Level Seven)	standards in eHealth such as HL7v2, CDA release 2 or FHIR

this alignment CASforEU ensures continuity and recognition with the international level and benefit of the up-to-date standards. Note that these standards and profiles have a large coverage including processes, organizations, semantic and technical aspects (see Table 5.2).

At the European level, the European Interoperability Framework (eEIF) described principles that apply in Europe. All these inputs are used directly on the specifications of the EURO-CAS test plan (CASforEU CATP).

Based on the recommendations of the European Commission on a selection of 27 profiles, the test plan identifies

- The interoperability use cases;
- The profiles specifications, implementation guidelines;
- The test scripts that will be used to test the conformity of the system to the identified actors;
- The test tools mostly the simulators and validators. Most of them are developed by IHE services and used at the Connectathon or for the IHE Conformity Assessment Scheme (IHE CAS).

The CASforEU CATP provides also recommendations on

- How to extend the scope;
- How the laboratory can access to the test plans and test methods;
- The uniform templates of test reports that include detailed and summary test reports.

One of the expectations is to encourage alignment with the international level and more specifically with the IHE Conformity Assessment Scheme (IHE CAS) and the Continua Alliance certification. This is why the test plan reuses the test methods developed by those organizations for their own needs.

Table 5.3 Use cases examples

Scale	Use case	Short description
International/Cross Border	Patient Summary exchanging across international borders	Providing medical background and history of a patient to a Healthcare Professional in another country
Cross Border	ePrescription and eDispensing exchanging across borders	To support the processes of prescription and dispensation through the electronic exchange for citizens travelling in Europe
National and regional	Discharge report of the patient from secondary care	Providing all relevant medical information of the patient to GP after a treatment in hospital
	Request and results sharing workflow for laboratory	Providing laboratory results and reports to the prescriber
	Request and results sharing workflow for radiology	Providing radiology reports to the prescriber
At home	Remote monitoring and care of people at home or on the move using sensor devices	Collecting information from devices at home to healthcare application
	Involvement of chronic patients in electronic documentation of healthcare information	Registration and monitoring of patient-generated health parameters

When the EURO-CAS organization will be set up, agreements with the IHE international CAS committee will be discussed in order to mutualize efforts for mutual recognition among the issued seals.

The test plan is the heart of the CASforEU and identifies requirements from a selection of use cases (see Table 5.3), applicable profiles and standards, test cases and test methods that are used to test products and ICT solutions.

The initial scope was validated during a meeting held in Paris in June 2017. The stakeholders (National centers of competencies, vendor associations, end-users, SDOs) select a set of profiles and standards that support use cases described on the Antilope Refined ehealth Interoperability framework and available in the use case data repository (Use case repository, see https://usecase-repository.ihe-europe.net) (Fig. 5.10).

The applicable profiles for the first version of the EURO-CAS Test Plan supporting such use cases were selected according their current deployment in several countries in Europe. They cover.

- Security aspects and more specifically confidentiality, integrity and traceability with

  - IHE CT Consistent Time
  - IHE ATNA audit Trail and Node Authentication

- Patient demographic information

  - IHE PDQ Patient Demographics Query
  - IHE PIX Patient Identifier Cross referencing
  - IHE XCPD Cross Community Patient Discovery

Use Case Repository

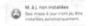

Welcome !

This use case repository provides an easy access to the use cases and their related scenarios that were defined in the
refined eHealth Interoperability Framework (eEIF) developed in Antilope in Antilope project (www.Antilope-project.eu)
and its extension developed in eStandards project (www.estandards.project.eu)

The framework describes an initial set of interoperability *use cases* that can be used as the basis for european/national/regional deployment.
Wherever applicable and useful, several variants of these use cases are given, to support the different deployment scales, Also, concrete
realisation scenarios, based on available profiles and standards, are specified for each of these use cases. The linking to standards and
profiles in these realisation scenarios provides guidance upon which to build localisation and interoperable implementations.

The framework increases consistency where possible, across eHealth projects in Europe, reducing project risks, giving higher quality with
reused test tools, and offering a broader choice of compatible solutions.

#	Medical domain	Description	Scale
1	Medication	e-Prescription and e-Dispensing	1a) Cross-border 1b) National / Regional 1c) Intra organisational

Fig. 5.10 Use case data repository

- Cross community infrastructure
  - IHE XDS.b Cross Enterprise Document Sharing
  - IHE XDR Cross Enterprise reliable Interchange
  - XDS-I.b Cross Community Imaging Sharing
  - IHE XCA Cross Community Access

- At home
  - Personal Health Devices Interface
  - Services Interface
  - Health Information System Interface

Finally, the CASforEU requests that the testing of products shall be performed by an accredited ISO/IEC 17025 test laboratory in order to increase the liability of the results of the testing and therefore increase the trust and confidence on those products having passed the conformity assessment.

The test plan was elaborated taking into account existing international conformity assessment such as IHE CAS[21] and certification process from PCHA with the objectives to align their processes for better adoption of the interoperability specifications in eHealth. The alignment covers also the use of same testing tools and test plan at the two levels, European and international to enforce closed relationships.

The next step will be the establishment of a mutual recognition between the International Conformity Assessment and the European one. It will allow any product has been assessed at the European level to be recognized as assessed for the international level for the benefit of the vendor and buyers.

---

[21] https://www.ihe.net/testing/conformity-assessment/.

5.6   Benefits for the eHealth Stakeholders

The benefits are presenting by categories of stakeholders *(from Euro-Cas project)*

- Healthcare Professionals and patient:
  - Having applications that are compliant on interoperability specifications and tested, will provide better quality of clinical data, for their treatment and usability by increasing confidence and trust;
  - Better time to market of innovative solutions;
  - Enhanced patient's engagement and mobility through innovative solutions;

- Vendors and IT companies:
  - Reduction of effort in interoperability testing: having one conformity assessment scheme over Europe allow vendors to sell products that integrate the European interoperability specifications in all European countries (see Fig. 5.11);
  - The investments will be redirected to innovative features;
  - Broaden market opportunities in a European Digital Single Market (and beyond);

- ehealth initiatives, policy makers, procurers, payers:
  - Provide an independent benchmark;
  - Provide reduced effort and expenses in specification and testing;
  - Conform to the European regulation.

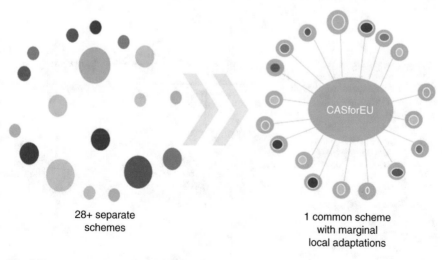

28+ separate
schemes

1 common scheme
with marginal
local adaptations

Fig. 5.11   CAsforEU in Europe. (From EURO-CAS)

5.6.1 Certification vs Conformity Assessment

Based on ISO 9001:2000 (or ISO 9001:2008) and ISO 14001:2004, certification could be defined as an independent accredited external body issuing written assurance (the "certificate") that has audited and verified the product or software is conformed to the specified requirements." [HITCH, 2011]. The conformity assessment demonstrates that specified requirements related to a product, process, system or body are fulfilled [ISO/IEC 17000].

EURO-CAS does not define a certification scheme but organizes the interoperability assessment of the products. This best practice identifies on one side the test laboratory that provides the assessment report and on the other side the body issuing the certificate at the European or national level.

EURO-CAS is complementary to the certification body: the validation test reports provided by the test laboratory can be sent and used by an identified certification body that will issue the certificate after review according to the requirements, with the validation test reports. Each organization has a clear role that avoids any conflict of interest. The certification body follows the policy and rules defined by the authority generally a governmental authority, seeking to submit products to certification (Fig. 5.12).

Clinical Pearls
EURO-CAS is a means to increase interoperability among products in Digital health. It gives more confidence and trust on those products implemented with profiles and standards. To facilitate the understanding of the end-users requirements to procure such products, EURO-CAS provides a set of use cases that are supported by the CASforEU test plan. A first draft was published in 2019 and will be maintained

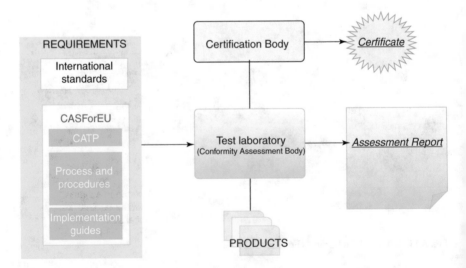

Fig. 5.12 Certification and Conformity Assessment best practices

by extending the current test plan with new use cases that healthcare professionals, authorities, vendors and other actors of the ecosystem will choose with consensus following the governance and the maintenance process.

CASforEu provides for clinicians and patients.

- More transparency when procuring or choosing healthcare products or solutions: when procurers specify the tender for specific products or solutions; at first, they will review the set of use cases available on the CASforEU test plan and select the one corresponding to their needs and secondly request for profiles, standards and their conformity validation test report according the specifications that the CASforEU covers. Finally, the vendors are able to answer to the tender with the proof of their conformity by providing their validation test report (or the certification seal if any) and when available the integration statement of their products;
- For vendors it provides solutions and a clear direction on the future development of the Digital Health allowing vendors to invest in interoperability with less risks: knowing what the interoperability demands are and what the requirements are that the products shall be compliant with, vendors are able to anticipate their development roadmap, which is often called "interoperability by design".

Acronyms

DMP: Dossier Médical Partagé (Electronic Health Record)
EHR: Electronic Health Record
GSPS: Grayscale Softcopy Presentation State
IAB: Internet Architecture Board
IEEE: IEEE Advancing Technology for Humanity
IETF: Internet engineering Taskforce
ISOC: Internet Society
MRI: Magnetic Resonance Imaging
PACS: Picture Archive and Communication System

Review Questions

1. You are working on your tender because you are building an EHR repository that will support exchanges of patient summaries among Healthcare Professionals (GPs, Hospitals, etc) in your region. Describe your use case (see examples on the use case repository: https://usecase-repository.ihe-europe.net)
2. Best practices are now available on the implementation of such an EHR repository. Analyze them and identify the main profiles that are implemented. What do those profiles cover in terms of functionalities?
3. Many of the projects presented in this chapter agreed that testing the conformity to profiles is one of the key elements for the success of the project. What are the main testing tools which are needed for your project (see https://gazelle.ihe.net/content/gazelle-user-guides)?
4. How can you compare products that will be offered by various vendors, what can you include in your tender as a means of validation. Explain why this appraoch will provide more confidence to the products that will be selected.

Answers

1. Use the template provided by the Antilope project. Example is given in the use case repository
   The sections to be filled are

   (a) Purpose: describe in one sentence the use case
   (b) Relevance: why this use case has to be deployed in your environment
   (c) Domain: Patient Summary
   (d) Scale: regional
   (e) Context: describe with sentences your use case, ecosystem and context. It will allow any end-user the functional requirements of the use case for validation
   (f) Information: provide the set of data needed to realize the use case (for example, Patient demographics, patient identifier, allergies, current prescription medication, etc)
   (g) Participants: Patient, GPs, other HCPs
   (h) The functional process workflow: describe the interaction between human actors using systems, for example the GP is requesting the last patient summary for his patient that was admitted at the emergency setting of the regional hospital

2. Examples provided in this paper demonstrates that this use case is currently broadly deployed in many countries. A common set of profiles are used in various projects over the world. See for example Table 5.1.

   In synthesis, the main profiles are CT, ATNA, XDS, EUA, PIX and PDQ and CDA r2 for structuring the documents. Terminology should be chosen by clinicians. In the case of cross community, XUA and XCA are also used. The profile XDS (Cross Border Document Sharing) manages the exchange of documents between Healthcare organization. ATNA (Audit Trail Node Authentication) defines security audit logging and secured network. PIX (Patient identification Cross Referencing) provides the means to cross identify a patient. PDQ (Patient demographics Query) allows queries by patient demographics. The EUA profile enables single sign-on inside an enterprise. See https://wiki.ihe.net/index.php/Profiles for more information.

3. The testing tools that can be used are (list non exhaustive). More information at https://gazelle.ihe.net/content/gazelle-user-guides

Type	Testing tool	Description
Validators	Gazelle External Validation Front-end (EVS)	To allow the user to use a user-friendly interface to access to validator
	HL7 Validator	Web services to validate HL7v2 and HL7v3 messages exchanged in the IHE context
	Schematron based validator	Web service to validate xml documents
	Gazelle Object checker	Web service to validate a large set of CDA documents using a model-based architecture
	XDS metadata validator	Web service to validate metadata of XD* profiles
Simulators	Patient Manager	Emulates actors for PIX/PDQ
	XD* Client	Emulates the initiating actors of XD* profiles

4. An organization which provides a Scheme on conformity validation will maintain
   (a) A test plan that users can refer to in their tender;
   (b) A public website where products having passed the conformity assessment
       and will be available (see for example https://conformity.ihe.net/summary-
       reports for IHE CAS);
   (c) A list of accredited test laboratories enables users to test products against the
       test plan in a neutral and rigorous environment.
       It will allow procurers to have a better overview on the interoperability
       functionalities and capabilities of the products (more transparency) with con-
       fidence and it provides an easy way to compare products. In counterparty, the
       procurer and his team should maintain their skills on interoperability archi-
       tecture and IHE specifications to better address their needs.

Acknowledgements The authors use existing IHE and EURO-CAS project documentations including images to provide proper content to this chapter and would like to thank warmly all the contributors that were involved in these documentations. Images may be reproduced and/or distributed, totally or in part, irrespective of the means and/or the formats used only, without prior permission, provided that the respective copyright holder is always acknowledged as the source of the material. Such acknowledgement must be included in each copy of the material.

Glossary

CDA Clinical Documentation Architecture
CEN European Standards Organisation
Conformance The level of adherance to an agreed rule or standard
Connectathons Planned events by IHE to test new implementations
DICOM Digital Imaging and Communications in Medicine
DMP Dossier Médical Partagé (Electronic Health Record)
EHR Electronic Health Record
epSOS European Patients—Smart Open Service
European Interoperability Framework Four layers of interoperability
   (Foundational, structural, semantic, and organizational) are the foundation of the
   framework
FRAND FAIR, Reasonable and Non-Discriminatory
GSPS Grayscale Softcopy Presentation State
HIE Health Information Exchange
HIT Health Information Technology
HL7 Health Level Seven
HPD Healthcare provider directory
IAB Internet Architecture Board
IEEE IEEE Advancing Technology for Humanity
IETF Internet engineering Taskforce
IHE Integrating the Healthcare Enterprise

ISA Interoperability Standards Advisory
ISO International Organization for Standardization
ISOC Internet Society
LOINC Logical Observation Identifiers Names and Codes
Mandation A term that groups categories of mandatory, condition, or optional
Metadata Information that provide facts about one or more aspects of a data element
MPI Master Patient Index
MRI Magnetic Resonance Imaging
OASIS Organization for the Advancement of Structured Information Standards
PACS Picture Archive and Communication System
PCC Patient Care Co-ordination
Projectathon Projectathon, when deploying IHE profiles at the project level,
the IHE Gazelle test platform is used at the Projectathon which is a type of
Connectathon but dedicated to the specifications-based profiles of the eHealth
project. The Projectathon has the same role as the Connectathon: it provides sup-
port, training and expertise to vendors that are selected for the project deployment
SDO Standards Development Organisation
Standard A rule that enables consistent and repeatable use, performance, and
outcomes
Use Case An integration profile used as a guideline for implementation of a specific
process called use case. The use case provides precise definitions of how standards can be implemented to meet specific clinical needs for a specific purpose.
For example, integration profiles organize and leverage the integration capabili-
ties that can be achieved by coordinated implementation of communication standards, such as DICOM, HL7, W3C and security standards in Digital Health
VA United States Department of Veteran Affairs
W3C World Wide Web Consortium
XCPD Cross community patient discovery

References

2020–2025 Federal Health IT Strategic Plan. Office of the National Coordinator for Health Information Exchange (ONC). 2020. https://www.healthit.gov/topic/2020-2025-federal-health-it-strategic-plan.

Bourquard K, Le Gall F, Cousin P. Standards for interoperability in Digital Health: selection and implementation in eHealth project. Berlin: Springer; 2014.

Commission implementing regulation (EU) 2018/292 of 26 February 2018. https://eur-lex.europa.eu/legal-content/EN/TXT/?uri=uriserv:OJ.L_.2018.055.01.0034.01.ENG.

Commission recommendation on a European Electronic Health Record exchange format (C(2019)800) of 6 February 2019 [database on the Internet]. 2019. https://ec.europa.eu/digital-single-market/en/news/recommendation-european-electronic-health-record-exchange-format.

Communication on enabling the digital transformation of health and care in the Digital Single Market; empowering citizens and building a healthier society. 2020. https://ec.europa.eu/digital-single-market/news-redirect/624248.

Definition of interoperability. 2020. Dedicated website for a Definition of Interoperability at interoperability-definition.info. Copyright AFUL under CC BY-SA.

Digital health progressing towards more interoperability for the digital cross border exchange of health data in Europe. 2020. https://ec.europa.eu/health/sites/health/files/ehealth/docs/2019_bucarest_en.pdf.

European Interoperability Framework for pan-European eGovernment Services. Version 1.0. 2004. ISBN 92-894-8389-X

Gazelle simulators. 2020. https://gazelle.ihe.net/content/simulators.

Health and care in the digital single market - ICPerMed. 2020. https://www.icpermed.eu/en/Health-Care-Digital-Single-Market.php.

Hoerbst A, Ammenwerth E. Quality and certification of electronic health records: an overview of current approaches from the US and Europe. Appl Clin Inform. 2010;1(2):149–64. https://doi.org/10.4338/ACI-2010-02-R-0009.

IHE Conformity Assessment Scheme. 2014. https://www.ihe.net/testing/conformity-assessment/.

IHE Conformity Reports. 2020. http://conformity.ihe.net/summary-reports.

IHE Domains. 2020. https://www.ihe.net/ihe_domains/.

IHE Member Organizations. 2020. https://www.ihe.net/Member_Organizations/.

IHE Process. 2020. https://www.ihe.net/about_ihe/ihe_process/.

IHE Product Registry. 2020. https://product-registry.ihe.net/PR/home.seam.

IHE User handbooks. 2020. https://www.ihe.net/resources/user_handbooks/.

New European Interoperability Framework. 2017. Promoting seamless services and data flows for European public administrations. 2017. https://joinup.ec.europa.eu/collection/nifo-national-interoperability-framework-observatory/eif-european-interoperability-framework-0.

Rosemberg A, Plaut O, Sepulchre X, Spahni S. ["MonDossierMedical.ch": an efficient tool for sharing medical data between patients and doctors]. Rev Med Suisse. 2015;11(474):1069–73. French.

Slater T. "What is interoperability?", Network Centric Operations Industry Consortium – NCOIC. 2012. https://www.ncoic.org/what-is-interoperability/.

Spahni S, Guardia A, Boggini T, Geissbuhler A. Design and implementation of a shared treatment plan in a federated health information exchange. Stud Health Technol Inform. 2013;192:1090.

Transformation of health and care in the digital single market. 2019. https://ec.europa.eu/digital-single-market/en/european-policy-ehealth.

What is HIE?|HealthIT.gov. 2020. https://www.healthit.gov/topic/health-it-and-health-information-exchange-basics/what-hie.

What is interoperability in Healthcare?. 2013. https://www.himss.org/what-interoperability.

Witting K. Health information exchange: integrating the Healthcare Enterprise (IHE). London: Springer; 2015. https://doi.org/10.1007/978-1-4471-2999-8_6.

Chapter 6
Health Informatics Standards

Pamela Hussey and Margaret Ann Kennedy

Abstract This chapter introduces readers to the world of health information standards and standards development organizations. The chapter provides insight into the relationship between standards and nursing practice and how they relate to evidence in practice. The definitions and purpose of standards are explored, as well as the development and approval processes of international standards development organizations. Conformance and relevance to nursing practice are also covered from an international perspective.

Keywords Nursing · Informatics · eHealth · Standard · Interoperability
Electronic health record · Terminology

Learning Objectives for the Chapter
1. Articulate the value of standards for Health Informatics and for nursing practice.
2. Identify and access standards that are relevant to their context (clinical practice, education, informatics, etc.).
3. Use appropriate standards to assess conformance of Health Informatics practices, processes and applications.
4. Participate in standards development, conformance assessment and review.

Electronic Supplementary Material The online version of this chapter (https://doi.org/10.1007/978-3-030-58740-6_6) contains supplementary material, which is available to authorized users.

P. Hussey (✉)
School of Nursing Psychotherapy and Community Health, Dublin City University, Dublin, Ireland
e-mail: pamela.hussey@dcu.ie

M. A. Kennedy
Centre of Excellence, Gevity Consulting Inc, Vancouver, BC, Canada
e-mail: mkennedy@gevityinc.com

© Springer Nature Switzerland AG 2021
P. Hussey, M. A. Kennedy (eds.), *Introduction to Nursing Informatics*, Health Informatics, https://doi.org/10.1007/978-3-030-58740-6_6

6.1   Introduction

Nursing informatics and health informatics are no longer the domain of specialists. As this book demonstrates, information management and the use of information and communication technology (ICT) are an integral part of the delivery of quality health care. In future, ICT will become even more essential for the delivery of affordable health and nursing care, as the number of people living with multiple chronic conditions increases and the number of qualified nurses continues to fall.

The integration of health informatics (HI) practice with nursing practice is a key theme of this chapter on HI standards. Standards for nursing practice and standards for the information and communication technologies (ICT) that support nursing practice are intertwined, each dependent on the other to help nurses deliver safe, effective care and to communicate across boundaries.

This chapter represents a revision of a chapter, authored by Anne Casey, RN, MSc, FRCN, which appeared in a previous edition of this book. In this chapter, the nature of standards in health informatics is explained and key concepts such as conformance and consensus are explored. Table 6.1 provides definitions of relevant terms, some of which are also explained in the text. HI standards are described in the context of clinical nursing. Examples of standards from different countries are used to demonstrate how standards guide practice and support interoperability. Many of the examples are standards published by the International Organization for Standardization (ISO). These are referred to by number and not fully referenced.

Examples of HI standards are mostly drawn from the UK partly because the author is more familiar with these but also to encourage readers to look beyond local policies and state or national standards to international sources. This is not only necessary, given that there are significant gaps in national standards portfolios, but also relatively easy to do with the potential of internet searching to identify appropriate resources from across the globe.

In the final section of the chapter, the standards lifecycle is described and approaches to standards development and review are explained. Readers are encouraged to consolidate their understanding by reviewing relevant additional resources on the topic, for example the educational materials produced by ETSI (ETSI 2020)

6.2   Defining Standards and Related Concepts

6.2.1   What Is a Standard?

Standards are relevant to every aspect of our daily lives, from the way we drive, to the food we eat. International standards are especially important. Consider the Automatic Teller Machine (ATM): people can use a personalized card to obtain money almost anywhere in the world because the banking systems have all adopted relevant international standards. In contrast, when travelling abroad, people have to carry an adaptor plug because different countries do not have the same standard for electricity power points.

Table 6.1 Terms and descriptions

Term	Description
Clinical guideline	Systematically developed statements to assist practitioners and patient decisions about appropriate health care for specific circumstances (Feild and Lohr 1990)
Compliance	Used interchangeably with 'conformance' but with a flavour of a mandatory regulation. Conformance implies some degree of choice whereas compliance suggests sanctions for not complying.
Conformance	Degree to which the requirements in a standard specification are met
Conformity assessment	Process used to show that a product, service or system meets specified requirements (ISO 2020a)
De facto standard	Way of doing things or artefact that is widely accepted as best practice/gold standard even though it has not been officially recognised or documented by a recognized body
HI standard	Document, established from evidence and by consensus and approved by a recognized body, that provides rules, guidelines or characteristics for activities or their results, in the field of information for health, and health information and communications technology
Information Governance	Framework of policies and procedures for handling personal health information in a confidential, secure and accurate manner to appropriate professional, ethical and quality standards
Interoperability	Ability of two or more systems or components to exchange information and to use the information that has been exchanged (United Nations 2020)
Mandation	Term that groups the categories of conformance requirement specified in standards: 'mandatory', 'conditional' and 'optional'
Recognized body	Legal or administrative entity that has specific tasks and composition, with acknowledged authority for publishing standards (ISO. 5 2020)
Regulation	Legal or professional rule or principle that directs activities or their results; also known as 'regulatory standard'
Standard	Document established by consensus and approved by a recognized body that provides for common and repeated use, rules, guidelines or characteristics for activities or their results, aimed at the achievement of the optimum degree of order in a given context (ISO. 1 2020)

Aside from personal convenience, international standards benefit us in numerous ways.

They:

- Help businesses reduce costs, better meet the needs of customers, and improve environmental performance.
- Open up access to new markets and reduce barriers to international trade.
- Provide a basis for better regulation, both nationally and internationally (ISO 2020b).

ISO defines a standard as:

A document established by consensus and approved by a recognized body that provides for common and repeated use, rules, guidelines or characteristics for activities or their results, aimed at the achievement of the optimum degree of order in a given context. (International Electrotechnical Commission 2020)

Put more simply, a standard is *'an agreed way of doing something'* (BSI 2020).

In order to understand HI standards we need to consider both their purpose and their 'functional usage', particularly conformance assessment (Chap. 5 demonstrated through the Euro CAS project, which completed in 2018, how conformance may be acheived (European Commission 2020)).

Before discussing these topics however, there is one other aspect of standards that needs to be considered. ISO views a standard as a set of guidelines presented in a **document**; people on the other hand often view standards as **things**. For example: 'the Braden scale is the standard assessment tool for pressure ulcer risk in our organization'; 'we use a standard terminology in our electronic record system'; 'the X monitor is the standard device for measuring blood pressure in neonates'. In these examples, the Braden scale, the terminology and the device have been adopted by a clinical team, an organization or other body as their standard approach. In order to ensure quality and consistency, staff would be expected to use only these artefacts in the situations for which they have been adopted.

This meaning of the word 'standard' (i.e. as a descriptor that gives an artefact additional status) is not covered further in this chapter—here we focus on standards as documents that state 'rules, guidelines or characteristics'. Interestingly, many standards support the selection of artefacts for preferred use by describing the characteristics that make them safe, effective and useful. For example, ISO/IEEE 11073 Medical/Health Device Communication Standards represent a family of standards for interoperability between medical devices, such as blood glucose monitors.

6.2.2 Purpose of HI Standards

At a general level, HI standards support clinical practice and the management, delivery, and evaluation of health services. More specifically, their purpose is to promote interoperability between independent systems (as discussed in Chap. 5).

In all healthcare settings around the World, we need to be able to exchange information reliably and then interpret and use it effectively: interoperability is essential. Reducing duplication of effort and redundancy are also important goals, as are making manufacture, supply and trade easier. However, there is something missing from this list of purposes for HI standards—the safe, effective integration of information management and ICT into clinical practice. This purpose fits well with definitions of nursing informatics, which emphasise the integration of the science and art of nursing with information management and ICT (American Nurses Association 2014).

This leads to the conclusion that HI standards have two main purposes: to support interoperability and to guide safe, effective HI practice. However, it is their 'functional usage' which is perhaps most important—we use standards to guide what we do and to measure conformance.

6.2.3 Conformance

In the same way that we use practice standards to audit the quality of nursing care, we use HI standards to ensure that HI systems and the way we use them conform to agreed 'best practice'. The word 'conform' is key: a standard is something against which conformance or compliance can be measured—see Table 6.1.

Closely related to conformance is the idea of 'levels of mandation'—a term that groups the categories of 'mandatory', 'conditional' and 'optional'. Mandatory statements in a standard are those that must be complied with. Conditional ones must be complied with if certain specified conditions are met and optional ones are recommended but not required for conformance. An example is given below from the Palliative Care Co-ordination Information Standard published by NHS Digital in the UK (NHS Digital 2020a)

This standard specifies the content of electronic palliative care co-ordination systems (EPaCCS). One of the requirements in the standard is that *Clinical governance and IT safety leads in each organisation where the standard is implemented MUST ensure that the editing rights for specified clinical content elements are limited to the appropriate clinicians.* This mandatory (MUST) requirement aims to ensure that only the lead clinician records or amends critical information such as Do Not Attempt Cardiopulmonary Resuscitation orders. Some content elements such as person name are mandatory in each record. Others should be recorded once the person has made a decision (conditional), for example, 'Preferred place of death'.

There are some similarities between these levels of mandation and the way we talk about professional standards. In health care, we use terms like 'requirements', 'recommendations' and 'principles' which are found in Regulations, Clinical Guidelines and Practice Guidance. Regulations are legal or professional requirements for practising nurses mainly aimed at protecting the public. In the US, education and licensure requirements are set by the State Boards of Nursing (NCSBN 2020) and a Code of Ethics for Nurses is published by the American Nurses Association (American Nurses Association 2020a).

In the UK, the Nursing and Midwifery Council is the regulatory body established in law that sets standards for education, conduct, performance and ethics (Nursing and Midwifery Council 2020a).

In contrast, clinical guidelines are:

systematically developed statements to assist practitioners and patient decisions about appropriate health care for specific circumstances. (Feild and Lohr 1990, p. 38)

'Systematically developed' means that a systematic literature search and review of research evidence have been undertaken using agreed criteria and rigor. Practice guidance is generally evidence based but has not been systematically developed, depending rather on consensus among practice experts. The terms guideline, guidance, practice standard, practice parameter, quality standard and others are frequently used interchangeably. They are all standards in that they are 'agreed ways of doing something'. No matter what they are called, the important thing is to know how they were developed and who approved or endorsed them so that users can decide whether to comply with the recommendations made.

All nurses must comply with relevant regulations if they are to continue to practice. However, the degree to which a nurse is expected to comply with clinical guidelines or practice guidance will depend on national and local polices but it often comes down to (a) the strength of the evidence that supports the recommendations and (b) the authority of the organization that has published or adopted the standard.

Continuing the example of End of Life Care, all clinicians would be expected to comply with the *End of life care for adults* quality standard, published by the English National Institute for Health and Clinical Excellence (NICE) (National Institute for Health and Care Excellence 2020a). NICE has the same kind of authority as the US Agency for Healthcare Research and Quality (AHRQ) (Agency for Healthcare Research and Quality 2020a)—clinicians would have to give a very good reason for not complying with guidelines from these organizations, for example, in a court of law or fitness-to-practise hearing.

Standards produced by less well known organizations can be equally authoritative provided the evidence cited is strong enough and the recommendations fit with nursing principles and best practice. The Registered Nurses' Association of Ontario's guideline on *End-of-life care during the last days and hours* (Registered Nurses' Association of Ontario 2020) has good research evidence for many of its recommendations with the remainder being supported by consensus from leading experts in palliative care nursing. This balance of evidence and consensus is required in many areas of nursing where there is little empirical research to guide recommendations. However, as can be seen in the ISO definition of a standard in the introduction to this chapter, consensus rather than evidence seems to be the basis for the development of HI standards.

6.2.4   Consensus or Evidence?

Most international HI standards organizations prepare new standards through a process of consensus by experts, technical committees and national standards bodies. The initial drafting process also includes consideration of evidence such as what standards already exist in the area under consideration and how effective these are. Many standards are developed using the experience and lessons from applications that are well advanced in some settings. For example, the ISO standard for patient health card medication data (ISO 21549-7) was agreed among a number of countries that had implemented and evaluated health cards. The standard is therefore based on consensus underpinned by experience of what works but not necessarily from formal evaluation studies or other empirical evidence. For other applications and supporting processes there is less experience, and consensus may be more difficult to obtain. For example, as Personal Health Records (PHRs) are not yet widespread in most countries, ISO's Health Informatics Technical Committee (TC215) published a Technical Report (TR) (ISO/TR 14292) to summarise current knowledge on this topic and establish some definitions and principles. An International Standard may be developed for PHRs when more is known about any interoperability, safety or other requirements that would benefit from standardization.

If there is insufficient support for a full standard (International Standard or Technical Report), ISO's experts may agree to publish a Technical Specification (TS)—unlike a TR this can be used as a standard but only has consensus within the Technical Committee, not across all the national standards organizations. For example, ISO/TS 21547 specifies principles for security requirements for archiving electronic health records—these have been adopted by a number of countries. The TS was reviewed and updated in 2017 and therefore remains current. However, it is possible that the TS will be promoted to a full standard based on feedback from practical use.

After a published standard has been in use for several years it will be reviewed. Evidence is collated on how it is being used, whether it is achieving its objectives and whether it needs to be revised or withdrawn. Previously, fitness for purpose and implement evaluation may not have been sufficiently accounted for in the consensus approach to development and review of HI standards. More attention is now being paid to questions such as cost and outcomes of standards implementation, implications for staff, patients, application providers and others.

A combination of consensus and evidence should be used for the development and review of HI standards but there is still a question about how they are approved and adopted i.e. who are the HI standards 'authorities' equivalent to AHRQ and NICE?

6.2.5 'Recognized Body'

One of the greatest challenges in the standards world is that there are multiple sources for standards. Many different 'recognized bodies' and other organizations publish rules, guidelines and 'agreed ways of doing things', even in the specialised field of health informatics. Governments, health departments, regulators and others adopt or develop their own HI standards for use in their countries and regions. Other organizations, such as the World Health Organization (WHO) and the International Council of Nurses (ICN), produce artefacts that are adopted as HI standards. For example, the WHO International Classification of Functioning Disability and Health (ICF) has been adopted in a number of countries as the standard to describe and measure health and disability (World Health Organization 2020).

A small but growing number of HI standards are developed by national and international professional bodies. Where no authoritative standard is available, the practice that is in common use may become known as the 'default standard' or 'de facto' i.e. it is widely accepted as best practice even though it has not been officially recognised or documented by a recognized body.

The most widely known HI SDOs are listed in Table 6.2 but perhaps more relevant to readers of this chapter are the national standards organizations in each country, which contribute on their behalf to international developments and decide which standards should be adopted and promoted in their country. ANSI, the American National Standards Institute, is a good example of a national 'recognized body'. Founded in 1918, ANSI is 'the voice of the US standards and conformity assessment system' (American National Standards Institute 2020).

Many national organizations of this kind will develop standards for their own country, but then share these internationally when other countries identify a similar need. The standards produced by different organizations may be entirely consistent, differing only in presentation such as when different versions are published for technical experts and for clinicians. Unfortunately, there are inconsistencies across SDOs. A trivial example is the spelling of the word 'organisation'. The European standards organisation (CEN) uses 's' whereas ISO uses 'z'. There are similar examples specific to health informatics: the HI technical committee of ISO is labelled TC 215—the equivalent committee in Europe is labelled TC 251. At best, multiple HI standards lead to confusion; at worst they result in wasted resources and increase the risk of poor communication and unsafe practice and, concomitantly, risk to patient safety. To address existing inconsistencies and to prevent development of new competing standards, international HI standards organizations have established the Joint Initiative Council for Global Health Informatics Standardization (see Table 6.2) (Joint Initiative Council 2020).

Members of SDOs comprise mainly HI experts and industry representatives. However, there is recognition that clinicians and health consumers should also be part of standards development activity.

ISO has recognised the importance of consumer participation, for example in their own learning materials: '*a "good" standard means one that creates a good product—a product that you will want to use because it is safe, fit for purpose, and easy to operate*' (ISO. 2 2020).

This sounds exactly what nurses, patients and public want from the systems and applications they use in health care. It is therefore essential that organizations representing, nurses, other clinicians and patients are an integral part of the 'recognised bodies' that develop, approve and adopt HI standards.

In the US, the Interoperability Standards Advisory (ISA) provides a framework for the Office of the National Coordinator for Health Information Technology (ONC) to identify, evaluate and raise awareness on standards to support interoperability. Stakeholders are encouraged by ONC to implement and test existing and emerging standards identified in the ISA. Standards that are relevant to nursing practice include those relating to:

Table 6.2 Standards Development Organizations

Acronym	Organization	Description
ISO	International Organization for Standard (also known as the International Standards Organization) www.iso.org	ISO is an independent, non-governmental organization made up of members from the national standards bodies of 164 countries. It has published more than 23,188 International Standards and has 784 technical committees and subcommittees developing standards. Technical Committee TC 215 is responsible for ISO Health Informatics standards. ISO standards can be purchased from the online ISO store or through the national standards body.
CEN	European Committee for Standardization www.cen.eu	CEN is an international non-profit association based in Brussels. It has 34 members (national standards bodies) who develop voluntary European Standards (ENs), which are then adopted as national standards in the member countries. It has formal arrangements for working with ISO to avoid duplication and promote harmonisation. Technical Committee TC 251 is responsible for CEN Health Informatics standards. CEN standards can be purchased from national member bodies.
JIC	JIC for Global Health Informatics Standardization www.jointinitiativecouncil.org	The Joint Initiative Council for Global Health Informatics Standardization was formed to address gaps, overlaps, and counterproductive HI standardization efforts. Members include ISO TC215, CEN TC 251, HL7, CDISC, GS1, DICOM, SNOMED International and IHE.
HL7	Health Level Seven International www.hl7.org	Health Level Seven International is a not-for-profit, ANSI-accredited SDO providing a framework and standards for the exchange, integration, sharing, and retrieval of electronic health information that supports clinical practice and the management, delivery and evaluation of health services. HL7 has over 1600 members from over 50 countries. Membership is open to individuals and organizations for a fee—with a special low cost for health care professionals. HL7 standards are free to members and can be purchased from the HL7 online store.
openEHR	Open EHR Foundation www.openehr.org	The openEHR Foundation is a not-for-profit company providing 'an open domain-driven platform for developing flexible e-health systems'.
CDISC	Clinical Data Interchange Standards Consortium www.cdisc.org	CDISC is a global, multidisciplinary, non-profit organization developing standards to support the acquisition, exchange, submission and archive of clinical research data and metadata. CDISC standards can be downloaded for free from the CDISC website.

(continued)

Table 6.2 (continued)

Acronym	Organization	Description
ANSI	American National Standards Institute www.ansi.org	ANSI facilitates the development of National Standards (ANS) by accrediting the procedures of SDOs—groups working cooperatively to develop voluntary national consensus standards. It is the US national standards body member of ISO and encourages the adoption of international standards as national standards where they meet the needs of the user community. Membership is open to individuals and organizations. ANSI standards can be purchased from the online store.

- Representing Clinical/Nursing Assessments—https://www.healthit.gov/isa/representing-clinicalnursing-assessments.
- Representing Patient Problems for Nursing—https://www.healthit.gov/isa/representing-patient-problems-nursing.
- Representing Nursing Interventions—https://www.healthit.gov/isa/representing-nursing-interventions.
- Representing Outcomes for Nursing—https://www.healthit.gov/isa/representing-outcomes-nursing.

A range of contexts, and their accompanying standards, are also included in the ISA standard for care plans that might be relevant to nursing (https://www.healthit.gov/isa/care-plan).

6.2.6 Definition of an HI Standard

From the preceding discussion, we can adapt the ISO definition of a standard, and extend it with notes about purpose and functional usage as follows:

An HI standard is a document, established from evidence and by consensus and approved by a recognized body, that provides rules, guidelines or characteristics for activities or their results, in the field of information for health, and Health Information and Communications Technology (ICT).

The purpose of an HI standard includes to:

- *Support safe, effective HI practice*
- *Promote interoperability between independent systems*
- *Enable compatibility and consistency for health information and data*
- *Reduce duplication of effort and redundancies.*

HI standards should meet the needs of users, be practical to implement and be sufficiently well specified to enable assessment of conformance. Standards should have a clear and defined development lifecycle or development process. Clinicians and consumers of health care should be involved in the development, implementation and review of HI standards.

6.3 HI Standards

6.3.1 The Scope of Standards

In this section, we consider the 'rules, guidelines and characteristics of activities or their results' that are needed to integrate information management and ICT into health care, particularly into nursing practice. For this purpose, the scope of health informatics can be considered as covering all aspects of the health system (ISO. ISO/TC 215 2020).

HI also covers the use of information and ICT by patients, clinicians, managers, researchers and others. Many standards will be common to all, for example, anyone providing health care could be expected to have some level of competence in using technology, in accessing, understanding and using information to make decisions and in the secure management of information. Other chapters in this book go into more detail about specific topics such as education and competence, clinical and administrative applications, documentation systems, security, etc. and the focus here will be on the standards that are available to support clinicians in their everyday practice, including their support for healthcare consumers.

6.3.2 HI Standards for Clinicians

As indicated the introduction to this chapter, HI standards are closely related to clinical practice standards. Take the example of record content standards, which specify what must or should be recorded about the care of a patient in a particular context. It is impossible to talk about standardizing the content of a document used for handing over care between shifts, for example, without first defining best practice for shift handover. In the same way it is impossible to have a standard for recording falls risk assessment without reference to the evidence based guideline for assessing a person's risk for falls.

Examples of HI standards for nurses and other clinical staff are given below, organised into a number of HI themes (NHS Networks 2020):

- Protection of individuals and organisations
- Data, information and knowledge
- Communications and information transfer
- Health and care records
- Clinical coding and terminology
- Clinical systems and applications
- The future direction of healthcare

Protection of Individuals and Organisations

Around the World, laws (including practice acts), regulations and codes require nurses to ensure confidentiality, privacy and security of information, irrespective of whether it is held and communicated on paper or electronically. The International Council of Nurses (ICN) requires National Nursing Associations to 'incorporate issues of confidentiality and privacy into a national code of ethics for nurses' (International Council of Nurses 2012).

Health departments and professional associations are the main sources of practice standards associated with information governance. Such guidance documents range from statements of law and principles through to example templates and other tools to support implementation of these standards in practice. For example, the Royal College of Nursing provides a summary of the scope of the conversation that should be had with the patient regarding their health record, including:

- the kinds of information that is being recorded and retained
- the purposes for which the information is being recorded and retained
- the protections that are in place to ensure non-disclosure of their information
- the kinds of information sharing that will usually occur
- the choices available to them about how their information may be used and disclosed
- their rights to access and where necessary to correct the information held about them on paper or electronic records (Royal College of Nursing 2009, p. 3).

When and how to share patient information with others is a major issue for clinicians, including sharing with law enforcement and other non-health agencies. Legal requirements for obtaining consent to disclose patient information and for disclosing without consent differ between and even within countries, leading to confusion and communication failures. Failure to share information can result in significant harm. Table 6.3 lists examples of standards for information sharing as well as for maintaining privacy and confidentiality.

Table 6.3 Examples of practice standards—Confidentiality, privacy and information security

Organization	Title and year	URL
Centre for Disease Control (CDC) and the US Department of Health and Human Services	HIPAA Privacy Rule and Public Health (2003)	http://www.cdc.gov/mmwr/preview/mmwrhtml/m2e411a1.htm
British Columbia College of Nursing Professionals	Privacy and Confidentiality	https://www.bccnp.ca/Standards/RN_NP/PracticeStandards/Pages/privacy.aspx
Sutter Health	Privacy of Information	https://www.sutterhealth.org/pamf/health/teens/sexual/privacy-of-information
Royal College of Nursing (UK)	Consent to access, share and create eHealth records (2008)	https://www.rcn.org.uk/-/media/royal-college-of-nursing/documents/policies-and-briefings/uk-wide/policies/2008/0908.pdf

The International Standard *ISO 22857 Provides guidelines on data protection to facilitate trans-border flows of personal health information*. This kind of standard brings together practice and technical aspects but at a general level so that countries can extend the international provisions with content relevant to their different legal and professional jurisdictions (Table 6.3).

Although guidance may be available for seeking consent for information sharing, there do not appear to be any standards for recording consent or refusal, a necessary precursor for designing appropriate structure and content for electronic recording. However, ISO TC215 has been collating international best practice and is developing a Technical Specification (not yet a standard) for *Principles and data structures for consent in the Collection, Use, or Disclosure of personal health information—Patient consent* (ISO/AWI TS 17975).

Data, Information and Knowledge

Nurses and other clinicians access and use data, information and knowledge in every aspect of their work, from checking the normal range of a laboratory result to performing an organizational audit or carrying out a nationwide research study. There is a vast array of standards to support these activities, most of them not specific to health informatics.

Health information literacy for clinicians is one area that has been extensively developed, recognising firstly that they must be lifelong learners and secondly that they cannot retain all the information and knowledge required to practise health care in the modern age. Specifications of information literacy competencies by national organizations (including health library science organizations) provide default standards for healthcare staff in the various roles they may fulfil, including researchers and managers. Health information literacy is related to digital literacy which is discussed is Chap. 3.

Standards for the data that are required to monitor healthcare quality and manage services are one of the most common HI standards available at local and national levels. These dataset specifications are another example of how HI standards cannot be divorced from practice standards if they are to be an accurate reflection of care and outcomes and, most importantly, if the data are to be extracted from care records—the 'record once, use many times' principle. The UK Tissue Viability Society (TVS) publication *Achieving Consensus in Pressure Ulcer Reporting* (Tissue Viability Society 2012) is a good example.

Tissue viability specialist nurses had recognised that data about pressure ulcer incidence *'has little value if it is not collected in a rigorous and practical way, and that comparisons between organizations are pointless as there is no standardised data set used across the country'* (Tissue Viability Society 2012, p. 6). The TVS proposed a UK standard using the definitions agreed by the US and EU Pressure Ulcer Advisory Panels i.e. a practice standard. Integrating the reporting of pressure ulcers with adverse event reporting and root cause analysis is a key part of the TVS standard, which specifies what should be reported, when and how. Being able to report and then to access, interpret and use data of this kind for quality improvement are core competencies for all qualified nurses.

Another core competency is supporting patients and health consumers to access, understand and use health related information. Nurses are frequently described as 'information brokers'. This means that nurses must themselves have the skills needed for example to critique the accuracy, quality and authority of health-related websites.

There a number of standards and guidelines for ensuring the quality, readability and usability of health information. Specifications of the characteristics of good health information are used by accrediting organizations to indicate that the information itself or the organization producing the information meets specified quality standards. In 1999, the Agency for Healthcare Quality and Research (AHQR) in the U.S. identified seven quality criteria to guide evaluation of health information on the internet (Agency for Healthcare Research and Quality 2020b) which have been the basis for standards set by other organizations since then. These are:

- *Credibility*: includes the source, currency, relevance and editorial review process
- *Content*: accuracy and completeness
- *Disclosure*: informs the user of the purpose of the site, as well as any profiling or collection of information associated with using the site
- *Links*: evaluated according to selection, architecture, content, and back linkages
- *Design*: accessibility, logical organization (navigability) and internal search capability
- *Interactivity*: feedback mechanisms and means for exchange of information among users
- *Caveats*: whether site function is to market products and services or is a primary information content provider (Agency for Healthcare Research and Quality 2020b).

Table 6.4 lists examples of standards guiding practice related to information literacy (for clinicians and consumers) and to information quality. Note that

Table 6.4 Examples of practice standards—Information literacy and information quality

Organization	Title and year	URL
DISCERN (UK)	Quality criteria for consumer health information	http://www.discern.org.uk/
National Library of Medicine. MedlinePLus	Evaluating Internet Health Information: A Tutorial from the National Library of Medicine	https://medlineplus.gov/webeval/webeval.html
New Zealand Nurses Organization	Health Literacy (2011)	https://www.nzno.org.nz/LinkClick.aspx?fileticket=vL8p8cbHY-o%3D&tabid=109&portalid=0&mid=4918
US Department of Health and Human Services	Health Literacy (includes guide to improving the usability of health information)	https://health.gov/our-work/health-literacy/health-literacy-online

information literacy of health consumers is one part of wider 'health literacy' as discussed in Chap. 2.

Communication and Information Transfer

One of the most basic goals of nursing is that patients and those who care for them experience effective communication. The importance of good communication and information transfer is demonstrated when things go wrong, as almost every review of sentinel events/critical incidents illustrates. Good quality information about care and treatment must be communicated to patients so they can make sense of what is happening and participate in decision-making and self care. Staff must communicate effectively with each other to ensure continuity, safety and quality of health care for all. These principles are enshrined in laws, regulations and codes and in national and international standards and benchmarks (Casey and Wallis 2011).

Alongside face-to-face and telephone conversations, nurses are now using a greater range of communication tools such as SMS texting, social media and video links. Standards for use of these technologies to communicate with patients and with other clinicians are considered below in the section on applications and clinical systems.

There has been a focus for many years on hand-off/handover communications involving the transfer of information between shifts, between agencies and between professionals when a patient is transferred from one setting to another, for example, from hospital to home or from the critical care unit to the operating room. In these circumstances, incomplete or delayed information can compromise safety, quality and the patient's experience of health care (British Medical Association 2004). A number of principles have emerged that inform guidance for nurses and others on safe handover. These include:

- A standardized approach to handover communication
- Use of a structured format for the information to be handed over [WHO recommends the SBAR (Situation, Background, Assessment, and Recommendation) technique] (World Health Organization 2007)
- Allocation of sufficient time for communicating and a location where staff won't be interrupted
- Limiting the information to that which is necessary to provide safe care.
- Use of technologies and methods that can improve handover effectiveness, such as electronic records
- Ensuring that processes, which use electronic technology are interactive and allow for questions or updates (British Medical Association 2004; World Health Organization 2007; Joint Commission Center for Transforming Healthcare 2020).

In 2012, the Cochrane Collaboration began a systematic review of the growing literature on handover, specifically focused on the *Effectiveness of different nursing handover styles for ensuring continuity of information in hospitalised patients* (Smeulers et al. 2014). Disappointingly the review found insufficient robust

Table 6.5 Examples of practice standards—Communication and information transfer

Organization	Title and year	URL
Royal Pharmaceutical Society	Keeping patients safe when they transfer between care providers—getting the medicines right (2012)	https://www.rpharms.com/Portals/0/RPS%20document%20library/Open%20access/Publications/Keeping%20patients%20safe%20transfer%20of%20care%20report.pdf
World Health Organization	Communication During Patient Hand-Overs (2007)	https://www.who.int/patientsafety/solutions/patientsafety/PS-Solution3.pdf

evidence to make any conclusions about effectiveness of different handover styles and studies with greater methodological rigour are needed.

There are more examples of practice standards for good communication and information transfer than could be listed in this chapter. A selection is provided in Table 6.5.

Health and Care Records

Nurses are required to maintain clear and accurate records and to ensure that all records are kept securely (Nursing and Midwifery Council 2020b).

They must be able to record elements of the nursing process in a manner that reflects nursing practice including:

- the patient's views, expectations and preferences
- results of assessments
- judgments about the patient's needs and problems
- decisions made
- care planned and provided
- expected and actual outcomes
- communications with patients and carers and other professionals/agencies (Wang et al. 2011).

Records should reflect core nursing values such as being patient focused, supporting patient decision making and self care. Their primary purpose is to support high quality care, effective decision-making and communication. Record keeping by nurses is supposed to be an integral part of practice, not 'an optional extra to be fitted in if circumstances allow' (NHS Digital 2020b, p. 3). However, many studies have identified that there is room for improvement in the quality of nursing documentation (Wang et al. 2011).

This will not happen unless records are valued and used rather than being viewed as a 'necessary evil' in case of litigation (Casey and Wallis 2011). Although nurses are blamed for poor record keeping, it may be that the records themselves need to become more useful and usable as communication tools, a challenge for health informatics. A number of the studies cited in the review by Wang et al. (2011) indicate that electronic applications and standardized documentation systems had the potential to improve documentation. However, a Cochrane Review of nursing record systems (Urquhart et al. 2018) concluded that there is a fundamental problem to be solved before both paper and electronic records can be improved: *'there needs to be more work with the nursing professions to understand exactly what needs to be recorded and how it will be used'* (Urquhart et al. 2018, p. 2).

The development of standards for the nursing content of patient records is a challenge that must be taken up by the profession, with support from informatics and terminology specialists.

Knowledge of standards for both record keeping practice and record content are essential for informatics specialists as these dictate the regulatory and professional requirements that must be incorporated into applications supporting record keeping and communication. Where national or regional standards exist, they provide a good basis for improving the quality of nurses' record keeping and for supporting the design of applications. It should be noted that uni-disciplinary standards are becoming less relevant as more provider organizations move to single patient records. Professional bodies and others who set practice standards need to collaborate more widely to ensure that there are clinical record standards common to all specialties and clinical disciplines. According to a UK joint professional working group, multi-professional standards: *'will provide the foundation upon which to base the collection, storage, communication, aggregation and reuse of structured clinical information across organizational boundaries throughout health and social care'* (Royal College of Physicians 2020).

Standards for recording, storing and retention/destruction of records are not further addressed in this chapter. Instead we will now focus on the major gap in standards related to record keeping, that is: record content—the 'what' of record keeping, as distinct from the 'how, when and by whom'.

Nurses know in principle what they should be recording but may struggle with exactly what makes a good care record, either on paper or in electronic systems. In some countries, there are national requirements for what nurses should record but these are often at too high a level to direct practice. For example, Håkonsen et al. reported in 2012 that the Danish national guideline at that time listed twelve areas about which nurses must document but it does not specify exactly what they have to document: *'It is an empty framework where nurses themselves must assess what is relevant to document … in the specific patient situations'* (Håkonsen et al. 2012).

As well as supporting best practice, detailed record content standards are needed to inform the design of electronic records and communications. As the UK Joint Working Group noted, technical standards alone do not ensure the communication of interpretable health data; professionally agreed 'standard representations' for content are also needed (Royal College of Physicians 2020). Record content standards specify information elements that <u>must</u> and <u>should</u> be present for a specified record or communication context e.g. a discharge summary. Interestingly, these record content specifications can be found in some clinical practice guidelines. For example, a clinical guideline for managing head injury includes 'minimum acceptable documented neurological observations' such as: Glasgow coma score; pupil size and reactivity; limb movements; respiratory rate; heart rate; blood pressure;

Table 6.6 Examples of information elements that could be part of a content set for a discharge summary

Heading	Description
Information/advice given to the patient	Detail of the verbal or written information or advice given to the patient and the patient's preferred form for such information. May be in the form a structured list of patient information leaflets or web links for a specific clinical context.
Advance decisions about treatment	List of and location of advance decisions i.e. written documents completed and signed when a person is legally competent, that explain a person's wishes in advance, allowing someone else to make treatment decisions on his or her behalf late in the disease process.

temperature and blood oxygen saturation (National Institute for Health and Care Excellence 2020b).

Another example is the RCN's guidance on weighing infants and children in hospital which includes a section on standards and quality criteria for recording their weight (Royal College of Nursing 2020). If the recording practice standard were to be included routinely in practice guidelines there would be less need for separate content standards.

When content standards are separately specified, each information element in a record content set usually has a heading and a description with examples to ensure consistent use—Table 6.6 illustrates the structural (heading) and indicative content which may be a list of terms, numerical values or free text.

In summary, content standards:

- Are based on best/evidence based clinical practice and Regulatory Standards.
- May (and should) be integrated with clinical practice guidelines
- Define structural headings and may describe indicative content to populate the headings; they may define restricted content sets, for example, a list of terms and codes.
- May take account of what data is required for analysis (for example, to monitor and improve quality) but this is secondary to the primary purpose of supporting clinical care, communication and decision making.
- Are specified or endorsed by clinical professional organizations.
- Are the basis for related technical standards or specifications that support content design for clinical applications (see examples in Table 6.7).

Replicating paper record formats in electronic systems is not good user interface design therefore most content standards do not specify a layout of the content on a page, template or screen as these depend on the context of use and on good user interface design/standards. Where necessary for safety or consistency, standards may specify a standard layout or include examples to demonstrate good practice. Wherever possible, content standards should also be independent of any specific technical or clinical implementation context. Again, a standard may reference good practice examples and implementation resources/audit tools. To date, there are

Table 6.7 Examples of professional record content standards

Organization	Title and year	URL
Patient Safety Organization Privacy Protection Center (US)	Common formats for event reporting—hospital version 1.2 (2020)	https://www.psoppc.org/psoppc_web/publicpages/commonFormatsV1.2
Professional Records Standards Body (UK)	PRSB Standards for the Structure and Content of Health and Care Records (2018)	https://www.rcplondon.ac.uk/file/10682/download
NHS Digital (England)	SCCI1580: Palliative Care Co-ordination: Core Content (2015)	https://digital.nhs.uk/data-and-information/information-standards/information-standards-and-data-collections-including-extractions/publications-and-notifications/standards-and-collections/scci1580-palliative-care-co-ordination-core-content
Academy of Medical Royal Colleges, Royal College of Nursing, British Pharmaceutical Society (UK)	Standards for the design of hospital in-patient prescription charts (2011)	https://www.aomrc.org.uk/reports-guidance/standards-design-hospital-prescription-charts-0411/

professional standards for the structure and content of records—examples are provided in Table 6.7.

A number of related standards are required as building blocks for content standards and their related technical specifications, including terminologies, data dictionaries, data sets and detailed clinical models as well as interoperability resources such as terminology subsets and message specifications.

Clinical Coding and Terminology

Nursing has a relatively long history of terminology development and use. The American Nurses' Association (ANA) was among the first to highlight the importance of standardised terminologies for supporting nursing practice, education, management and research (Rutherford 2008); ANA formally recognized early in their adoption a number of nursing-specific terminologies, multi-disciplinary terminologies and datasets. Nurses in other countries have adopted terminologies developed in the US or have established their own to meet the specific needs of their populations. The International Council of Nurses has contributed to these efforts through the International Classification for Nursing Practice (ICNP) in order to develop a 'common language for nursing practice' (Rutherford 2008).

A systematic review in 2006 suggested that use of standardised terminology improved documentation (Muller-Staub and Lavin 2006) but there has been no systematic review of the effect of standardized terminology on patient outcomes and experience of care.

However, the International Journal of Nursing Terminology and Classification and other publications do provide good examples of how standardised terminologies are used, and the ways in which they could benefit nursing and patients. There are also examples of the positive effects of national initiatives to standardise the terminology used in practice instruments such as assessment scales, such as the Canadian Health Outcomes for Better Information and Care (C-HOBIC) (C-HOBIC 2020).

In recent years, the main challenge for terminology developers and application designers has been to incorporate adequate representations of nursing care into computer and digital applications. It is this aspect of terminology which concerns us here but it should be noted that any professionally-endorsed terminology can add value to the ongoing work to develop and maintain the advanced terminological systems required in current and future healthcare applications. Many of the nursing terminologies previously recognised by ANA have informed the integration of nursing content into major international multi-disciplinary terminological resources such as the Unified Medical Language System (UMLS), Clinical LOINC and SNOMED Clinical Terms.

In 2018, ANA reaffirmed its support, through a position statement, of the use of recognized terminologies to support nursing practice and facilitate interoperability between systems (American Nurses Association 2020b).

In the position statement, ANA more closely aligned its support with data representation and exchange and interoperability standards included in the US Interoperability Standards Advisory (ISA) (described previously in this chapter). It recommended to each setting type the adoption of a standard terminology 'that best suits their needs and and select that terminology for their EHR, either individually or collectively as a group' (American Nurses Association 2020b). However, except in cases where settings are using the same terminology, ANA recommended that when exchanging data with another setting, SNOMED Clinical Terms (for problems, interventions and observation findings) and LOINC (for nursing assessments and outcomes) should be used. In some cases this might require mapping from the source nursing terminology to either SNOMED CT or LOINC. SNOMED CT and LOINC are designed to support the entry and retrieval of clinical concepts in electronic record systems and their communication in messages. They are built using logical definitions, rather than definitions drawn from practice knowledge and evidence, and are intended for use in computer applications.

Several international standards developed by ISO TC215 focus on terminological resources for health informatics applications. For example, ISO/TR 12300 *Principles of mapping between terminological resources* provides guidance on mapping between different terminologies and ISO/TS 21564 *Terminology resource map quality measures (MapQual)* provides guidance on how to assess the quality and utility of mappings.

Clinical Systems and Applications

Guidance and training for nurses in the use of specific applications has traditionally been the responsibility of the supplier or the employing organization. However, the spread and variety of applications means that it is now possible to draw together practice principles that build on evidence and lessons learnt from evaluations of system implementations. There are many gaps in this relatively new area of standards development but where they exist, nurses and provider organizations can use agreed standards or adapt them (with caution) for their local context. This will help prevent duplication and ensure consistency and safety. Approaches to system safety and risk management are perhaps the most important standards for both informatics specialists and clinical nurses when considering clinical systems and applications.

Risk management and patient safety processes are core aspects of all clinical practice. Any new intervention, device or health technology will have undergone rigorous testing up to and including formal clinical trials. It is surprising then that HI technologies have not generally been subjected to the same evidence based/risk management approaches. Serious harm can arise from the way systems are designed or the way they are used in practice, and any risk of harm must be identified and managed.

ISO has published a classification of safety risks from health software (TS 25238) citing concerns about the growing potential for harm to patients as the number, variety and sophistication of applications increases. Initial concerns focused on decision support systems with their obvious risks of errors, but have now spread to all types of health software.

The NHS in England requires all healthcare organizations to comply with its standards for the application of clinical risk management to deployment and use of health IT systems (NHS Digital 2020b). Note that in April 2020, it was agreed that due to the COVID-19 pandemic, organisations were able to defer full compliance with (NHS Digital 2020b), but there was an expectation that they would adhere to the fundamental principles of the standard and work towards compliance.

There is a related standard for those who design and manufacture systems, including processes for handover of responsibility for clinical safety when a system is deployed or upgraded (NHS Digital 2020c).

The principle behind these standards is that proactive safety risk management will help to reduce the likelihood of adverse events. According to the standard for manufacturers:

- The health care organisation must nominate a suitably qualified lead for clinical safety (a clinician).
- Manufacturers must have a documented clinical risk management process (approved by the clinical safety lead).
- Manufacturers must implement a clinical risk analysis process, including hazard identification with risk estimation, with ongoing monitoring and reporting (NHS Digital 2020c).

Table 6.8 Examples of professional standards and guidance for use of clinical systems and applications

Organization	Title and year	URL
College of Registered Nurses of Nova Scotia	Telenursing Practice Guidelines (2019)	https://cdn1.nscn.ca/sites/default/files/documents/resources/Telenursing.pdf
National Council of State Boards of Nursing (NCSBN) (US)	A Nurse's Guide to the Use of Social Media (2018)	https://www.ncsbn.org/3739.htm
Royal College of Nursing (UK)	Using text messaging services (2012)	https://www.rcn.org.uk/-/media/royal-college-of-nursing/documents/publications/2012/may/pub-004230.pdf
TEC Quality (UK)	TEC Quality Standards Framework (2020)	https://www.tsa-voice.org.uk/standards/

This last point is essential if nurses are to protect patients and fulfil the requirements of their ethical codes; if they have concerns about the safety of clinical systems and applications or the way these are being used they have a duty to act on their concerns (Nursing and Midwifery Council 2020b). This responsibility extends to those who work for the companies that design and supply systems.

Safety standards apply to all systems and applications and are supplemented by specific standards and guidance for integrating mobile technology (mHealth), telehealth applications, social media, SMS text messaging, decision support and other clinical systems into practice. Examples of these types of standards, written for practitioners rather than informatics specialists, are given in Table 6.8. Over the coming years we should see more examples where telehealth and other applications are integrated into clinical practice guidelines as just another kind of intervention or mode of care delivery.

The Future Direction of Healthcare

Given the widespread use of ICT in health care, in order to support contemporary nursing practice and the future direction of healthcare, a natural assumption is that all national and international standards of nursing proficiency or competence include the knowledge and skills necessary to manage information and to use ICT in daily clinical practice. Well known examples of such standards include the American Nurses' Association's *Nursing Informatics: Practice Scope and Standards of Practice* (American Nurses Association 2014), the TIGER (Technology Informatics Guiding Educational Reform) Initiative competencies (HIMSS 2020) and the Canadian Association of Schools of Nursing (CASN) Entry-to-Practice Nursing Informatics Competencies (Canadian Association of Schools of Nursing 2012).

However, in this rapidly evolving area of practice where new terms like big data and mHealth rapidly become broadly recognized in everyday use, it is doubtful that faculty everywhere will have the skills to successfully integrate new technologies and the latest standards into their programs. In common with other organisations, the National League for Nursing for example provides an Informatics Teaching resource (National League for Nursing 2020). However, not all such resources cite national or international HI standards. Raising awareness of HI standards is one way that informatics specialists could help to improve the education of non-specialists such as students and faculty.

6.3.3 Consumer Health Information Standards

The concept of consumer health informatics has been around for some time. It has been defined as "the branch of medical informatics that analyses consumers' needs for information; studies and implements methods of making information accessible to consumers; and models and integrates consumers' preferences into medical information systems." (Eysenbach 2000).

A number of consumer-specific standards have been developed ranging from the international definition, scope and context for personal health records (ISO/TR 14292) to guidance for nurses on how to support patients using technology (Royal College of Nursing 2012) and guidance for patients on keeping their online records safe and secure (BCS/NHS 2013). As more people engage with health information applications, they are becoming more involved with the development of standards and dissemination to fellow consumers. We are already seeing a move away health professionals and industry partners defining these standards and towards development in collaboration with patient organizations, as well as consumer-led developments. However, there is an ongoing a need for further national and international regulation and standardization.

6.3.4 HI Standards for Informatics Specialists

In 2017, the top three job responsibilities for nursing informatics specialists were:

1. Systems implementation—including preparing users, training and providing support
2. System optimisation
3. Systems development (HIMSS 2017).

It is interesting to note that responsibilities around regulatory initiatives also featured strongly.

Health informatics specialists support improvements in health outcomes, healthcare system performance and health knowledge discovery and management, through the application of technology (Australian Health Informatics Education Council 2011).

In order to fulfil their responsibilities, HI specialists need to be clinical professionals and meet the standards of education and competence set by their professional organizations or government agencies. They also need to be familiar with standards that support safe use of clinical systems and applications in order to educate and support their clinical colleagues.

These include standards for:

- Semantic content—covering the structure and content of HI terminologies through standards. For example, ISO 18104 *Categorial structures for representation of nursing diagnoses and nursing actions in terminological systems*
- Data structures—covering data types, record architecture, reference information models, detailed clinical models and other information components. For example, ISO 18308 *Requirements for an electronic health record architecture*
- Data interchange—covering the format of messages used to exchange health data electronically. For example, HL7 *Fast Healthcare Interoperability Resources (FHIR®)*
- Security—For example, ISO 27799 *Information security management in health using ISO/IEC 27002*
- Safety—For example, IEC 82304-1 *Health software—Part 1: General requirements for product safety.*

6.4 Standards Development and Review

Structured development processes always begin with statement of need or requirements, i.e. what is the problem, who is affected by it and what is needed to solve it. Standards development is no different and begins with industry or other stakeholders identifying a gap in the standards portfolio that needs to be filled at a national or international level. In this section, the steps in the ISO standards lifecycle are summarised, including the essential steps of dissemination and review. A useful summary of the process is provided on the ISO site: https://www.iso.org/developing-standards.html. Other standards developers follow similar pathways involving multiple stakeholders in a consensus process based on expert opinion.

Challenges for HI standards development are discussed before moving on to the final section which considers how nurses can participate in the many activities required to promote safe, effective HI practice, the development of safe usable systems and to support interoperability.

6.4.1 The ISO Standards Lifecycle

The ISO standards lifecycle can be divided into 7 main stages, given below:

1. Proposal
2. Preparatory stage

3. Committee stage
4. Enquiry stage
5. Approval and publication
6. Implementation
7. Review

Proposal

This stage begins with the identification of stakeholders who can contribute to clarifying the requirement and the scope and purpose of a standard. A global scan is also undertaken to identify what standards already exist and where there is recognised expertise in the area under discussion. At the end of this stage a decision is made whether to:

- **Adopt** or **adapt** an existing international or national standard OR
- **Develop** a new standard, drawing on what is already known to work.

The adopt/adapt/develop decision is an important ISO principle: standards should not duplicate each other and should build on what is already known. ISO may adopt a standard produced by CEN, HL7 or another standards body through a fast track process; joint working across standards development organizations is common. For example, work on ISO 18104 began in CEN as ENV 14032 *System of concepts to support nursing*. It was moved to ISO under an arrangement called the Vienna Agreement, a formal route for cooperation between ISO and CEN (ISO/CEN 2001). Ensuring harmonisation across all HI standards is the goal of the Joint Initiative Council for Global Health Informatics Standardization which now coordinates standards strategies and plans with the aim of making all future standards available through ISO (Joint Initiative Council 2020).

If a decision is made to adapt or develop a standard, an expert group then begins a preliminary draft document and puts a proposal forward to the governance structures of the standards organization. At ISO, a new work item proposal is submitted to the relevant Technical Committee (TC 215 for health informatics) where a vote by TC members determines whether this should become an ISO programme of work. The TC seeks a clear international justification that reflects the benefits of implementing the proposed standard and/or the loss or disadvantage if a standard is not made available. At least five 'P-members' must commit to provide active support for the work in order for it to be approved (P- or Participating members are national member bodies rather than organizations with ISO Observer status—'O-members').

Countries that put forward experts usually have a domestic standards infrastructure that mirrors ISO working groups. For example, ANSI's HI Technical Advisory Groups (TAGs) manage US contributions, including ballot responses (American National Standards Institute (ANSI) 2020). They also promote the use of US standards internationally, advocating US policy and technical positions so that international and regional standards are more likely to align with domestic requirements.

Similar structures exist in all member countries so that, for example, health informatics experts in the Japan can actively engage with relevant work items and send delegations to TC 215 working group meetings to represent consensus views from that country. In the US and UK, these experts are normally volunteers from industry, government, academia or healthcare provider organizations. The success of standards efforts is therefore dependent on the willingness of these bodies to commit the resources required for experts to participate.

Preparatory Stage

The nominated experts from five (or more) supporting countries form the core of a working group/task force to prepare a working draft of the standard with a volunteer leader/convenor to plan and coordinate the work. Development is open so the working group will often involve other experts. For ISO 18104, stakeholders that were involved from the beginning included the International Council of Nurses (ICN), the Nursing Specialist Group of the International Medical Informatics Association (IMIA-NI) and ACENDIO, the Association for Common European Nursing Diagnoses, Interventions and Outcomes. Once the experts are satisfied with the draft, it goes as a Committee Draft (CD) to the parent working group and then to the TC for the consensus-building phase. At this stage the document must be structured according to ISO rules with sections for Definitions, Normative References and Normative Content, and Conformance requirements. Explanatory information, discussion, implementation examples, additional references etc. are contained in Informative Annexes i.e. they are not included in the Normative (mandatory) provisions of the standard.

Committee Stage

The Committee Draft is registered by the ISO Central Secretariat and distributed for comment and voting within the TC by its P-members. Successive Committee Drafts may be considered until consensus is reached on the technical content. Once consensus has been attained, the text is finalized for submission as a Draft International Standard (DIS). The voting process is limited to ISO's national member bodies (i.e. P-members); other stakeholders, such as the three international nursing groups mentioned (i.e. O-members) above have no formal role in the commenting and voting rounds (although it is hoped that their feedback would be considered).

ISO and many other SDOs use a structured approach to feeding back comments. This requires the country making the comments to categorise them to indicate whether they are editorial (such as spelling and format) or technical (e.g. errors in definitions or unclear/unsupported Normative content) and to include a suggested amendment to the relevant part of the document. The expert group is required to respond to every comment made and must provide a rationale for each response (including suggested amendments that are not accepted). Any contentious issues are taken back to the wider TC so that other experts can provide input and reach consensus before the enquiry stage.

Enquiry Stage

The Draft International Standard (DIS) is circulated outside the TC to all ISO member bodies by the ISO Central Secretariat for voting and comment. It is approved for submission as a Final Draft International Standard (FDIS) if a two-thirds majority of the votes are in favour and not more than one-quarter of the total number of votes cast are negative. If the approval criteria are not met, the text is returned to the originating TC for further work following which a revised document will be sent out voting and comment again as a Draft International Standard.

Approval and Publication

In the last development stage, the FDIS is circulated to all ISO member bodies requesting a final Yes/No vote within a period of two months. If further technical comments are received during this period, they are not considered but are registered for consideration during a future revision. The document is approved as an International Standard again if a two-thirds majority of the members is in favour and not more than one-quarter of the total number of votes cast are negative. And once again, if these approval criteria are not met, the standard is referred back to the originating TC for reconsideration. Once the FDIS has been approved, only minor editorial changes are permitted before the final text is sent to the ISO Central Secretariat for translation into the three official languages of ISO (English, French and Russian) and publication.

Implementation

Regions and countries have different approaches to the adoption and implementation of International Standards. For example, while every country uses ISO 3166 *Country codes* exactly as it is published, the UK takes ISO/IEC 5218 *Codes for the representation of human sexes* as the basis for a more extensive entry in the NHS data dictionary that defines 'person sex' for use in all health data reporting data sets.

In some European countries, CEN standards automatically become national standards whereas in the UK a decision will be made whether or not to adopt a standard as a mandatory/contractual requirement for those supplying HI solutions to the NHS. The specification of relevant standards in national laws/regulations (e.g. medical devices regulations) and vendor contracts are the major implementation drivers. For other standards, a number of approaches may be required including: endorsement by organizations such as professional associations; awareness raising; education; supported change management; and incentives.

Some organizations support a coherent, user driven approach to implementing proven standards. One example is IHE which brings together users and developers of healthcare applications in a four-step process:

1. Clinical and technical experts define critical use cases for information sharing
2. Technical experts create detailed specifications for communication among systems to address these use cases, selecting and optimizing established standards
3. Industry implements these specifications called IHE Profiles in their systems
4. IHE tests vendors' systems (Integrating the Healthcare Enterprise 2020).

Review (Confirmation, Revision, Withdrawal)

International Standards are reviewed at least every five years and a decision made by a majority vote of the P-members on whether the standard should be confirmed, revised or withdrawn. Countries are asked to indicate whether they use the standard and if they have any issues with it that would require revision or withdrawal. Revised standards follow a similar pathway with an expert group steering the work through ballot/voting stages, seeking international consensus, approval and publication.

Some reviews will elicit more concrete technical requirements, based on live use of a standard in multiple systems or settings. For example, EN/ISO 13940 *System of concepts to support continuity of care* was referenced by the NHS Data Dictionary in England. This work validated the provisions of the standard and confirmed its value but also identified a number of issues with relationships between data elements as they were specified in the standard. These were taken forward to the next version.

6.4.2   Standards Development Challenges

The core principles for national and international standards development are that this activity is voluntary, open to all, consensus based and stakeholder driven. However, there are a number of challenges with achieving these goals, particularly at the international level. The 'open standards' process must balance the interests of those who will implement the standard with the interests and voluntary cooperation of experts who may own intellectual property rights (IPR) associated with it. The word 'open' does not imply free—there may be a need for some form of licensing to protect IPR and often there is a fee to obtain a copy of the standard which offsets the costs of the development and maintenance process.

Volunteer effort sometimes limits the level and type of expertise available and means that a standard can take longer to develop than is required in a rapidly developing field like health informatics. Organizations such as HL7 have made significant advances in the way it engages stakeholders and develops standards in an effort to be more responsive to the urgent demands of the industry. However, end users of health informatics standards such as health professionals and health care consumers are still not actively engaging to the extent that ISO would expect. In 2008, a multi-disciplinary task group led by nursing members of TC 215 made a number of recommendations for improving clinical stakeholder engagement in international HI standards development and review, and embodied these within a TR (ISO/TR 11487). The recommendations within the TR still hold, including:

- Establish communications with international health professional organizations, particularly those that have a health informatics profile/component. This could include regular information exchanges and invitation for liaisons to attend TC 215 meetings
- Explore mechanisms by which input of such international stakeholder organizations can be recognized within formal TC215 processes, including lessons from other ISO domains (engineering, chemical, etc.)
- Require that proposers of new work items identify relevant clinical and other stakeholder groups, their input to the proposal and how they may be involved in the work item
- Request national member bodies to report on the measures being taken to engage and facilitate the participation of clinical stakeholders at the domestic level as a basis for further action and to identify models of good practice that other members could adopt.

Participation of developing countries and non-English speaking members in HI standards development has also been limited, although this is changing slowly. In 2004, a survey of participation in ISO's standards development processes reported that Western Europe represented '*almost half the voting base in ISO's standards development work, despite representing approximately six percent of the world's population*' (92, p. 2), although there has been increased engagement of non-European countries such as Korea, Japan and China in TC215 meetings in recent years.

Given these challenges, it is no surprise that there are significant gaps in the HI standards portfolio. International policy making organizations such as the European Union (EU), the Joint Initiative Council and WHO have all identified the need for improved and coherent action to address the healthcare interoperability requirements of the future.

The high profile of HI standards and the huge amount of national and international standards-related activity presents a particular challenge for nursing as we will see in the final section below.

6.4.3 Participation in Standards Development and Review

There are a number of routes and opportunities for nurses to engage in the development of HI standards. Researchers, practising nurses, policy leaders and others can collaborate to influence what standards get developed, creating and collating evidence to support standard/guideline development and promoting their use, for example through education. Individual nurses can engage by contacting their professional organizations some of which may need to be made aware of the need for HI standards but may welcome interested volunteers.

Participating in the development and review of national and international HI standards themselves is not straightforward. There are very few clinicians involved in general and too few nurses in particular. Those who are involved come in several guises:

- The practising clinician who has an interest in a specific aspect of health information and participates on a part time basis. Many of these people do this work in their own time although some employers recognise the value of this activity and provide varying levels of support to attend events and undertake development/review work
- The health informatics specialist i.e. someone who has developed a career in health informatics. This person can have a significant role in helping technical people understand the clinical world and vice versa. However, unless he/she maintains clinical networks, this person may become distanced from the world of practice
- The practising clinician who becomes involved for a short time on a particular project. Facilitation of this input can result in new skills for this person who could be encouraged to participate further.

A major area of interest for nurses is terminology and content standards, but only a few are involved in this kind of international standards activity, mainly at HL7, ISO and CEN. It is a complex world for new members to enter at any level; and time and support are needed to develop sufficient understanding to participate effectively. Efforts to recruit and develop new participants have had little success for a number of reasons including:

- Lack of time and financial support to participate—some countries provide funding but this is often limited to national delegates
- Perceived lack of relevance to nursing practice and therefore to managers
- Perceived complexity of the domain: jargon, technical knowledge requirements, etc.
- Lack of awareness of the need or of how to get involved.

Entry-level material is available on the websites of the major SDOs with information on need, relevance and development processes. Each country that has a participating organization will include on its website information about how to participate and many provide online training opportunities. Willing volunteers are usually welcomed with open arms. However, there may be a fee to join some organizations, and before signing up it is important to consider whether support is available (such as for time to undertake reviews and attend meetings, payment of expenses, peer support, etc.).

6.5   Conclusion

Information and communications technology are central to the future of health and social care. To support the rapid advances needed for future solutions, health information standards are being developed and implemented across the globe. These will have a profound impact on nursing, patient care and outcomes. HI standards are needed to support integration of information management and ICT into clinical practice. They provide guidance for clinicians, patients and public on how to make best use of information and technology and are closely linked to standards for practice, including record keeping. Specialist HI standards are also required to ensure that applications are safe, usable and fit for purpose. They must support interoperability between systems so that information that is communicated electronically can be accurately interpreted and used for decision-making, continuity of care and other purposes.

Although the number of nurses working in health informatics roles is increasing, the number participating in standards development and review is, if anything, decreasing. Health informatics specialists need to work with their clinical colleagues, professional organizations and developers of clinical guidelines to produce, maintain and measure conformance to HI standards. They should also engage with national and international HI standards organizations, helping to fill gaps in the standards portfolio and promoting the use of standards in their own organizations. New approaches to participation that do not involve expensive and time consuming travel must be found so that nursing can continue to have an active, leadership role in this important activity.

6.6   Clinical Pearls

- Nurses are required to maintain clear and accurate records and to ensure that all records are kept securely
- HI standards provide a foundation so that nurses can have more confidence in the systems they use in practice.

6.7   Review Questions

6.7.1   Questions

1. Describe the role that HI standards play in nursing practice.
2. Identify the aspects of nursing practice that are covered by HI Standards.
3. Describe the lifecycle of an HI standard.

6.7.2 Answers

1. HI standards support the integration of information management and ICT into clinical practice. They provide guidance for clinicians, patients and public on how to make best use of information and technology and are closely linked to standards for practice, including record keeping. Specialist HI standards are also required to ensure that applications are safe, usable and fit for purpose. They must support interoperability between systems so that information that is communicated electronically can be accurately interpreted and used for decision-making, continuity of care and other purposes.
2. It might be useful for respondents to present the answer to this review question as a set of use cases drawn from their own practice. They may also find it useful to refer also to generic use cases, for example, those developed for eHealth by ETSI (https://www.etsi.org/deliver/etsi_tr/103400_103499/103477/01.01.0 1_60/tr_103477v010101p.pdf).
3. A useful approach to framing the HI standards lifecycle is by describing the 7 stages of the approach taken in ISO:
Proposal
Preparatory stage
Committee stage
Enquiry stage
Approval and publication
Implementation
Review

Acknowledgments As indicated in the front matter of this 5th edition, this chapter represents a revision of a chapter, authored by Anne Casey, RN, MSc, FRCN, and revised with the support of Prof Nick Hardiker, which appeared in a previous edition of this book. The authors gratefully acknowledge Ms Casey's original chapter and Prof Hardiker's contributions and review of this chapter for this 5th edition.

Glossary

AHQR Agency for Healthcare Research and Quality
ANA American Nurses Association
ANSI American National Standards Institute
CEN European Standards Organisation
Consumer Informatics The use of modern computers and telecommunications to support consumers in obtaining information, analyzing unique health care needs and helping them make decisions about their own health
Clinical guidelines Systematically developed statements to assist practitioners and patient decisions about appropriate health care for specific circumstance
HI standard A document, established from evidence and by consensus and approved by a recognized body, that provides rules, guidelines or characteristics

for activities or their results, in the field of information for health, and Health Information and Communications Technology (ICT)

HIPAA Health Insurance Portability and Accountability Act of 1996

HL7 Health Level Seven

HL7 RIM Reference Information Model Represent an approach to clinical information exchange based on a model driven methodology that produces messages and electronic documents expressed in XML syntax

ICF International Classification of Functioning Disability and Health

ICN The International Council of Nurses

ICNP International Classification of Nursing Practice

ISA Interoperability Standards Advisory (ISA) is a process which represents the model by which the Office of the National Coordinator for Health Information Technology (ONC) will coordinate the identification, assessment, and determination of "recognized" interoperability standards and implementation specifications for industry use to fulfill specific clinical health IT interoperability needs.

ISO International Organization of Standardization

ISO defines a standard as A document established by consensus and approved by a recognized body that provides for common and repeated use, rules, guidelines or characteristics for activities or their results, aimed at the achievement of the optimum degree of order in a given context

JIC Joint Initiative Council

LOINC Logical Observation Identifiers Names and Codes

NHS National Health Service

RIM Reference Information Model

SMS Short Message Service

SNOMED Clinical Terms Systematized Nomenclature of Medicine a systematic computer processable collection of medical terms in human and veterinary medicine

TVS Tissue Viability Society

UMLS Unified Medical Language System

Usability The extent to which a product can be used by specified users to achieve specified goals with effectiveness, efficiency and satisfaction in a specified context of use

WHO World Health Organisation

XML Extensible Mark Up Language is a computer markup language that defines a set of rules for encoding documents in a format that is both human-readable and machine-readable

References

Agency for Healthcare Research and Quality. Agency for healthcare research and quality. [Online] [Cited: 18 May 2020a]. https://www.ahrq.gov/.

Agency for Healthcare Research and Quality. Assessing the quality of internet health information. [Online] [Cited: 19 May 2020b]. https://archive.ahrq.gov/research/data/infoqual.html.

American National Standards Institute. American national standards institute. [Online] [Cited: 19 May 2020]. https://www.ansi.org/.

American National Standards Institute (ANSI). Introduction to ANSI. [Online] [Cited: 19 May 2020]. www.ansi.org/about_ansi/introduction/introduction.aspx.

American Nurses Association. Nursing informatics: Scope and standards of practice. 2nd ed. Silver Spring, MD: American Nurses Association, Inc; 2014.

American Nurses Association. View the code of ethics for nurses. [Online] [Cited: 18 May 2020a]. https://www.nursingworld.org/practice-policy/nursing-excellence/ethics/code-of-ethics-for-nurses/.

American Nurses Association. Inclusion of recognized terminologies supporting nursing practice within electronic health records and other health information technology solutions. [Online] [Cited: 19 May 2020b]. https://www.nursingworld.org/practice-policy/nursing-excellence/official-position-statements/id/Inclusion-of-Recognized-Terminologies-Supporting-Nursing-Practice-within-Electronic-Health-Records/.

Australian Health Informatics Education Council. Health informatics: scope, careers and competencies. Australia: Australian Health Informatics Education Council; 2011. https://www.ahiec.org.au/docs/AHIEC_HI_Scope_Careers_and_Competencies_V1-9.pdf

BCS/NHS. Keeping your online health and social care records safe and secure. London, England: Department of Health; 2013. https://www.nhs.uk/nhsengland/thenhs/records/healthrecords/documents/patientguidancebooklet.pdf

British Medical Association. Safe handover: safe patients. guidance on clinical handover for clinicians and managers. London, England: British Medical Association; 2004. https://www.rcpch.ac.uk/sites/default/files/2018-02/bma_handover_college_tutors.pdf

BSI. What is a standard. [Online] [Cited: 18 May 2020]. https://www.bsigroup.com/en-GB/standards/Information-about-standards/what-is-a-standard/.

Canadian Association of Schools of Nursing. Nursing informatics entry-to-practice competencies for registered nurses. Ottawa, Canada: Canadian Association of Schools of Nursing; 2012. https://www.casn.ca/wp-content/uploads/2014/12/Infoway-ETP-comp-FINAL-APPROVED-fixed-SB-copyright-year-added.pdf

Casey A, Wallis A. Effective communication: principle of nursing practice E. Nurs. Stand. 2011;25(32):35–7.

C-HOBIC. Inclusion of nursing-related patient outcomes in electronic health records. [Online] [Cited: 19 May 2020]. https://www.cihi.ca/en/c-hobic-infosheet_en.pdf.

ETSI. Understanding ICT standardization: principles and practice. [Online] [Cited: 18 May 2020]. https://www.etsi.org/images/files/Education/Understanding_ICT_Standardization_LoResPrint_20190125.pdf.

European Commission. EU eHealth interoperability conformity assessment scheme. [Online] [Cited: 18 May 2020]. https://cordis.europa.eu/project/id/727028.

Eysenbach G. Consumer health informatics. BMJ. 2000;320:1713.

Feild MJ, Lohr KN, editors. Clinical practice guidelines: directions for a new program. Washington, DC: National Academies Press; 1990.

Håkonsen S, Madsen I, Bjerrum M, Pedersen U. Danish national framework for collecting information about patients' nutritional status. Nursing minimum dataset (N-MDS). Online J. Nurs. Inform. 2012;16(3) http://ojni.org/issues/?p=2044

HIMSS. TIGER initiative for technology and health informatics education. [Online] [Cited: 19 May 2020]. https://www.himss.org/tiger-initiative-technology-and-health-informatics-educatio.

HIMSS. HIMSS 2017 nursing informatics workforce survey. Chicago, IL: HIMSS; 2017. https://www.himss.org/sites/hde/files/d7/2017-nursing-informatics-workforce-full-report.pdf

Integrating the Healthcare Enterprise. IHE process. [Online] [Cited: 19 May 2020]. https://www.ihe.net/about_ihe/ihe_process/.

International Council of Nurses. The ICN code of ethics for nurses. Geneva, Switzerland: International Council of Nurses; 2012. https://www.icn.ch/sites/default/files/inline-files/2012_ICN_Codeofethicsfornurses_%20eng.pdf

International Electrotechnical Commission. International standards (IS). [Online] [Cited: 18 May 2020]. https://www.iec.ch/standardsdev/publications/is.htm.

ISO. Certification & conformity. [Online] [Cited: 20 May 2020a]. https://www.iso.org/conformity-assessment.html.

ISO. Benefits of standards. [Online] [Cited: 18 May 2020b]. https://www.iso.org/benefits-of-standards.html.

ISO. 1. Standards in our world. [Online] [Cited: 20 May 2020]. https://www.iso.org/sites/ConsumersStandards/1_standards.html.

ISO. 2. How standards benefit consumers. [Online] [Cited: 19 May 2020]. https://www.iso.org/sites/ConsumersStandards/2_benefits.html.

ISO. 5. Glossary of terms and abbreviations. [Online] [Cited: 20 May 2020]. https://www.iso.org/sites/ConsumersStandards/5_glossary.html.

ISO. ISO/TC 215. [Online] [Cited: 19 May 2020]. https://www.iso.org/committee/54960.html.

ISO/CEN. Agreement on technical co-operation between ISO and CEN. ISO/CEN, 2001. https://isotc.iso.org/livelink/livelink/fetch/2000/2122/3146825/4229629/4230450/4230458/01__Agreement_on_Technical_Cooperation_between_ISO_and_CEN_(Vienna_Agreement).pdf?nodeid=4230688&vernum=-2.

Joint Commission Center for Transforming Healthcare. Hand-off Communications. [Online] [Cited: 19 May 2020]. https://www.centerfortransforminghealthcare.org/improvement-topics/hand-off-communications/.

Joint Initiative Council. Joint initiative council for global health informatics standardization. [Online] [Cited: 19 May 2020]. http://www.jointinitiativecouncil.org/.

Muller-Staub M, Lavin M. Nursing diagnoses, interventions and outcomes—application and impact on nursing practice: systematic review. J. Adv. Nurs. 2006;56(5):514–31.

National Institute for Health and Care Excellence. End of life care for adults. [Online] [Cited: 18 May 2020a]. https://www.nice.org.uk/guidance/qs13.

National Institute for Health and Care Excellence. Head injury: assessment and early management. [Online] [Cited: 19 May 2020b]. https://www.nice.org.uk/guidance/cg176.

National League for Nursing. Informatics teaching. [Online] [Cited: 19 May 2020]. http://www.nln.org/professional-development-programs/teaching-resources/toolkits/informatics-teaching.

NCSBN. About NCSBN. [Online] [Cited: 18 May 2020]. https://www.ncsbn.org/about.htm.

NHS Digital. SCCI1580: palliative care co-ordination: core content. [Online] [Cited: 18 May 2020a]. https://digital.nhs.uk/data-and-information/information-standards/information-standards-and-data-collections-including-extractions/publications-and-notifications/standards-and-collections/scci1580-palliative-care-co-ordination-core-content.

NHS Digital. DCB0160: clinical risk management: its application in the deployment and use of health IT systems. [Online] [Cited: 19 May 2020b]. https://digital.nhs.uk/data-and-information/information-standards/information-standards-and-data-collections-including-extractions/publications-and-notifications/standards-and-collections/dcb0160-clinical-risk-management-its-application-in-the-deployment-and-use-of-health-it-systems.

NHS Digital. DCB0129: clinical risk management: its application in the manufacture of health IT systems. [Online] [Cited: 19 May 2020c]. https://digital.nhs.uk/data-and-information/information-standards/information-standards-and-data-collections-including-extractions/publications-and-notifications/standards-and-collections/dcb0129-clinical-risk-management-its-application-in-the-manufacture-of-health-it-systems.

NHS Networks. eICE resources available. [Online] [Cited: 19 May 2020]. https://www.networks.nhs.uk/nhs-networks/national-nursing-informatics-strategic-taskforce/news/eice-resources-available.

Nursing & Midwifery Council. Nursing midwifery council. [Online] [Cited: 18 May 2020a]. https://www.nmc.org.uk/.

Nursing & Midwifery Council. The code. [Online] [Cited: 19 May 2020b]. https://www.nmc.org.uk/standards/code/.

Registered Nurses' Association of Ontario. End-of-life care during last days and hours. [Online] [Cited: 19 May 2020]. https://rnao.ca/bpg/guidelines/endoflife-care-during-last-days-and-hours.

Royal College of Nursing. e-Health and nursing practice: consent to access, share, and create e-Health records. London, England: Royal College of Nursing; 2009. https://www.rcn.org.uk/-/media/royal-college-of-nursing/documents/policies-and-briefings/uk-wide/policies/2008/0908.pdf

Royal College of Nursing. Personal health records and information management. London, England: Royal College of Nursing; 2012. https://www.rcn.org.uk/-/media/royal-college-of-nursing/documents/policies-and-briefings/uk-wide/policies/2012/1612.pdf

Royal College of Nursing. Standards for the weighing of infants, children and young people in the acute health care setting. [Online] [Cited: 19 May 2020]. https://www.rcn.org.uk/professional-development/publications/pub-006135.

Royal College of Physicians. Developing standards for health and social care records. [Online] [Cited: 19 May 2020]. https://www.rcplondon.ac.uk/projects/outputs/developing-standards-health-and-social-care-records.

Rutherford M. Standardized nursing language: what does it mean for nursing practice? Online J. Issues Nurs. 2008;13(1) http://ojin.nursingworld.org/MainMenuCategories/ThePracticeofProfessionalNursing/Health-IT/StandardizedNursingLanguage.html

Smeulers M, Lucas C, Vermeulen H. Effectiveness of different nursing handover styles for ensuring continuity of information in hospitalised patients. Cochrane Database Syst. Rev. 2014;6:CD009979. https://doi.org/10.1002/14651858.CD009979.pub2.

Tissue Viability Society. Achieving consensus in pressure ulcer reporting. Benefits of standards. Roos, Englane: Tissue Viability Society; 2012. https://tvs.org.uk/wp-content/uploads/2013/05/TVSConsensusPUReporting.pdf

United Nations. Interoperability. [Online] [Cited: 20 May 2020]. http://tfig.unece.org/contents/interoperability.htm.

Urquhart C, Currell R, Grant MJ, Hardiker NR. Nursing record systems: effects on nursing practice and healthcare outcomes. Cochrane Database Syst. Rev. 2018, Issue 5. Art. No.: CD002099. DOI: https://doi.org/10.1002/14651858.CD002099.pub3.

Wang N, Hailey D, Yu P. Quality of nursing documentation and approaches to its evaluation: a mixed-method systematic review. J. Adv. Nurs. 2011;67(9):1858–75.

World Health Organization. Communication during patient hand-overs. Geneva, Switzerland: World Health Organization; 2007. https://www.who.int/patientsafety/solutions/patientsafety/PS-Solution3.pdf

World Health Organization. International classification of functioning, disability and health (ICF). [Online] [Cited: 18 May 2020]. https://www.who.int/classifications/icf/en/.

Chapter 7
Nursing Documentation in Digital Solutions

Loretto Grogan, Angela Reed, and Orna Fennelly

Abstract Information plays a vital role in the nursing process. The information aggregated by registered nurses in a wide range of records across the breadth of practice underpins and can bring about services that will support global populations into the next decade and beyond.

Nurse leaders need to be able to translate, synthesise, interpret and manage that information into measurable outcomes. The impact of knowledgeable and enthusiastic Executive Nurses who provide and develop informatics leadership is essential to build both the art and science of nursing into the next decade.

In terms of how nursing data is captured and structured to effectively do that, no one type of clinical data will accommodate the spectrum of nursing and midwifery practice for every scenario but in determining the most appropriate type of data or combination of data types, the advantages and disadvantages of each should be considered, as well as the workflows and downstream effects of capturing data.

Much work has been completed in the last 20 years to advance thinking around the use of nursing Standardised Terminologies. The findings from the identified studies cited demonstrate benefits of using Standardised Terminologies although it is difficult to determine whether STs impact directly on patient outcomes or the time efficiency of end-users. The careful implementation, education and support of nurses and midwives to utilise STs as well as a well-designed, user-friendly EHCR system contributes to its use and the benefits derived.

Electronic Supplementary Material The online version of this chapter (https://doi.org/10.1007/978-3-030-58740-6_7) contains supplementary material, which is available to authorized users.

L. Grogan (✉)
Health Service Executive, Dublin 8, Ireland

Five Country Nursing and Midwifery Digital Leadership Group, Belfast, Ireland
e-mail: loretto.grogan1@hse.ie

A. Reed
Northern Ireland Practice and Education Council for Nursing and Midwifery, Belfast, UK

Five Country Nursing and Midwifery Digital Leadership Group, Belfast, UK

O. Fennelly
ICHEC, Irish Centre for High-End Computing, Dublin, Ireland

© Springer Nature Switzerland AG 2021
P. Hussey, M. A. Kennedy (eds.), *Introduction to Nursing Informatics*, Health Informatics, https://doi.org/10.1007/978-3-030-58740-6_7

Keywords Nursing documentation · Nursing data · Nursing practice · Nursing leadership · Data collection · Clinical information capture · Data types · Structured data · Unstructured data · Coded data · Semi-structured data · Standardised terminologies

Overview
This chapter is presented in two sections.

The first section sets a professional context for nursing documentation, the impact of nursing data and the nursing imperative for efficient and appropriate processes for current and future data collection including the impact of dynamic knowledgeable and nursing leadership to leverage appropriate data collection.

The second section discusses capturing nursing data. It focuses on clinical data types namely unstructured data, structured data, coded data and semi-structured data, their application and the advantages and disadvantages of each type. Standardised nursing terminologies and their impact on practice are also discussed.

Learning Objectives for the Chapter

Section 1—To gain an understanding of:

1. The imperative for and impact of effective professional record keeping practice in nursing.
2. The importance of nursing data to underpin and bring about services that will support global populations into the next decade and beyond.
3. The impact of Executive Nurses who provide and develop leadership in the informatics area of practice in their organisations for digital practice and the knowledge age.

Section 2—To gain an understanding of:

1. Clinical data types namely unstructured data, structured data, coded data and semi-structured data.
2. The application of clinical data types and the advantages and disadvantages of each type.
3. Standardised Nursing Terminologies and their impact on practice.

7.1 Recording and Evidencing Nursing Practice

In their study of innovation across 152 differing health systems globally, Braithwaite et al. (Braithwaite et al. 2018), identified five principles for optimising future health and social care underpinned by four success factors. Across those elements, digital practice and the meaningful use of data were significant levers for change including: development of sustainable systems; digital innovation; and recognition of the need to situate models of care as near to the person's own home or community; underpinned by: evaluative activity using appropriate measures (Braithwaite et al. 2016); transformation of data into information and then intelligence to continually create an evidence base (Braithwaite et al. 2018); authentic collaboration between multiple stakeholders; and person-centredness (Braithwaite et al. 2017). Nursing is well placed to leverage the future service change required that will support global populations into the next decade and beyond. The levers and success factors for change identified by Braithwaite et al. (Braithwaite et al. 2018) should be the stimulus for nursing leadership to renew and redouble focus on meaningful use of data, efficient digital practice and interoperability across systems and places of care, recognising appropriate evaluative activity, across global health economies.

7.2 The Nursing Imperative

In this global context and that of nursing practice in the twenty-first century, where services are under increasing pressure (Kelly et al. 2016), populations are rising with predicted large numbers of over 65 year olds many living with complex co-morbidities and associated conditions of ageing (Amalberti et al. 2016), the profession is evolving, to take on a broader scope of practice, improving the quality and person centric nature of models of care (Kennedy and Moen 2017). The largest percentage of the professional healthcare workforce nursing occupies 50% of the total headcount for many countries (World Health Organisation 2016a). Simultaneously, there is a wealth of evidence demonstrating the impact of registered nurses on healthcare outcomes for populations across a range of roles (Dick et al. 2017; Griffiths et al. 2016). Working across programmes of care and service delivery environments, the need for high quality information from this significant section of the health care workforce is an imperative to drive future change harnessed through the professions' ability to collect data at the point of care.

The imperative for registered nurses to make accurate records of their interactions with staff and people, regardless of where they work, falls under a number of obligations within statutory, regulatory and contractual frameworks, and not least the requirement to evidence the professional impact and quality of their daily work. More usually, advice and guidance across organisations emanate from local policy and standards set by national or regional bodies, which have led to a range of views often differing in emphasis, rather than a clear national strategy to nursing and midwifery data.

Like many nursing and midwifery regulatory bodies globally, those in the United Kingdom (UK) and Ireland make explicit reference to the necessity for high quality professional records in their codes of practice (Nursing and Midwifery Council 2018; Nursing and Midwifery Board Ireland 2014) drawing attention to the need for timely, accurate record keeping that demonstrates decision making and service provision to populations. Whilst it is well discussed that accurate and complete records providing a detailed account of a person's journey through health and social care services can protect both patient and registrant (Prideaux 2011), a common cause of legal claim arises from a breakdown in communication between health professionals particularly related to incomplete or inadequate records (Wood 2010). Evidence exists of variance of the quality of nursing information reflected in records (Saranto et al. 2014); incomplete records demonstrating a lack of information on the effect of nursing measures (Jeffries et al. 2012) and considerable deficiencies in quality of information (Gomes et al. 2019). Additionally, studies have demonstrated that when staffing issues impact on a care environment, documentation of nursing care is one of the safety critical activities which is often missed (Thomas-Hawkins et al. 2020; Ball et al. 2018). 'Good' records put the patient at the centre of care, demonstrate clinical decision-making and goals of care, allow audit of practice, support quality improvement and evidence co-production, safety and efficacy over time.

7.3 The Information Future of Nursing Practice

Increasingly nurses are being invited to expand their scope of practice in service models, to purportedly enable a holistic response to evolving needs, rurality of populations and Social Determinants of Health (SDH) (Mason et al. 2015; Nelson-Brantley et al. 2018). Whilst the nursing profession is often well placed to implement new models of service delivery, a change in ways of working is required to engage with the increasing complexity of care for populations and impact of SDH (Mason et al. 2015). Enhanced ways of working for nurses to match future service models linked to demographic trends include: promoting population health literacy (McMurray et al. 2018); greater use of technologies and Electronic Health Care Records (EHCRs) with advanced coordination of multi-professions across care settings (Zaworsky and Bower 2016; Erikson et al. 2017); and collaborative partnership with service users and their families to negotiate individualised person-centred outcomes. Whilst such service models obviously require investment to maximise the shift in demand from populations through development of the profession to support them (Leahy-Warren et al. 2017), early findings from global nursing exemplars have demonstrated positive outcomes such as reduction of hospital admissions, improved experience of care and cost reductions (McMurray et al. 2018; Maeung et al. 2013). In these practice prototypes, meaningful real-time data has been identified as a crucial enabler for efficient services to make best use of available nursing time (McMurray et al. 2018).

Evidence on the impact of documenting in EHCRs in terms of contribution to sustainability and efficacy of global health services varies, ranging from positively preventing hospitalisations (Burnel 2018) to reported 'weak empirical evidence in relation to increasing efficiency and improving medical care' (Bolous-Rødje 2019, p. 3). Furthermore, the necessary integration across organisational boundaries to communicate and share data seamlessly has not been achieved (Fitzpatrick and Ellingsen 2013). These issues are of particular importance when considering the intention to focus efforts on providing future nursing practice models, co-producing plans of care and supporting individuals in their own homes (Braithwaite et al. 2018), as movement of data across primary, secondary and community locations will be required to facilitate nursing and other members of professional teams. Accessible, reliable integrated systems are essential to the success of maximising digital nursing record keeping practice across organisations. Inefficient design and technical issues have been evidenced to impact on care delivery (Staggers et al. 2018), where nurses struggle to access systems to input relevant data across organisational boundaries and buildings. Poorly designed technology that fails to capture the essence of nursing practice and decision making, along with systems wrought with technical issues have been demonstrated to frustrate nurses, who will resort to printing documents to manually include information (Staggers et al. 2011). All too often, design flaws arise from the simple translation of paper documents into digital forms, rather than investment in system designs that map nursing workflows, capture nursing decision making through appropriate terminologies and enable point of care nursing data entry.

In addition, undoubtedly, as person-centred approaches evolve along with a focus on co-production, the use of citizen portals linking to EHCRS will increase, as populations become more digitally enabled across health economies. The sparse evaluative evidence on the efficacy of citizen portals demonstrates the value of a mixed approach model of both professional and digital contact (Zanaboni et al. 2018) and as the profession with the highest level of constancy with populations (All Party Parliamentary Group on Global Health (APPG) 2016), nursing has undoubtedly the greatest opportunity to influence the uptake and therefore utility of this digital partnership, therefore unlocking the potential of new approaches to health outcomes for populations, including those underpinned by self-care.

7.4 Evidencing Impact and Supporting Nursing Practice

The importance of evidencing the impact of registered nurses on population health outcomes, given the opportunity from the breadth and scale of the workforce, should be a driver for a strengthened professional focus in a world that is increasingly digitally driven and data saturated. Nurses, as the largest regulated profession with continuous contact with the public to impact on population health (All Party Parliamentary Group on Global Health (APPG) 2016) generate the greatest volume of healthcare data (Englebright and Caspers 2016). It is imperative, therefore, that this data is meaningfully structured and captured (Hussey et al. 2015), for the purposes of analysis and sharing (Ricciardi and Boccia 2017), evidencing and assuring the contribution of nursing.

The development of the emerging discipline of nurse informaticians has been growing on a global scale over the last 30 years (Liu et al. 2015), if somewhat driven by interested enthusiasts rather than a determined workforce decision to value and grow such roles. This piecemeal development of the discipline appears counterintuitive, the digital knowledge and skills of the nursing workforce, including those required to meaningfully use and evaluate information, evidently requiring a focus for investment in the current global context of services to create a workforce that is appropriately equipped to expertly handle their own professional data.

Big data capabilities from EHCRs can now provide healthcare organisations with information that enables understanding and evaluation of care decisions, processes and outcomes. Founds (Founds 2018) welcoming the big data era, asserted that the individualised and public facing ethos of nursing practice positioned the profession well to adopt and promote this future enabler for sustainable service models. This in turn can help quantify the nursing contribution, underpinning evidence-informed practice with real-time data (Reid Ponte et al. 2016). Sadly, EHCRs can sometimes include scant data describing nursing interventions and outcomes, failing to adequately describe critical decision making. Learning over the years of implementation would suggest there is a danger in trying to compare nurse and physician use of an EHCR to apply the same terminologies (Rogers et al. 2013). Evidence demonstrates that the 'checklist' medical system of recording within current EHCRs does not always capture relevant nursing information, leading to a lack of nursing narrative, particularly around psychosocial needs, often devoid of critical data on the performance of the largest professional workforce (Green and Thomas 2008).

Current data capture processes globally have varying degrees of efficacy to realise the future potential of the profession. Much of the vast volumes of nursing data captured, even when in digital format, are not structured or coded in a standardised way to allow linkages to be made across data elements (Khokar et al. 2017). There is also recognition that nurses spend considerable amounts of time recording high volumes of data of questionable utility (Lodhi et al. 2016; Leary et al. 2017). Great possibilities exist through the wealth of information gathered via the constancy of nursing including the potential to monitor real-time nursing assessments, interventions, processes and outcomes across care continuums (Welton and Harper 2016). Coupled with the opportunity to connect with and gather health data from populations through wearable technologies, cloud computing, smartphone mobile technologies and social media (Lokuge et al. 2018), there has never been such an era of opportunity to study and evaluate linkages to create knowledge for the purposes of improvement of professional practice, Personalised Medicine and population health outcomes (Higgins et al. 2018). This presents unprecedented prospects to advance the scientific knowledge and discover new opportunities for emphasis on aspects of nursing practice that effect improved predicted outcomes of care (Lodhi et al. 2016). The reality however is that adoption is slow, systems not fully understood (Gee et al. 2012) and funding to support development hard won, mainly due to the risk of failure which has been significant in the past within the United Kingdom (UK) (Campion Awaad et al. 2014). Barriers to technology adoption and therefore meaningful use include: misconceptions about evidence based practice; lack of leadership support; lack of time and mentorship; poor information literacy; and challenges with financial investment (Fulton et al. 2014).

7.5 Leading Digital Transformation of Nursing Information Practice

Some of the challenges to adoption could be positively leveraged through the influence and voice of nursing leadership globally, particularly those in executive roles. Whilst Kennedy-Page and Simpson (Kennedy-Page and Simpson 2016) asserted: 'Big data has the potential to elucidate the phenomena of nursing' (p. 272), other authors are more cautious in their prediction, understanding that it is dependent on strategic nursing leaders to recognise this potential and provide the necessary leadership for digital innovation to enhance nursing and develop an appropriately skilled and future facing workforce that includes the competence to manage information in an increasingly digital world (Jaimet 2016). Worryingly, the evidence suggests a lack of digital competence for nurse leaders in executive positions (Simpson 2013; Remus 2016). Those executive nurses who understand the value in providing and developing leadership in this area of practice in their organisations however, positively impact professional development processes for digital practice and the knowledge age (Remus 2016; Clarke and Mitchell 2014). Understanding and representing the experience of nurses, ensuring that technology appropriately captures, rather than impairing, burdening or eroding critical thinking and practice, is a new and important area of competence for executive nurses (Burkosi 2019).

Linking executive responsibilities, Kennedy-Page and Simpson (Simpson 2013) asserted that a critical component of the Executive Nurse leadership role is the meaningful capture and use of nursing data to drive quality practices across organisations. This included ability to transform raw data into information and then subsequently knowledge that could underpin the 'art and science of nursing practice' (Simpson 2013, p. 271). It is imperative, therefore, that executive nurses lead the development of nursing capabilities to capture, mine, collate and study data leading to relevant knowledge emerging directly in real-time rather than that gathered retrospectively (Khokar et al. 2017; Westra et al. 2017), including awareness of high volume data machine learning processes for predictive outcomes modelling (Obermeyer and Emanuel 2016). A critical future step for executive nurses is to push beyond current acceptance of physician-led EHCR design to data capture (Byrne 2012; Kerfoot 2015) reframing the purpose of nursing data collection from a focus on the legal and regulatory responsibilities to an opportunity to exponentially increase underpinning knowledge, advancing quality and the scientific practice of nursing (Kennedy-Page and Simpson 2016).

Key Points of Learning
1. Nursing is well placed to leverage the future change required to bring about services that will support global populations into the next decade and beyond.
2. Occupying 50% of the professional healthcare workforce globally, the need for high quality information is an imperative to drive future change harnessed through the professions' ability to collect data at the point of care.
3. Effective record keeping practice puts the patient at the centre of care, demonstrates clinical decision-making and goals of care, allows audit of practice, sup-

ports quality improvement and evidences co-production, safety and efficacy over time.

4. Future facing service prototypes have identified meaningful real-time data as a crucial enabler for efficient services to make best use of available nursing time.

5. The digital knowledge and skills of the nursing workforce, including those required to meaningfully use and evaluate information, requires a focus for investment to create a workforce that is appropriately equipped to expertly handle data.

6. Generating the greatest volume of healthcare data, it is imperative that nursing data is meaningfully structured and captured for the purposes of analysis and sharing evidencing and assuring the contribution of nursing.

7. Executive nurses who understand the value in providing and developing leadership in the informatics area of practice in their organisations, positively impact professional development processes for digital practice and the knowledge age.

7.6 Capturing Nursing Data in a Digital Environment

Development and implementation of Electronic Health Care Records (EHCRs) and other information technology (IT) offers tremendous opportunities to enhance nursing practice and capacity to capture and utilise patients' clinical information to improve healthcare. This enables multiple benefits including more timely access to health information which reduces duplication in work, improved end-user efficiencies and enables retrieval of pertinent information (e.g., patients on a specific medication) and aggregation of large data sets to enable service development and planning and new potential for research (Department of Health 2017; Nguyen et al. 2014; Kouroubali and Katehakis 2019; HIMSS 2019).

These benefits are extended via adjunct technologies such as clinical decision support (CDS) software and the Internet of Things (IoT) which respectively match patient clinical information with a computerised knowledge base to provide recommendations to the healthcare professional (HCP) and provide more comprehensive and accurate patient-generated information to the EHCR (Gartner 2019).

Access to more clinical data does not necessitate higher quality data and patient care, and we need to consider what are best practices to drive value from an EHCR as well as the adjunct technologies (Gartner 2019). At the same time, we must retain the overarching aim of capturing clinical information which is to track a patient's condition and communicate this to other members of the nursing and midwifery team in addition to the wider healthcare team to inform clinical decision-making (Kuhn et al. 2015; Mehta et al. 2016).

With nurses and midwives being responsible for a large amount of the data being entered into the EHCR or other digital systems it is vital that that nursing data is represented in a shareable manner which preserves its complexity, context and richness of patient care. These data can usually be entered in an unstructured, structured, coded or semi-structured format (HSE 2019).

7.7 Unstructured Data

Unstructured text refers to free or narrative text generated using a single window (i.e. similar to a word processing programme) which is often included in clinical notes, surgical records, medical reports or discharge summaries (Linder et al. 2012; Helgheim et al. 2019; Lardon et al. 2015). Unstructured free text entry of clinical data allows freedom of speech and expressivity (Lardon et al. 2015; Johnson et al. 2008), which facilitates documentation of complex presentations or impressions of a diagnosis which do not fit into predictable templates or quantifiable values (Rosenbloom et al. 2011; Crampton et al. 2016). It is also a critical factor in assisting management decisions and reflecting the training and perspective of the professional recording the data (Johnson et al. 2008; Siegler and Adelman 2009). Free text is often preferred and valued by HCPs due to its familiarity, speed and ease-of-use (Johnson et al. 2008; Rosenbloom et al. 2011; Shachak et al. 2013). For the reader, narrative text provides a greater and more comprehensive understanding of the patient compared with highly-structured data (Johnson et al. 2008; Rosenbloom et al. 2011). However, narrative text often contains large amounts of text, much of which may be redundant, which can obscure key information (Wrenn et al. 2010; Huang et al. 2018). Due to its unstructured format, it can also lead to omission of important information (Johnson et al. 2008; Wilbanks et al. 2018) and makes it difficult to effectively retrieve and use information for preventive care, disease management and quality improvement purposes (Shachak et al. 2013). These challenges may also be amplified where *copy-and-paste* or some *autofill* functions are utilised to duplicate unstructured narrative data from one note into the new current note (Wilbanks et al. 2018; Weis and Levy 2014).

Many of the intended benefits of EHCR systems such as clinical decision support (CDS) and automatic pull of data from one section of the EHCR to another (e.g., Smart Form), require automatic processing of clinical information which necessitates the use of controlled vocabulary as opposed to free text. Therefore, whilst free text may be more familiar to end-users (Lardon et al. 2015; Weis and Levy 2014; Bush et al. 2017; Campion et al. 2014; Joukes et al. 2018), it limits the extent and reliability to which computers can interpret and re-use the data (Johnson et al. 2008; Kalra 2006; Joukes et al. 2019). Conversion of free text into a structured format can be a time-consuming and difficult task (Kreimeyer et al. 2017) and thus, development of automated mechanisms for interpreting free text is of utmost importance (Helgheim et al. 2019). Artificial intelligence (AI) such as natural language processing (NLP) is a promising method for data extraction and retrieval from unstructured text (Rosenbloom et al. 2011; Ford et al. 2016). AI could be used by the HCP at the time of data entry to identify key terms from unstructured text and formulate structured text from it (Loui and Hollinshead 2016), or for secondary purposes (e.g., data retrieval for audits). However at present, challenges exist with the portability of NLP systems between clinical settings and its ability to recognise improper grammatical use, misspellings, local dialects, short phrases (e.g., BID) and clinical shorthand (e.g., D2M) (Rosenbloom et al. 2011; Helgheim et al. 2019; Sohn et al. 2017;

Pomares-Quimbaya et al. 2019). Overall, whilst unstructured data facilitates more comprehensive and flexible clinical documentation, it also comes with many challenges to optimising EHCR use which could affect patient safety and HCP productivity.

7.8 Structured Data

Structured data entry at the point-of-care, as opposed to post hoc structuring using NLP discussed above, includes: (1) Inputting data into structured forms/templates which divide components of the note into different sections (e.g., history of presenting illness); and (2) Selecting options from drop-down lists, tick boxes or radio buttons (Rosenbloom et al. 2011; Vuokko et al. 2017; California Healthcare Group 2010; Murray and Berberian 2011). Structured documentation templates often lend themselves to less complicated patient presentations (Mehta et al. 2016; Linder et al. 2012), computerised provider order entry (CPOE) systems (Siegler and Adelman 2009; Seidling and Bates 2016), registry forms, research forms dates (Krumm et al. 2014), social information, biological data measures and biological investigation results (Lardon et al. 2015; Helgheim et al. 2019). Whereas check boxes, radio buttons and drop down lists suit aspects which have limited options (Rosenbloom et al. 2011; Kreimeyer et al. 2017; Murray and Berberian 2011) such as yes/no and patient-reported outcome measures (Busack et al. 2016; Zhang et al. 2019). Until large scale NLP can accurately produce structured data from dictated and free text reports, structured data entry will be an essential input method to enable data retrieval for reports and analytics as well as CDS software (Linder et al. 2012).

For the author, entering data into structured templates in the EHCR can reduce data omission, as checklists can act as 'memory joggers' to assist HCPs to comply with best practice (Johnson et al. 2008; Rosenbloom et al. 2011; Linder et al. 2012; O'Donnell et al. 2018; Lorenzetti et al. 2018; Saranto et al. 2014). Additionally, structured data facilitates automated population of data fields (i.e., autofill) from other sections of the EHCR (Johnson et al. 2008; Helgheim et al. 2019; Linder et al. 2012) and from EHCR-integrated devices (Plastiras and O'Sullivan 2018) (e.g., bar code medication administration), improving overall efficiency in clinical documentation as well as reducing errors in the transfer of data between systems (Lawrence et al. 2018). Additionally, for the reader, structured templates are easier to read and locate information, whilst administrative staff benefit from the ability to easily aggregate and retrieve structured data (Joukes et al. 2018). However, whilst end-user efficiency may be improved when taking into account secondary uses of clinical data such as content importing technology (e.g., SmartForms), entering structured data at point-of-care requires more effort on the part of the end-user (Johnson et al. 2008; Rosenbloom et al. 2011; Bush et al. 2017; Campion et al.

2014; Joukes et al. 2018) and can negatively affect system usability (O'Donnell et al. 2018; Ajami and Bagheri-Tadi 2013; Kruse et al. 2016). It also imposes restrictions on HCPs in terms of how they document (Kalra 2006; Vuokko et al. 2017) and how they critically think and make decisions, which can risk the depersonalisation of healthcare (Nguyen et al. 2014; Saranto et al. 2014) and the incorrect identification of patients as having a certain condition due to lack of room for ambiguity (Johnson et al. 2008; Crampton et al. 2016).

To negate these risks, it has been recommended that the EHCR system does not mandate end-users to check a box if not appropriate, and that structured templates should never replace the clinical narrative (Kuhn et al. 2015). Unprecedented challenges have also been identified with structuring and standardising certain types of data such as psychosocial and emotional information, and whilst their importance is recognised, according to the literature, the best format for recording these data needs to be explored further (Busack et al. 2016). It is recommended that the design of structured templates involves a multi-disciplinary task force, workflow analysis (including downstream effects) and ongoing evaluation and comparisons of pre and post templates (Cao et al. 2017). Fundamental to any discussion of structured documentation is patient care (California Healthcare Group 2010), as well as recognition of the minimum dataset which needs to be collected to support patient care (Hakonsen et al. 2019). Additionally, whilst structure needs to be balanced with flexibility, developers should be mindful that the addition of too many options within the structured template could result in no meaningful data being collected (Rosenbloom et al. 2011). Even after following this process, a structured template will not suit every patient presentation, especially the more complicated patients (California Healthcare Group 2010). Therefore, personalisation which enables end-users to customise how data is input and viewed is recommended to allow some flexibility and improve end-user satisfaction with structured templates (Parent 2017; KLAS 2018; Hine et al. 2008).

7.9 Coded Data

Clinical information can often be tacit, context-bound, and ambiguous (Ben-Zion et al. 2014), and without a 'shared tongue', communication between HCPs can be significantly impaired (Sundling and Kurtycz 2019). Therefore, standardised terminologies (STs) have been developed which are associated with codes and represent defined aspects of clinical practice (Williams et al. 2017; World Health Organisation 2016b; Bronnert et al. 2012). For example, traditionally several terms are utilised to describe high cholesterol but with STs everyone uses the same term, and these are mapped to a code (e.g., ICD-10 code E78.0 represents Hypercholesterolemia). This multiples the benefits of structured data, as definitions are understood and synonyms can be aggregated (e.g., heart attack, myocardial infarct and MI) (California Healthcare Group 2010). Additional benefits include:

1. Improved data quality (Sundling and Kurtycz 2019; World Health Organisation 2016b; Health Information and Quality Authority (HIQA) 2014; SNOMED International 2017).
2. Terminology understood by all HCPs across organisations and geographical boundaries (irrespective of language) (Sundling and Kurtycz 2019; World Health Organisation 2016b; Health Information and Quality Authority (HIQA) 2014; SNOMED International 2017).
3. Patients benefit from HCPs utilising same term across clinical documentation to describe their condition (Sundling and Kurtycz 2019).
4. Improved quality of care (Sundling and Kurtycz 2019).
5. Semantic interoperability between information systems (Cao et al. 2017; Health Information and Quality Authority (HIQA) 2014; SNOMED International 2017).
6. Accurate and comprehensive searches to identify patients requiring follow-up or changes to treatment based on revised guidelines (Sundling and Kurtycz 2019; World Health Organisation 2016b; Health Information and Quality Authority (HIQA) 2014; SNOMED International 2017).
7. Monitoring of treatment effectiveness, patterns and trends (Vuokko et al. 2017; California Healthcare Group 2010; Saranto et al. 2014).
8. Use of CDS software (Vuokko et al. 2017; California Healthcare Group 2010; Saranto et al. 2014).
9. Additional research opportunities (Sundling and Kurtycz 2019; World Health Organisation 2016b; Health Information and Quality Authority (HIQA) 2014; SNOMED International 2017).

Whilst many STs have been developed, no single terminology has been accepted as a universal standard (Rosenbloom et al. 2006). Three different types of coding sets exist:

7.9.1 Aggregation Terminologies (or Administrative Code Sets)

Enable classification of concepts using simple hierarchy relationships for administrative purposes such as reimbursement (Williams et al. 2017; Bronnert et al. 2012; Health Information and Quality Authority (HIQA) 2014). As these codes were designed to either group diagnoses and procedures or to contain broad categories with administrative technical terms, aggregation terminologies can be restrictive and prevent concepts from having multiple parents (Williams et al. 2017). Where HCPs are forced to use these code sets to capture clinical data, there is potential for inaccuracies and loss of the clinical intent (Williams et al. 2017; Bronnert et al. 2012). Examples of aggregation terminologies include International Classification of Diseases and related health problems (ICD), International Classification of Primary Care (ICPC), Read Codes and Office of Population Censuses and Surveys Classification of Interventions and Procedures (OPCS).

7.9.2 Reference Terminologies (or Clinical Code Sets)

Enable more sensitive and specific terms to be collected as they are concept-based and controlled clinical terminologies which maintain a common reference point in healthcare (Bronnert et al. 2012). Unlike aggregation terminologies, reference terminologies facilitate the combination of concepts (i.e., post-coordination) to create a more detailed or complex concept from a simple one (Williams et al. 2017; Rosenbloom et al. 2006). For example, the following terms may coexist: chest pain, substernal chest pain and crushing substernal chest pain. Reference terminologies are less restrictive, considered more usable and meaningful for HCPs, reduce time spent searching for terms and enable use of CDS software as well as aggregation of data (Bronnert et al. 2012; Rosenbloom et al. 2006; van der Kooija et al. 2006). Reference terminologies utilised at point-of-care include the Systematized Nomenclature of Medicine-Clinical Terms (SNOMED-CT) which capture all clinical notes including allergies, vitals, past history, family history, symptoms, clinical findings and diagnosis; the Logical Observation Identifiers Names and Codes (LOINC) which captures laboratory and clinical observations; and RxNorm which captures medication names (Bronnert et al. 2012; Health Information and Quality Authority (HIQA) 2014; SNOMED International 2019). To balance the more usable reference terminology with the more rigorous aggregation terminologies which may be needed for national audits or reimbursement, reference terminologies can be mapped to an aggregation terminology e.g., ICD (The Office of the National Coordinator for Health Information Technology 2017).

7.9.3 Interface Terminology

To capture more granularity and clinical intent in the documentation, a third type of standardised terminology has been developed referred to as interface terminologies (Bronnert et al. 2012). These interface terminologies are often discipline-specific such as standardised nursing terminologies (The Office of the National Coordinator for Health Information Technology 2017; Vivanti et al. 2018), institution-specific (Rosenbloom et al. 2013) or speciality-specific (Sundling and Kurtycz 2019). Whilst large-scale reference terminologies attempt to represent every possible entity, interface terminologies reduce the need for post-coordination (e.g., combination of "acute" and "pain") as they represent the common terms utilised in the specific practice its employed in (Bronnert et al. 2012; Rosenbloom et al. 2013; Berger 2013). Additionally, this decreases time spent searching for codes and facilitates documentation of more comprehensive, accurate and relevant clinical information (Bronnert et al. 2012; Rosenbloom et al. 2013; Berger 2013). Interface terminologies can be also be used to gain a deeper understanding of care approaches during evaluations, as well as having potential to improve patient outcomes (Saranto et al. 2014; The Office of the National Coordinator for Health Information Technology

2017; Macieira et al. 2017; Tayyib et al. 2015). Therefore, interface terminologies are important for problem lists (Bronnert et al. 2012) and these can then be mapped to the reference and aggregation terminologies where required for health information exchange, administrative or secondary use (Bronnert et al. 2012; The Office of the National Coordinator for Health Information Technology 2017; Westra et al. 2008).

7.10 Standardised Terminologies in Nursing Practice

Since the 1970s, there has been a concerted effort to promote STs within nursing and midwifery practice (Hardiker 2011) with the pioneering of the first standardised nursing language or terminology NANDA International (NANDA-I), formerly known as North American Nursing Diagnosis Association (Jones et al. 2010; Oreofe and Oyenike 2018). These standardised nursing terminologies commonly systematically group, define and encode nursing care as nursing diagnoses, interventions and outcomes (Kieft et al. 2018; Warren et al. 2015; Hellesø 2006; Bernhart-Just et al. 2010) and link nursing diagnoses with evidenced-based interventions and outcomes (Clancy et al. 2006). This is seen as the pathway for making the nursing process more useable and visible (Oreofe and Oyenike 2018) which promotes good communication, provides the basis for care planning and identification of patient problems (Dykes et al. 2009) and improves data quality for research and service development planning (da Costa and da Costa Linch 2018).

The American Nurses Association (ANA) have approved twelve terminology sets that support nursing practice for use within the ECHR which includes both nursing-specific and multi-disciplinary terminologies (Table 7.1) (Gencbas et al.

Table 7.1 American Nurses Association (ANA)-approved terminology sets

Standardised terminology	Content
Nursing outcomes classification (NOC)	Nursing outcomes
NANDA-I	Nursing diagnoses
Nursing intervention classification (NIC)	Nursing interventions
Clinical care classification (CCC) system	Nursing diagnoses, interventions, outcome ratings
Perioperative nursing data set (PNDS)	Perioperative nursing diagnoses, interventions, outcomes
Omaha system	Nursing diagnoses, interventions, outcomes ratings
International classification for nursing practice (ICNP®)	Nursing diagnoses, interventions, outcome
Nursing minimum data set (NMDS)	Nursing clinical data elements
Logical observation identifiers names and codes (LOINC®)	Assessments, outcomes
ABC codes	Billing codes
Systematized nomenclature of medicine-clinical terms (SNOMED-CT®)	Diagnoses, interventions, outcomes, findings

2018; The Office of the National Coordinator for Health Information Technology 2017). Additionally, a recent review commissioned by the Five Country Nursing and Midwifery Digital Leadership Group identified that in addition to the STs outlined in Table 7.1, nurses and midwives have also used locally-controlled and other medical and/or multi-disciplinary STs (Fennelly et al. 2020). These STs are in utilisation across at least 26 different countries (Fennelly et al. 2020) but although both the UK and Ireland have adopted the use of SNOMED-CT (Health Information and Quality Authority (HIQA) 2014; Sheerin 2003; Arnot-Smith and Smith 2010), their utilisation of nursing-specific STs has been more sporadic (Sheerin 2003; Murphy et al. 2018).

Initially, the deployment of STs in nursing and midwifery practice has been uncoordinated with little convergence towards a unified nursing language system that can be integrated within the wider health-care language arena (Cho and Park 2006). It is now acknowledged that these STs need to be integrated and understood within the broader healthcare system to support interoperability and data continuity across community and acute settings (Oreofe and Oyenike 2018; Martin et al. 2011; Kim et al. 2014). However, many of the nursing-specific STs have been developed, utilised and evaluated in a specific clinical setting such as the Omaha System and CCC in primary care, and the ICNP and PNDS in secondary care (Fennelly et al. 2020). Consideration, therefore, needs to be given to the advantages and disadvantages of a large comprehensive multi-disciplinary ST versus a discipline or institution-specific ST, and the purpose of using the ST. Although the multi-disciplinary ST may facilitate communication between professions and settings (Jukes et al. 2012), searching for the correct code to match a patient's diagnosis from a long list can also be time-consuming (Vuokko et al. 2017). Whereas nursing-specific STs offer more granularity, help to distinguish nursing care (Estrada and Dunn 2012) and enable the linkage of nursing diagnoses with evidence-based interventions which have potential to improve clinical decision-making skills (Wuryanto et al. 2017) and patient care (Zhang et al. 2018). However, they may not always fully comprehensive of the nursing and midwifery care provided (Cho and Park 2006) and have, at times, resulted in the availability of too many terms representing the same patient presentation (i.e., content duplication) (Morais et al. 2015; Monsen et al. 2011). Therefore, irrespective of the type of ST being used, its applicability, validity and reliability should be considered for the specific context it is being implemented in. Otherwise, it could jeopardise patient care and safety as well not as driving the full potential of using the ST.

Although the type and content of the ST is important, its implementation also drives its success. A usable ECHR interface in which the ST is searched or enters influences the use and acceptability of the ST amongst nurses and midwives (Cho and Park 2003; Hariyati et al. 2016). An interface which supports shortcuts such as searching mechanisms, display of the most frequently selected codes (for the given user) at the top of the list, i.e., 'favourites' (California Healthcare Group 2010) and/ or use of NLP techniques to suggest appropriate codes and expression (SNOMED International 2019; Hodge and Narus 2018) have been recommended. Additionally, when the ST is being used within a unstructured template compared to a drop down list, the education of nurses to use the ST has been shown to impact on the quality of the nursing documentation (Müller-Staub et al. 2007, 2008; Müller-Staub 2009). Although STs have been shown to facilitate retrieval and aggregation of data from clinical records and health information exchange (Tastan et al. 2014; Topaz et al. 2014), this also depended on the reporting and analytical capabilities built into the ECHR system and the format and file types used (Westra et al. 2010).

Overall, use of STs or coded data within the EHCR provide several benefits to end-users, patients, healthcare organisations and policy-makers, and it is likely that more than one type of terminology will be required in the EHCR to facilitate both administrative and clinical purposes. Decisions regarding the selection of these STs should be made prior to EHCR design as otherwise adaptations to the terminology in the EHCR are expensive and labour-intensive (Sundling and Kurtycz 2019). Each of these terminologies will come with a license fee and mapping of terminologies to one another will need to be maintained as changes and updates are made to the ST by the software developer, third-party vendor or the individual healthcare organisation (Kalra 2006; The Office of the National Coordinator for Health Information Technology 2017; Houser et al. 2013).

7.11 Semi-structured Data

Use of STs do not always easily accommodate for diagnostic uncertainty (Ford et al. 2016) and are not always sensitive and specific to the condition in question (e.g., depression could present symptomatically as insomnia, fatigue, malaise) (McBrien et al. 2018). Therefore, the option to enter free text in conjunction with the ST is often allowed within the ECHR (Ford et al. 2016) to allow additional context or further clinically-relevant information to be added (Wilbanks et al. 2018; California Healthcare Group 2010; Sundling and Kurtycz 2019). This hybrid model of unstructured, structured and coded data is known as semi-structured data (California Healthcare Group 2010; Murray and Berberian 2011). Additionally, within the structured elements of the EHCR, options to input narrative data are often provided where end-users cannot find an appropriate structured concept or code (Rosenbloom et al. 2011). However, this can risk end-users overusing the free text box rather than searching for the appropriate code and thus, end-users need to understand the benefits of using coded and structured data in combination with unstructured data. Overall, semi-structured clinical data combines the benefits associated with the flexibility of unstructured data with the downstream benefits of using coded and structured data.

7.12 Key Findings for Nursing on Clinical Data Types

No one type of clinical data will accommodate nursing and midwifery documentation of every clinical scenario and/or secondary use of the data and thus, it is likely that a combination of those will be utilised (Arrendale 2018). In determining the

Table 7.2 Summary of clinical data types in the electronic health record

	Unstructured	Structured	Coded	Semi-structured
Definition	Free or narrative text	Templates divided into defined sections, checklists, drop-down lists or radio buttons	Standardised terminologies with definitions which are associated with codes	Combination of unstructured, structured and coded data
Advantages	• Flexible • Easy-to-use • Fast • More comprehensive	• Easier to read and navigate • Prompts HCP to ask questions • Enables autofill function • More comprehensive searches and data retrieval	• Consistent meaning and value associated with terms • Facilitates: – Interoperability – Data retrieval – CDS – Autofill	Allows some flexibility whilst retaining the benefits associated with structured and coded data
Disadvantages	• Large amounts of text obscuring key information • Omission of information • Difficult to retrieve specific information • Difficult for computer to process	• Restrictive for HCPs • Can be more time-consuming to enter • Risk of losing individualised patient information capture	• Restrictive for HCPs • Can be more time-consuming to search for codes • Costs associated with licence fees	Risk of overuse of free text form as opposed to searching for appropriate code/structured element
Recommended uses	Where a clinical presentation does not lend itself to a predefined template	CPOE, birth date, biological data measure or biological investigation results, limited possible answers (yes/no) etc.	Diagnostic codes, laboratory results, procedure codes etc.	Where HCP may need to expand on the coded and structured data using free text

Source: HSE (HSE 2019)

most appropriate type of data or combination of data types, the advantages and disadvantages of each should be considered (Table 7.2), as well as the workflows and downstream effects of capturing data in this format.

Key Points of Learning

1. With nurses and midwives being responsible for a large amount of the data being entered into the EHCR or other digital systems it is vital that that nursing data is represented in a shareable manner which preserves its complexity, context and richness of patient care. These data can usually be entered in an unstructured, structured, coded or semi-structured format.

2. No one type of clinical data will accommodate nursing and midwifery documentation of every clinical scenario and/or secondary use of the data and thus, it is likely that a combination of those will be utilised

3. In determining the most appropriate type of data or combination of data types, the advantages and disadvantages of each should be considered as well as the workflows and downstream effects of capturing data in this format.

4. Use of Standardised Terminologies or coded data within the EHCR provide several benefits to end-users, patients, healthcare organisations and policy-makers, and it is likely that more than one type of terminology will be required in the EHCR to facilitate both administrative and clinical purposes.

5. There has been a concerted effort to promote Standardised Terminologies within nursing and midwifery practice. These standardised nursing terminologies commonly systematically group, define and encode nursing care as nursing diagnoses, interventions and outcomes and link nursing diagnoses with evidenced-based interventions and outcomes

6. Decisions regarding the selection of these STs should be made prior to EHCR design as otherwise adaptations to the terminology in the EHCR are expensive and labour-intensive

Review Questions
Questions

1. Describe what you consider to be the core requirements for delivery of good records in nursing care documentation?

Answer
'Good' records put the patient at the centre of care, demonstrate clinical decision-making and goals of care, allow audit of practice, support quality improvement and evidence co-production, safety and efficacy over time.

2. What do you consider to be the key barriers to technology adoption in your area of clinical practice?

3. Do they reflect all, one or some of the key barriers listed in this chapter. Select one of the barriers from the list of items below and expand using supporting evidence.

(a) Misconceptions about evidence based practice;
(b) Lack of leadership support;
(c) Lack of time and mentorship;
(d) Poor information literacy;
(e) Challenges with financial investment

Refhttps://indiana.pure.elsevier.com/en/publications/faculty-and-organizational-characteristics-associated-with-inform

4. This chapter explains the importance of representing nursing data in EHCRs or other digital systems in a shareable manner which preserves its complexity, context and richness of patient care. Discuss the different types and formats of data that can usually be entered in an EHCR.

Answer

EHCR data can usually be entered in an unstructured, structured, coded or semi-structured format. We briefly provide some of the key points from the chapter on the different type of data formats.

Unstructured text refers to free or narrative text generated using a single window. Unstructured free text entry of clinical data allows freedom of speech and expressivity, which facilitates documentation of complex presentations or impressions of a diagnosis which do not fit into predictable templates or quantifiable values. However, narrative text often contains large amounts of text, much of which may be redundant, which can obscure key information. Due to its unstructured format, it can also lead to omission of important information and makes it difficult to effectively retrieve and use information for preventive care, disease management and quality improvement purposes.

Structured data entry at the point-of-care, as opposed to post hoc structuring using Natural Language Processing (NLP), includes: (1) Inputting data into structured forms/templates which divide components of the note into different sections (e.g., history of presenting illness); and (2) Selecting options from drop-down lists, tick boxes or radio buttons. Structured documentation templates often lend themselves to less complicated patient presentations, computerised provider order entry (CPOE) systems, registry forms, research forms dates, social information, biological data measures and biological investigation results. For the author, entering data into structured templates in the EHCR can reduce data omission, as checklists can act as 'memory joggers' to assist HCPs to comply with best practice. It also imposes restrictions on HCPs in terms of how they document and how they critically think and make decisions, which can risk the depersonalisation of healthcare and the incorrect identification of patients as having a certain condition due to lack of room for ambiguity.

Coded data and standardised terminologies (STs) have been developed which are associated with codes and represent defined aspects of clinical practice. For example, traditionally several terms are utilised to describe high cholesterol but with STs everyone uses the same term, and these are mapped to a code (e.g., ICD-10 code E78.0 represents Hypercholesterolemia). This multiples the benefits of structured data, as definitions are understood and synonyms can be aggregated (e.g., heart attack, myocardial infarct and MI).

A semi structured hybrid model of unstructured, structured and coded data is known as semi-structured data. Additionally, within the structured elements of the EHCR, options to input narrative data are often provided where end-users cannot find an appropriate structured concept or code. However, this can risk end-users overusing the free text box rather than searching for the appropriate code and thus, end-users need to understand the benefits of using coded and structured data in combination with unstructured data. Overall, semi-structured clinical data combines the benefits associated with the flexibility of unstructured data with the downstream benefits of using coded and structured data.

Glossary

ABC Billing Codes
CCC Clinical Care Classification
CDS Clinical Decision Support
EHCR Electronic Health Care Record
HCP Health Care Professional
ICD International Classification of Diseases
ICNP International Classification for Nursing Practice
ICPC International Classification of Primary Care
IoT Internet of Things
LOINC Logical Observation Identifiers Names and Codes
NANDA North American Nursing Diagnosis Association
NANDA I North American Nursing Diagnosis Association International
NIC Nursing Intervention Classification
NLP Natural Language Processing
NOC Nursing Outcome Classification
OPCS Office of Population Censuses and Surveys Classification of Interventions and Procedures
PNDS Peri Operative Nursing Dataset
SDH Social Determinants of Health
SNOMED CT Systematized Nomenclature of Medicine—Clinical Terms
ST Standardised Terminologies

References

Ajami S, Bagheri-Tadi T. Barriers for adopting electronic health records (EHRs) by physicians. Acta Inform Med. 2013;21(2):129–34.

All Party Parliamentary Group on Global Health (APPG). Triple Impact. How developing nursing will improve health, promote gender equality and support economic growth. APPG. 2016. https://www.who.int/hrh/com-heeg/digital-APPG_triple-impact.pdf.

Amalberti R, Nicklin W, Braithwaite J. Preparing national health systems to cope with the impending tsunami of ageing and its associated complexities: towards more sustainable health care. Int J Qual Health Care. 2016;28(3):412–4.

Arnot-Smith J, Smith AF. Patient safety incidents involving neuromuscular blockade: analysis of the UK National Reporting and Learning System data from 2006 to 2008. Anaesthesia. 2010;65(11):1106–13.

Arrendale D. Transcription trends: self-documentation challenges. For The Record. 2018;30(8):28.

Ball JE, Bruynell L, Aiken LH, Sermeus W, Sloane DM, Raffert AM, et al. Post-operative mortality, missed care and nurse staffing in nine countries: a cross-sectional study. Int J Nurs Stud. 2018;78(Feb):10–5.

Ben-Zion R, Pliskin N, Fink L. Critical success factors for adoption of electronic health record systems: literature review and prescriptive analysis. Inf Syst Manag. 2014;31(4):296–312.

Berger M. Classification, diagnosis and datasets: towards an approach for clinical psychology services and electronic records. British Pscyhological Society (BPS). 2013.

Bernhart-Just A, Lassen B, Schwendimann R. Representing the nursing process with nursing terminologies in electronic medical record systems: a Swiss approach. Comput Inform Nurs. 2010;28(6):345–52.

Bolous-Rødje N. Tactics for constructing visions about electronic health records (EHRs). CJC. 2019;44:1–22.

Braithwaite J, Matsuyama Y, Mannion R, Johnson J, Bates DW, Hughes C. How to do better health reform: a snapshot of change and improvement initiatives in the health systems of 30 countries. Int J Qual Health Care. 2016;28(6):843–6.

Braithwaite J, Mannion R, Matsuyama Y, Shekelle P, Whittaker S, Al-Adawi S. Accomplishing reform: successful case studies drawn from the health systems of 60 countries. Int J Qual Health Care. 2017;29(6):880–6.

Braithwaite J, Mannion R, Matsuyama Y, Shekelle PG, Whittaker S, Al-Adawi S. Healthcare systems: future predictions for global care. Florida: CRS Press; 2018.

Bronnert J, Masarie C, Naeymi-Rad F, Rose E, Aldin G. Problem-centered care delivery: how Interface terminology makes standardized health information possible. J AHIMA. 2012;83(7):30–5.

Burkosi V. Nursing leadership in the fully digital practice realm. Nurs Leadersh. 2019;32(SI):9–15.

Burnel P. The introduction of electronic medical records in France: more progress during the second attempt. Health Policy. 2018;122:937–40.

Busack C, Daskalakis C, Rosen P. Physician and parent perspectives on psychosocial and emotional data entry in the electronic medical record in a pediatric setting. J Patient Exp. 2016;3(1):10–6.

Bush RA, Kuelbs C, Ryu J, Jiang W, Chiang G. Structured data entry in the electronic medical record: perspectives of pediatric specialty physicians and surgeons. J Med Syst. 2017;41(5):75.

Byrne MD. Informatics competence in the EHR era. J Perianesth Nurs. 2012;27(1):42–5.

California Healthcare Group. Clinical documentation: EHR deployment techniques. 2010.

Campion Awaad O, Hayton A, Smith L, Vuaran M. The national programme for IT in the NHS: a case history. MPhil Public Policy 2014, University of Cambridge. 2014. https://www.cl.cam. ac.uk/~rja14/Papers/npfit-mpp-2014-case-history.pdf.

Campion T, Johnson S, Paxton E, Mushlin A, Sedrakyan A. Implementing unique device identification in electronic health record systems: organizational, workflow, and technological challenges. Med Care. 2014;52(1):26–31.

Cao J, Farmer R, Carry PM, Goodfellow M, Gerhardt DC, Scott F, et al. Standardized note templates improve electronic medical record documentation of neurovascular examinations for pediatric supracondylar humeral fractures. JB JS Open Access. 2017;2(4):e0027.

Cho I, Park HA. Development and evaluation of a terminology-based electronic nursing record system. J Biomed Inform. 2003;36(4-5):304–12.

Cho I, Park HA. Evaluation of the expressiveness of an ICNP-based nursing data dictionary in a computerized nursing record system. J Am Med Inform Assoc. 2006;13(4):456–64.

Clancy TR, Delaney CW, Morrison B, Gunn JK. The benefits of standardized nursing languages in complex adaptive systems such as hospitals. J Nurs Adm. 2006;36(9):426–34.

Clarke JS, Mitchell MB. The CNE-CNIO partnership: improving patient care through technology. Nurse Lead. 2014;12(1):52–64.

da Costa C, da Costa Linch G. Implementation of electronic records related to nursing diagnoses. Int J Nurs Knowl. 2018;31(1):50–8.

Crampton NH, Reis S, Shachak A. Computers in the clinical encounter: a scoping review and thematic analysis. J Am Med Inform Assoc. 2016;23(3):654–65.

Department of Health. Sláintecare implementation strategy. Dublin, Ireland; 2017.

Dick TK, Patrician PA, Loan LA. The value of nursing care: a concept analysis. Nurs Forum. 2017;52(4):357–65.

Dykes PC, Kim HE, Goldsmith DM, Choi J, Esumi K, Goldberg HS. The adequacy of ICNP version 1.0 as a representational model for electronic nursing assessment documentation. J Am Med Inform Assoc. 2009;16(2):238–46.

Englebright J, Caspers B. The role of the chief nurse executive in the big data revolution. Nurse Lead. 2016;14(4):280–4.

Erikson CE, Pittman P, LaFrance A, Chapman S. Alternative payment models lead to strategic care coordination workforce investments. Nurs Outlook. 2017;65(6):737–45.

Estrada NA, Dunn CR. Standardized nursing diagnoses in an electronic health record: nursing survey results. Int J Nurs Knowl. 2012;23(2):86–95.

Fennelly O, Grogan L, Reed A, Hardiker N. Representing what we do as nurses and midwives – terminologies and standardised languages: systematic literature review and key considerations. Awating publication. 2020;

Fitzpatrick G, Ellingsen G. A review of 25 years of CSCW research in healthcare: contributions, challenges and future agendas. CSCW. 2013;22(4–6):609–65. https://doi.org/10.1007/s10606-012-9168-0.

Ford E, Carroll JA, Smith HE, Scott D, Cassell JA. Extracting information from the text of electronic medical records to improve case detection: a systematic review. J Am Med Inform Assoc. 2016;23(5):1007–15.

Founds S. Systems biology for nursing in the era of big data and precision health. Nurs Outlook. 2018;66:283–92.

Fulton CR, Meek JA, Hinton Walker P. Faculty and organisational characteristics associated with informatics/health information technology adoption in DNP programs. J Prof Nursing. 2014;30(4):292–9.

Gartner. Healthcare EHR and digital care delivery optimization primer for 2019. 2019.

Gee PM, Greenwood DA, Kim KK, Perez SL, Staggers N, De Von HA. Exploration of the e-patient phenomenon in nursing informatics. Nurs Outlook. 2012;60:E9–E16.

Gencbas D, Bebis H, Cicek H. Evaluation of the efficiency of the nursing care plan applied using NANDA, NOC, and NIC linkages to elderly women with incontinence living in a nursing home: a randomized controlled study. Int J Nurs Knowl. 2018;29(4):217–26.

Gomes PAR, Farah BF, Rocha RS, Friedrich DBC, Dutra HS. Electronic citizen record: an instrument for nursing care. Rev Fund Care Online. 2019;11(5):1226–35.

Green SD, Thomas JD. Interdisciplinary collaboration and the electronic medical record. Paediatr Nurs. 2008;34(3):225–40.

Griffiths P, Ball JE, Drennan J, Dall'Ora C, Jones J, Maruotti A, et al. Nurse staffing and patient outcomes: strengths and limitations of the evidence to inform policy and practice. A review and discussion paper based on evidence reviewed for the National Institute for Health and Care Excellence Safe Staffing guideline development. Int J Nurs Stud. 2016;63:213–25.

Hakonsen SJ, Pedersen PU, Bygholm A, Peters MD, Bjerrum M. Speaking the same language: development of a nutrition minimum data set for healthcare professionals in primary healthcare. Health Informatics J. 2019;26(1):248–63. https://doi.org/10.1177/1460458218824707.

Hardiker N. Developing standardised terminologies to support nursing practice. Boston: Jones and Bartlett Publishers LLC; 2011.

Hariyati RTS, Yani A, Eryando T, Hasibuan Z, Milanti A. The effectiveness and efficiency of nursing care documentation using the SIMPRO model. Int J Nurs Knowl. 2016;27(3):136–42.

Health Information and Quality Authority (HIQA). Recommendations regarding the adoption of SNOMED Clinical Terms as the Clinical Terminology for Ireland. Ireland; 2014.

Helgheim BI, Maia R, Ferreira JC, Martins AL. Merging data diversity of clinical medical records to improve effectiveness. Int J Environ Res Public Health. 2019;16(5):769.

Hellesø R. Information handling in the nursing discharge note. J Clin Nurs. 2006;15:11–21.

Higgins M, Simpson RL, Johnson WG. What about big data and nursing? Am Nurse Today. 2018;13(5):29–31.

HIMSS. Improving patient safety outcomes with health IT. 2019. https://www.himss.org/case-studies-improving-patient-safety-through-health-it.

Hine N, Petersen F, Pluke M, Sund T, editors. Standardization work on personalized eHealth systems. 30th Annual International IEEE EMBS Conference 2008; Vancouver, British Columbia, Canada.

Hodge CM, Narus SP. Electronic problem lists: a thematic analysis of a systematic literature review to identify aspects critical to success. J Am Med Inform Assoc. 2018;25(5):603–13.

Houser S, Morgan D, Clements K, Hart-Hester S. Assessing the planning and implementation strategies for the ICD-10-CM/PCS coding transition in Alabama hospital. Perspect Health Inf Manag. 2013;10:1a.

HSE. Clinical information capture in the electronic health record: literature review and key considerations. 2019. https://www.ehealthireland.ie/Strategic-Programmes/Electronic-Health-Record-EHR-/Information-Resources/Clinical-Information-Capture-in-the-EHR-Literature-Review-and-Key-Considerations.pdf.

Huang A, Hribar M, Goldstein I, Henriksen B, Lin W, Chiang M. Clinical documentation in electronic health record systems: analysis of similarity in progress notes from consecutive outpatient ophthalmology encounters. AMIA Annu Symp Proc. 2018;2018:1310–8.

Hussey P, Adams E, Shaffer FA. Nursing informatics and leadership, an essential competency for a global priority. Nurse Lead. 2015;13(5):52–7.

Jaimet K. Technology, demographics and new models of care: ready to embrace the future? Can Nurse. 2016;112(3):20–1.

Jeffries D, Johnson M, Nicholls D. Nursing documentation: how meaning is obscured by fragmentary language. Nurs Outlook. 2012;59(6):e6–e12.

Johnson SB, Bakken S, Dine D, Hyun S, Mendonca E, Morrison F, et al. An electronic health record based on structured narrative. J Am Med Inform Assoc. 2008;15(1):54–64.

Jones D, Lunney M, Keenan G, Moorhead S. Standardized nursing languages: essential for the nursing workforce. Annu Rev Nurs Res. 2010;28:253–94.

Joukes E, Cornet R, de Bruijne MC, de Keizer NF, Abu-Hanna A. Development and validation of a model for the adoption of structured and standardised data recording among healthcare professionals. BMC Med Inform Decis Mak. 2018;18(1):54.

Joukes E, de Keizer NF, de Bruijne MC, Abu-Hanna A, Cornet R. Impact of electronic versus paper-based recording before EHR implementation on health care professionals' perceptions of EHR use, data quality, and data reuse. Appl Clin Inform. 2019;10(2):199–209.

Jukes S, Cichero JA, Haines T, Wilson C, Paul K, O'Rourke M. Evaluation of the uptake of the Australian standardized terminology and definitions for texture modified foods and fluids. Int J Speech Lang Pathol. 2012;14(3):214–25.

Kalra D. Electronic health record standards. IMIA Yearbook of Medical Informatics. 2006;45:S136–44.

Kelly D, Lankshear A, Jones A. Stress and resilience in a post-Francis world – a qualitative study of executive nurse directors. J Adv Nurs. 2016;72(12):3160–8.

Kennedy MA, Moen A. Nurse leadership and informatics competencies: shaping transformation of professional practice. Forecasting informatics competencies for nurses in the future of connected health. Stud Health Technol Inform. 2017;232:197–206.

Kennedy-Page C, Simpson RL. Nurse leader challenges in data transparency: eyes to the future. Nurse Lead. 2016;14:271–4.

Kerfoot KM. Intelligently managed data: achieving excellence in nursing care. Nurs Econ. 2015;33(6):342–3.

Khokar A, Lodhi MK, Yao Y, Ansari R, Keenan G, Wilkie DJ. Framework for mining and analysis of standardized nursing care plan data. West J Nurs Res. 2017;39(1):20–41.

Kieft R, Vreeke EM, de Groot EM, de Graaf-Waar HI, van Gool CH, Koster N, et al. Mapping the Dutch SNOMED CT subset to Omaha system, NANDA international and international classification of functioning, disability and health. Int J Med Inform. 2018;111:77–82.

Kim TY, Hardiker N, Coenen A. Inter-terminology mapping of nursing problems. J Biomed Inform. 2014;49:213–20.

KLAS. Improving the EHR experience through personalization: Impact report. UK; 2018.

van der Kooija J, Goossena W, Goossen-Baremansa A, de Jong-Fintelmana M, van Beeka L. Using SNOMED CT codes for coding information in electronic health records for stroke patients. Stud Health Technol Inform. 2006;124:815–23.

Kouroubali A, Katehakis DG. The new European interoperability framework as a facilitator of digital transformation for citizen empowerment. J Biomed Inform. 2019;94, 103166

Kreimeyer K, Foster M, Pandey A, Arya N, Halford G, Jones SF, et al. Natural language processing systems for capturing and standardizing unstructured clinical information: a systematic review. J Biomed Inform. 2017;73:14–29.

Krumm R, Semjonow A, Tio J, Duhme H, Burkle T, Haier J, et al. The need for harmonized structured documentation and chances of secondary use - results of a systematic analysis with automated form comparison for prostate and breast cancer. J Biomed Inform. 2014;51:86–99.

Kruse CS, Kristof C, Jones B, Mitchell E, Martinez A. Barriers to electronic health record adoption: a systematic literature review. J Med Syst. 2016;40(12):252.

Kuhn T, Basch P, Barr M, Yackel T, Medical Informatics Committee of the American College of Physicians. Clinical documentation in the 21st century: executive summary of a policy position paper from the American College of Physicians. Ann Intern Med. 2015;162(4):301–3.

Lardon J, Asfari A, Souvignet J, Trombert-Paviot B, Bousquet C. Improvement of diagnosis coding by analysing EHR and using rule engine: application to the chronic kidney disease. Stud Health Technol Inform. 2015;210:120–4.

Lawrence JE, Cundall-Curry D, Stewart ME, Fountain DM, Gooding CR. The use of an electronic health record system reduces errors in the National Hip Fracture Database. Age Ageing. 2018;48(2):285–90.

Leahy-Warren P, Mulcahy H, Benefield L, Bradley C, Coffey A, Donohoe A, et al. Conceptualising a model to guide nursing and midwifery in the community guided by an evidence review. BMC Nurs. 2017;16:1–13.

Leary A, Tomai B, Swift A, Woodword A, Hurst K. Nurse staffing levels and outcomes – mining the UK national data sets for insight. Int J Health Care Qual Assur. 2017;30(3):235–47.

Linder JA, Schnipper JL, Middleton B. Method of electronic health record documentation and quality of primary care. J Am Med Inform Assoc. 2012;19(6):1019–24.

Liu CH, Lee TT, Mills ME. The experience if informatics nurses in Taiwan. J Prof Nurs. 2015;31(2):158–64.

Lodhi KM, Ansari R, Yao Y, Keenan GM, Wilkie DJ, Khokhar A. A framework to predict outcome for cancer patients using data from a nursing EHR. IEEE International Conference on Big Data. 2016:3387–95.

Lokuge S, Sedera D, Grover V, Xu D. Organizational readiness for digital innovation: development and empirical calibration of a construct. Inf Manag. 2018:1–17. https://doi.org/10.1016/j. im.2018.09.001.

Lorenzetti DL, Quan H, Lucyk K, Cunningham C, Hennessy D, Jiang J, et al. Strategies for improving physician documentation in the emergency department: a systematic review. BMC Emerg Med. 2018;18(1):36.

Loui RP, Hollinshead A. Efficient population of structured data forms for medical records using syntactic constraints and intermediate text. 2016 IEEE International Conference on Healthcare Informatics (ICHI), 2016. p. 317.

Macieira T, Smith M, Davis N, Yao Y, Wilkie D, Dunn Lopez K, et al. Evidence of progress in making nursing practice visible using standardized nursing data: a systematic review. AMIA Annu Symp Proc. 2017:1205–14.

Maeung D, Davis D, Tomcavage J, Graf T, Procopio K. Improving patient experience by transforming primary care: evidence from Geisinger's patient-centred medical homes. Pop Health Manag. 2013;16(3):157–63.

Martin KS, Monsen KA, Bowles KH. The Omaha system and meaningful use: applications for practice, education, and research. Comput Inform Nurs. 2011;29(1):52–8.

Mason DJ, Jones DA, Roy C, Sullivan CG, Woods LJ. Commonalities of nurse-designed models of health care. Nurs Outlook. 2015;63(5):540–53.

McBrien KA, Souri S, Symonds NE, Rouhi A, Lethebe BC, Williamson TS, et al. Identification of validated case definitions for medical conditions used in primary care electronic medical record databases: a systematic review. J Am Med Inform Assoc. 2018;25(11):1567–78.

McMurray A, Ward L, Johnson K, Yang L, Connor M. The primary health care nurse of the future: preliminary evaluation of the nurse navigator role in integrated care. Collegian. 2018;25:517–24.

Mehta R, Radhakrishnan NS, Warring CD, Jain A, Fuentes J, Dolganiuc A, et al. The use of evidence-based, problem-oriented templates as a clinical decision support in an inpatient electronic health record system. Appl Clin Inform. 2016;7(3):790–802.

Monsen K, Melton-Meaux G, Timm J, Westra B, Kerr M, Raman N, et al. An empiric analysis of Omaha system targets. Appl Clin Inform. 2011;2(3):317–30.

Morais SC, da Nobrega MM, de Carvalho EC. Convergence, divergence and diagnostic accuracy in the light of two nursing terminologies. Rev Bras Enferm. 2015;68(6):1086–92.

Müller-Staub M. Preparing nurses to use standardized nursing language in the electronic health record. Stud Health Technol Inform. 2009;146:337–41.

Müller-Staub M, Needham I, Odenbreit M, Lavin MA, van Achterberg T. Improved quality of nursing documentation: results of a nursing diagnoses, interventions, and outcomes implementation study. Int J Nurs Terminol Classif. 2007;18(1):5–17.

Müller-Staub M, Needham I, Odenbreit M, Lavin MA, van Achterberg T. Implementing nursing diagnostics effectively: cluster randomized trial. Journal of Advanced Nursing (Wiley-Blackwell). 2008;63(3):291–301.

Murphy S, Mc Mullin R, Brennan S, Meehan TC. Exploring implementation of the careful nursing philosophy and professional practice model© in hospital-based practice. J Nurs Manag. 2018;26(3):263–73.

Murray T, Berberian L. The importance of structured data elements in EHRs: Computer World; 2011.

Nelson-Brantley HV, Ford D, Miller KL, Bott MJ. Nurse executives leading change to improve critical access hospital outcomes: a literature review with research-informed recommendations. Online J Rural Nurs Health Care. 2018;18(1):148–79.

Nguyen L, Bellucci E, Nguyen LT. Electronic health records implementation: an evaluation of information system impact and contingency factors. Int J Med Inform. 2014;83(11):779–96.

Nursing and Midwifery Board Ireland. Code of professional conduct and ethics. Dublin: NMBI; 2014.

Nursing and Midwifery Council. The Code: Professional standards of practice and behaviour for nurses, midwives and nursing associates. London: NMC; 2018.

Obermeyer Z, Emanuel EJ. Predicting the future – big data, machine learning, and clinical medicine. N Engl J Med. 2016;375(13):1216–9.

O'Donnell A, Kaner E, Shaw C, Haighton C. Primary care physicians' attitudes to the adoption of electronic medical records: a systematic review and evidence synthesis using the clinical adoption framework. BMC Med Inform Decis Mak. 2018;18(1):101.

Oreofe A, Oyenike A. Transforming practice through nursing innovative patient centered care: standardized nursing languages. Int J Caring Sci. 2018;11(2):1319–22.

Parent C. How EHRs can give time back to docs. Health Management Technology. 2017.

Plastiras P, O'Sullivan D. Exchanging personal health data with electronic health records: a standardized information model for patient generated health data and observations of daily living. Int J Med Inform. 2018;120:116–25.

Pomares-Quimbaya A, Kreuzthaler M, Schulz S. Current approaches to identify sections within clinical narratives from electronic health records: a systematic review. BMC Med Res Methodol. 2019;19(1):155.

Prideaux A. Issues in nursing documentation and record-keeping practice. Br J Nurs. 2011;20(22):1450.

Reid Ponte P, Somerville JG, Adams JM. Assuring the capture of standardized nursing data: a call to action for chief nursing officers. Int J Nurs Knowl. 2016;27(3):127–8.

Remus S. The big data revolution: opportunities for chief nurse executives. Nurs Leadersh. 2016;28(4):18–28.

Ricciardi W, Boccia S. New challenges of public health: bringing the future of personalised healthcare into focus. Eur J Pub Health. 2017;27(4):36–9.

Rogers ML, Sockolow PS, Bowles KH, Hand KE, George J. Use of a human factors approach to uncover informatics needs of nurses in documentation of care. Int J of Med Inform. 2013;82:1068–74.

Rosenbloom ST, Miller RA, Johnson KB, Elkin PL, Brown SH. Interface terminologies: facilitating direct entry of clinical data into electronic health record systems. J Am Med Inform Assoc. 2006;13(3):277–88.

Rosenbloom ST, Denny JC, Xu H, Lorenzi N, Stead WW, Johnson KB. Data from clinical notes: a perspective on the tension between structure and flexible documentation. J Am Med Inform Assoc. 2011;18(2):181–6.

Rosenbloom ST, Miller RA, Adams P, Madani S, Khan N, Shultz EK. Implementing an interface terminology for structured clinical documentation. J Am Med Inform Assoc. 2013;20(e1):e178–82.

Saranto K, Kinnunen UM, Kivekas E, Lappalainen AM, Liljamo P, Rajalahti E, Hyppönen H. Impacts of structuring nursing records: a systematic review. Scand J Caring Sci. 2014;28(4):629–47.

Seidling H, Bates D. Evaluating the impact of health IT on medication safety. Stud Health Technol Inform. 2016;222:195–205.

Shachak A, Montgomery C, Dow R, Barnsley J, Tu K, Jadad AR, et al. End-user support for primary care electronic medical records: a qualitative case study of users' needs, expectations and realities. Health Syst (Basingstoke). 2013;2(3):198–212.

Sheerin F. NANDA and NIC: mediators to describe Irish intellectual disability nursing. Int J Nurs Terminol Classif. 2003;14:22.

Siegler EL, Adelman R. Copy and paste: a remediable hazard of electronic health records. Am J Med. 2009;122(6):495–6.

Simpson RL. Chief nurse executives need contemporary informatics competencies. Nurs Econ. 2013;31(6):277–88.

SNOMED International. SNOMED CT starter guide. 2017.

SNOMED International. SNOMED International: leading healthcare terminology worldwide 2019. http://www.snomed.org/.

Sohn S, Wang Y, Wi CI, Krusemark EA, Ryu E, Ali MH, et al. Clinical documentation variations and NLP system portability: a case study in asthma birth cohorts across institutions. J Am Med Inform Assoc. 2017;25(3):353–9.

Staggers N, Clark L, Blaz JW, Kasandoy S. Nurses' information management and use of electronic tools during acute care handoffs. West J Nurs Res. 2011;34(2):153–73.

Staggers N, Elias BL, Makar E, Alexander GL. The imperative of solving nurses' usability problems with health information technology. J Nurs Adm. 2018;48(4):191–6.

Sundling KE, Kurtycz DFI. Standardized terminology systems in cytopathology. Diagn Cytopathol. 2019;47(1):53–63.

Tastan S, Linch GC, Keenan GM, Stifter J, McKinney D, Fahey L, et al. Evidence for the existing American Nurses Association-recognized standardized nursing terminologies: a systematic review. Int J Nurs Stud. 2014;51(8):1160–70.

Tayyib N, Coyer F, Lewis PA. A two-arm cluster randomized control trial to determine the effectiveness of a pressure ulcer prevention bundle for critically ill patients. J Nurs Scholarsh. 2015;47(3):237–47.

The Office of the National Coordinator for Health Information Technology. Standard nursing terminologies: a landscape analysis. 2017.

Thomas-Hawkins C, Flynn L, Dillon J. Registered nurse staffing, workload and nursing care left undone, and their relationships to patient safety in hemodialysis units. Neph Nurs J. 2020;47(2):133–42.

Topaz M, Golfenshtein N, Bowles KH. The Omaha system: a systematic review of the recent literature. J Am Med Inform Assoc. 2014;21(1):163–70.

Vivanti A, Lewis J, O'Sullivan TA. The nutrition care process terminology: changes in perceptions, attitudes, knowledge and implementation amongst Australian dietitians after three years. Nutr Diet. 2018;75(1):87–97.

Vuokko R, Makela-Bengs P, Hypponen H, Lindqvist M, Doupi P. Impacts of structuring the electronic health record: results of a systematic literature review from the perspective of secondary use of patient data. Int J Med Inform. 2017;97:293–303.

Warren JJ, Matney SA, Foster ED, Auld VA, Roy SL. Toward interoperability: a new resource to support nursing terminology standards. Comput Inform Nurs. 2015;33(12):515–9.

Weis JM, Levy PC. Copy, paste, and cloned notes in electronic health records. Chest. 2014;145(3):632–8.

Welton JM, Harper EM. Measuring nursing care value. Nurs Econ. 2016;34(1):7–14.

Westra BL, Delaney CW, Konicek D, Keenan G. Nursing standards to support the electronic health record. Nurs Outlook. 2008;56(5):258–66.e1.

Westra BL, Oancea C, Savik K, Marek KD. The feasibility of integrating the Omaha system data across home care agencies and vendors. Comput Inform Nurs. 2010;28(3):162–71.

Westra B, Sylvia M, Weinfurter EF, Pruinelli L, Park J-I, Dodd D, et al. Big data science: a literature review of nursing research exemplars. Nurs Outlook. 2017;65:549–61.

Wilbanks BA, Berner ES, Alexander GL, Azuero A, Patrician PA, Moss JA. The effect of data-entry template design and anesthesia provider workload on documentation accuracy, documentation efficiency, and user-satisfaction. Int J Med Inform. 2018;118:29–35.

Williams R, Kontopantelis E, Buchan I, Peek N. Clinical code set engineering for reusing EHR data for research: a review. J Biomed Inform. 2017;70:1–13.

Wood S. Effective record-keeping. Pract Nurse. 2010;39(4):20–3.

World Health Organisation. Global strategic directions for strengthening nursing and midwifery 2016–2020. Geneva, WHO. 2016a.

World Health Organisation. International statistical classification of diseases and related health problems 10th revision (ICD-10)-WHO version. 2016b.

Wrenn JO, Stein DM, Bakken S, Stetson PD. Quantifying clinical narrative redundancy in an electronic health record. J Am Med Inform Assoc. 2010;17(1):49–53.

Wuryanto E, Rahayu GR, Emilia O, Harsono, APR O. Application of an outcome present test-peer learning model to improve clinical reasoning of nursing students in the intensive care unit. Ann Trop Med Public Health. 2017;10(3):657–63.

Zanaboni P, Ngangue P, Mbemba GIC, Schopf TR, Bergmo TS, Gagnon MP. Methods to evaluate the effects of internet-based digital health interventions for citizens: systematic review of reviews. J Med Internet Res. 2018;20(6):e10202. https://doi.org/10.2196/10202.

Zaworsky D, Bower K. Care coordination: using the present to transform the future. Nurse Lead. 2016;2016:324–8.

Zhang P, Xing FM, Li CZ, Wang FL, Zhang XL. Effects of a nurse-led transitional care programme on readmission, self-efficacy to implement health-promoting behaviours, functional status and life quality among Chinese patients with coronary artery disease: a randomised controlled trial. J Clin Nurs. 2018;27(5-6):969–79.

Zhang R, Burgess ER, Reddy MC, Rothrock NE, Bhatt S, Rasmussen LV, et al. Provider perspectives on the integration of patient-reported outcomes in an electronic health record. JAMIA Open. 2019;2(1):73–80.

Chapter 8
Connected Health and the Digital Patient

Shelagh Maloney and Simon Hagens

Abstract Technology has impacted every aspect of our lives, empowering us with more choice and more information upon which to make decisions. When it comes health care, most citizens want the same thing—they want to be empowered so they can take a more active role in managing their health. They want to understand their conditions and have access to digital tools to help manage their health and be involved in their care decisions.

This is important because the evidence is clear; when citizens are engaged in their health, they have better health outcomes. In Canada, there are many examples of how citizens have affected health policy and how they are using digital tools and services to empower them to play more active roles in their care. Telehomecare, which provides citizens with the ability to monitor their conditions while at home and patient portals, that provide citizens with access to their health information, are just two examples of how technology is changing the landscape of the health system by allowing citizens to become more engaged.

Digital health technology is also changing how clinicians deliver care. While progress has been relatively slower in health than in other industries and while Canada lacks behind other countries in some areas of digital health technology, we are making significant progress. The movement toward citizen-centred care and the digital patient is not without challenges and obstacles. Ensuring that personal health information is kept confidential and secure is a major concern for many. Similarly, we must be mindful of equity issues so that access to digital health and the benefits that accrue are available to all.

As the health professionals that are most accessible to patients, nurses can play a pivotal role in ensuring that they and their patients are equipped with the skills they need to be effective digital players in the health system.

Electronic Supplementary Material The online version of this chapter (https://doi.org/10.1007/978-3-030-58740-6_8) contains supplementary material, which is available to authorized users.

S. Maloney (✉) · S. Hagens
Canada Health Infoway, Toronto, ON, Canada
e-mail: smaloney@infoway-inforoute.ca; shagens@infoway-inforoute.ca

Keywords Digital health · Patient empowerment · Personal health information
Connected care · Telemedicine · Patient portals · Privacy

Learning Objectives for the Chapter
1. Understand what is meant by citizen-centric health care and the factors that contributed to its popularity.
2. Become familiar with the benefits of patient participation in their care and provide examples of how technology has empowered the digital patient.
3. Understand the Canadian and international landscape around citizen centred care and Canada's position relative to its international peers.
4. Understand the evolution of digital health technology among clinicians and their perceptions of the benefits.
5. Become familiar with the issues that must be considered as we move toward citizen-centric care and the role of the nurse in this evolution.

8.1 Technology Has Impacted Every Aspect of Our Lives

It is hard to believe just how quickly and pervasively technology has impacted our lives. The way we work, play, shop, learn, communicate—it has all been significantly impacted by technology. The advent of the internet, for example, has led to the democratization of knowledge such that information is readily available to all. Much in the same way the printing press facilitated the spread of information uniformly among the masses in the eighteenth century, the internet has allowed for the availability and dissemination of information to reach unprecedented levels. Today, the availability of online content far outnumbers the information published in every kind of print form. This increased access to information empowers people to inform themselves and reduces their dependence on experts.

In terms of pervasiveness, 86% of Canadians reported owning a smartphone, according to a 2019 survey conducted by the Consumer Technology Association. These mobile devices have made it possible for technology to disrupt entire industries. With vast amounts of computing power and so many apps, it has never been easier to call for a ride, order food, check the weather or order a new coat.

A 2020 survey of Canadians provides a snapshot of the expanding impact of technology.[1] As per Fig. 8.1 below, online shopping, navigation, money management and scheduling are the most common ways by which citizens are embracing having key information at their fingertips and migrating transactions from face-to-face experiences to virtual.

Question: How often do you use the following pieces of technology? January 2020

[1] Survey of Canadian Citizens, Environics, March 2020, Commissioned by Canada Health Infoway.

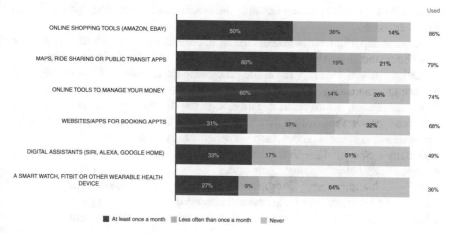

Fig. 8.1 Technology Use Among Canadians

8.1.1 Technology Has Changed the Experience and Expectations of Consumers

The primary benefits of technology are time savings and increased access to products and services.[2] Technology has changed the role and experience of the consumer. They now have choice, control and information.

Online shopping has literally 'opened the world' to consumers. Digital shopping has removed the analog constraints of time and distance. No longer limited to the bricks and mortar locations within a reasonable distance from their home, consumers now have access to products from around the globe. It is as convenient for them to see and access product details from large, global retailers as it is to check out the website of a small artisan. It is as convenient for them to shop for cheese at the local shop around the corner as it is to import cheese from France or Switzerland. This increased access to products and the ability to choose is a fundamental shift that has had a significant impact on how we shop.

Similarly, technology has given consumers more control and has put them in the driver's seat when it comes to making purchasing decisions. Consumers can now determine when they shop, no longer constrained by store hours. They are also no longer constrained by location—mobile devices make it possible to shop from home, while in transit, at a coffee shop or from a beach. If there is an internet connection, products and services can be purchased.

Finally, one of the biggest changes that consumers have seen is access to information that helps them make informed purchasing decisions. Information is usually available about the product as well as about the entire purchasing experience. While consumers contemplate their options, they can peruse detailed product specifications from the manufacturer, and they can read product reviews by other consumers like themselves. It is also worth noting that often consumer reviews include information beyond the quality of the product and address issues such as the ethical

---

[2] Survey of Canadian Citizens, Environics, March 2020, Commissioned by Canada Health Infoway.

scorecard of the seller, which expands the breadth of information upon which to base a decision.

Another important attribute about the digital consumer is their ability to rate their experience and share this information broadly. Because the digital age has vastly expanded consumer choice, the entire purchasing experience, not just the product, has become increasingly important. And consumers now have the power to share their experiences, positive and negative, with the digital world. This represents a significant power shift from sellers who controlled the message to consumers who are increasingly vocal about their experiences. And it matters; Northwestern University's Speigel Research Center reports that nearly 95% of shoppers read online reviews before making a purchase.

Why is this important? Consumers expectations have changed. They want the benefits of convenience, better access and improved decision making to extend to all aspects of their lives, including their interactions with the health system.

8.1.2   The Empowered Consumer as the Empowered Patient

Broadly stated, patient engagement is a term used to describe patients' ability and desire to being active participants in their health journey and being equipped, enabled, and empowered to do so.[3]

In the same way that the last decade has seen a shift in the role of the digital consumer, there has been an evolution in the role of the patient in healthcare. From a system where patients often had limited knowledge and limited voice, there have been a series of efforts at improvement, both from within the system and from patients themselves.

As early as 1998, the term "nothing about me without me" was coined and used as a rallying cry in the activist patient community to describe a global effort to help patients become equipped and educated so that they can participate as full members of their care team.

The patient safety movement also brought patient issues to the forefront and patient stories to the ears of policy makers. The Institute for Healthcare Improvement in the U.S. introduced the Triple Aim in 2008, which asserted the experience of the patient as critically important:

---

[3] Ferguson T. E-patients: how they can help us heal healthcare. 2007. http://e-patients.net/e-Patients_White_Paper.pdf Accessed March 15, 2015.

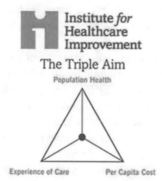

Improving the U.S. health care system requires simultaneous pursuit of three aims: improving the experience of care, improving the health of populations, and reducing per capita costs of health care. Preconditions for this include the enrollment of an identified population, a commitment to universality for its members, and the existence of an organization (an "integrator") that accepts responsibility for all three aims for that population.

A growing awareness and commitment to understanding the patient experience has brought insights and revealed concrete opportunities to do better. Patient-centred care has become a centre piece of legislation, and influenced thinking throughout health systems. There were many drivers for this change, led by a common understanding that it was the right thing to do.

Across Canada, patients and their families have played pivotal roles in shaping health policy, research and technology. For example, most health organizations and agencies have established patient and family advisory councils who influence or develop policies and processes. In 2014, The Change Foundation, an independent health policy think tank in Ontario, published *Patient/Family Advisory Councils in Ontario Hospitals: AT WORK, IN PLAY Part 3: Examples: What the Councils Changed.*[4] The report lists numerous projects where councils have had an impact. The examples are listed under five broad categories:

- Changes to hospital policy and/or programs affected by policy
- Initiatives to support infrastructure planning, re-design, signage and wayfinding
- Initiatives dealing with food
- Initiatives in staff orientation and public education
- Initiatives to create/update hospital informational materials

The Canadian Institute for Health Research[5] (CIHR) is another example of an organization that is embracing patient-centred care and research. Wanting to include patients as proactive partners in health research rather than passive receptors, CIHR launched Strategy for Patient-Oriented Research (SPOR). Patient oriented research

---

[4] https://changefoundation.ca/wp-content/uploads/2016/05/PFAC-Part3-FINAL-web.pdf.
[5] https://cihr-irsc.gc.ca/e/41204.html.

is about engaging patients as partners in the research process. This engagement helps to ensure that studies focus on patient-identified priorities, which ultimately leads to better patient outcomes.

In addition to healthcare organizations initiating patient groups, patients themselves, along with their caregivers and family members have formed grassroots patient organizations as well. *IMAGINE—Citizen Collaborating for Health,*[6] based in Alberta, for example, is a coalition of Albertans whose vision is: **a health system that is designed, and care that is delivered, in partnership with citizens, achieving the best possible experience and outcomes for patients.** IMAGINE, like most similar organizations, has four areas of strategic focus. The first is around citizen participation; connecting with citizens to create a collective voice. The second area of focus is to ensure that the citizen perspective is communicated effectively and shared extensively. A third focus for most patient organizations is the development of partnerships; collaborating with the health system to drive change. Finally, many groups have an evaluation and research component to their work; they collect and share information about best practice and/or improved patient experience.

8.1.3 Empowered Patients Have Better Health Outcomes

Patient engagement matters because there is growing evidence to suggest that engaged, empowered patients have better health outcomes. This is good for the patient and it is good for health system resources. Patients with access to their personal health information report feeling more confident and involved in managing their health and report having a better relationship with their primary care provider.[7] There is a significant association between engaged patient status and the use of digital health services; specifically, electronic personal health records and electronic prescription renewals.[8] The importance of the relationship between patient engagement and better health outcomes is nicely summarized in a 2012 quote by Leonard Kish, a health IT strategy consultant, when he wrote: *"If patient engagement were a drug, it would be the blockbuster drug of the century and malpractice not to use it"*.

Improving patient engagement and empowerment was the major driver in the global shift to providing citizens with access to their health information, according to a survey of member countries of the Global Digital Health Partnership (GDHP) (see Fig. 8.2). The GDHP is an international forum for global collaboration and sharing of evidence to guide the delivery of better digital health services within participant countries.

---

[6] https://imaginecitizens.ca/.

[7] https://infoway-inforoute.ca/en/what-we-do/blog/access-to-care/8439-meet-the-engaged-patients.

[8] https://infoway-inforoute.ca/en/what-we-do/blog/access-to-care/8439-meet-the-engaged-patients.

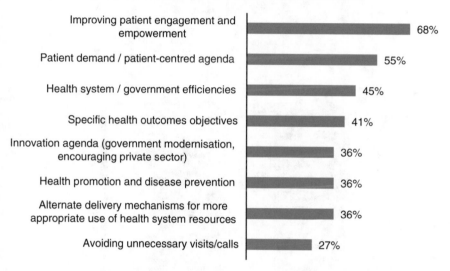

What were/are the MAJOR drivers, strategic goals or vision for value from providing citizen access to their personal health information?

Improving patient engagement and empowerment — 68%

Patient demand / patient-centred agenda — 55%

Health system / government efficiencies — 45%

Specific health outcomes objectives — 41%

Innovation agenda (government modernisation, encouraging private sector) — 36%

Health promotion and disease prevention — 36%

Alternate delivery mechanisms for more appropriate use of health system resources — 36%

Avoiding unnecessary visits/calls — 27%

Fig. 8.2 Drivers for providing citizens with access to their personal health information

Several countries—such as Estonia, Portugal, Uruguay and the Netherlands—focused on the philosophy of citizen ownership of data and centrality. Access by people to their information was described as an opportunity to address the power imbalance that exists between patients and clinicians. A number of countries that approach it as "the right thing to do" have focused on liberating the data for citizens as their primary objective, with the understanding that empowering patients is the starting point for a range of improvements. In other countries, access to information for patients is more focused on specific use cases or clinical objectives, such as post discharge care or management of chronic disease.

Other drivers for providing people with access to their personal health information include: improving the quality of care and patient experience (for example, reduction in adverse events, better coordination of care, reduced wait times, improved patient outcomes); reduction in health costs (for example, reduced duplicate testing, better self-management by patients); providing equity in access to clinical information; and ensuring patients their constitutional rights.

8.1.4 Health Care Technology: Empowering Patients

Technology is a significant driver of patient engagement. It provides patients with greater access to their health information and to digital tools that empower them to become more active members of their care team. Figure 8.3 shows results from a 2019 survey, in which nine of ten Canadians said it was important to have

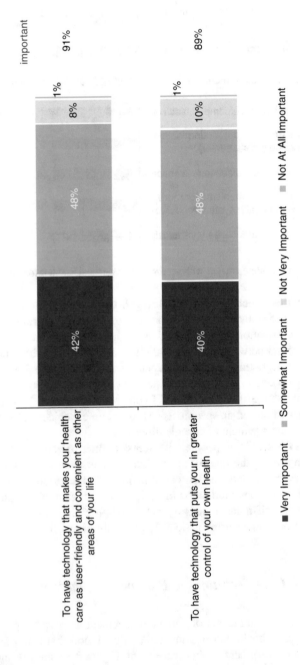

Fig. 8.3 Outcomes of digital health that are important to Canadians

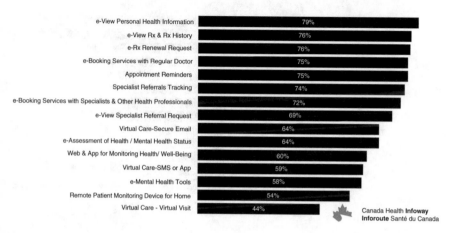

Fig. 8.4 Digital services of most interest to Canadians

technology that makes health care as convenient as other areas of their lives, and to have technology that puts them in greater control of their health (91 and 89%).[9]

Question: How important is it to you…? January 2020

Canada Health Infoway (Infoway) has been tracking Canadians' priorities and interests in digital health services for over a decade. The demand for digital health services has remained consistently high and the priorities that Canadians have identified as most important to them, are consistent over time and across geographies. Figure 8.4 below lists those digital tools and services most desired by Canadians. Not surprisingly, the benefits derived from the availability of the services listed reflect the same benefits listed by consumers: access to information, convenience (time savings), and control. Infoway has continued to test those market interests and trends and the demand remains strong for these top services, and when they are made available to them, Canadians will use them.

Question: Would you be interested in…?

8.1.5   Gap Between Desired Patient-Empowering Technology and Availability

In Canada, citizens are only beginning to experience digital health for themselves. In recent years, there has been great progress made in empowering patients with technology, however, there is a gap between the number of Canadians that want empowering technology that helps them manage their care and those that have it. In the Canadian context, "Understanding the gap between desire for and use of

---

[9] Survey of Canadian Citizens, Environics, March 2020, Commissioned by Canada Health Infoway.

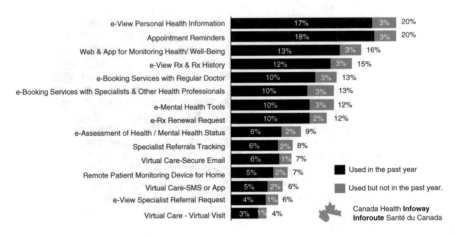

Fig. 8.5 Digital services most used by Canadians

consumer health solutions" published in 2014 presented this gap and reinforced the significant demand.[10]

A 2019 survey demonstrated that, while 79% of Canadians were interested in accessing their health information, only 20% of Canadians had done so. Similarly, while 75% expressed interest in e-booking an appointment with their regular care provider, only 13% had done so. Similar gaps exist for most services including electronically renewing a prescription (76% interest vs 12% who did) and virtual visits through email (64% interest vs 7% actual use). Figure 8.5, lists citizen utilization for selected digital health services.

Question: In the past year, did you? Have you ever?

8.1.6   International Progress

Internationally, the Commonwealth Fund International Health Policy Surveys collect experiences and perspectives from citizens and primary care physicians on a rotating basis. The data provide a sense of how the landscape is evolving across the ten or so participating countries on topics such as access to care, coordination of patient care, and use of information technology. The 2019 Commonwealth fund survey polled primary care doctors in 11 countries, including more than 2500 Canadian primary care physicians. This survey found that on average 37% of respondents across countries reported that their patients can view test results online, while 26% can view patient summaries[11] (see Fig. 8.6 below). Electronic booking

---

[10] https://www.longwoods.com/content/23871/healthcarepapers/understanding-the-gap-between-desire-for-and-use-of-consumer-health-solutions.

[11] https://www.cihi.ca/en/commonwealth-fund-survey-2019.

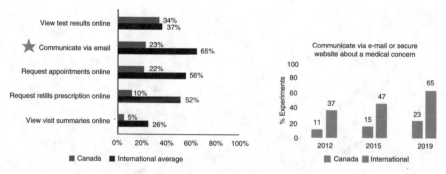

Fig. 8.6 Online services available to patients: comparison of Canada to international average

and prescription renewals are now becoming mainstream services, reportedly offered by more than half of respondents. These services are very popular because of the convenience they offer for patients; they also offer efficiencies for clinicians and administrative staff.[12]

The opportunity to communicate by email was the leading digital health tool that primary care physicians internationally report offering to their patients. For this metric, the question had been asked in previous waves of the survey, thus providing a snapshot of the rapid evolution of virtual visits. In 2012 it was a feature offered by 37% of respondents and by 2019 that number had increased to 65%. While this pace of change is slow in comparison to diffusion of many kinds of technology, health system change is demonstrably slower than in many other sectors. A closer examination of the simple exchange of messaging between patients and their care providers reveals the complexity of this change.

Availability of technology at both the patient and provider end is a necessity, but requires a higher bar for authentication, privacy and security than most electronic communications. The email citizens and providers use in day to day life is often not sufficient for the purpose. More importantly, clinical communication represents a very different approach to the processes by which clinicians assess health problems, arrive at diagnoses, determine treatment plans and work with patients to action those plans. Email is clearly appropriate only in some situations, and the evidence continues to evolve about how this kind of communication can be best used. Through this lens, the progress from 37% in 2012 to 65% internationally over 7 years should be viewed as a dramatic shift in healthcare delivery.

As per Fig. 8.6 below, Canada lags behind our international peers in making online services available for patients. While there are many reasons that have contributed to a slower uptake in Canada, clinician reimbursement for digital services for patients has been a challenge, with many physicians still paid based on the

---

[12] Doty, Michelle M., et al. "Primary Care Physicians' Role In Coordinating Medical And Health-Related Social Needs In Eleven Countries: Results from a 2019 survey of primary care physicians in eleven high-income countries about their ability to coordinate patients' medical care and with social service providers." Health Affairs 39.1 (2020): 115–123.

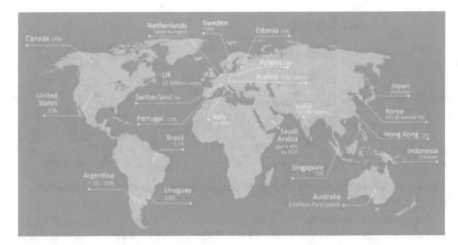

Fig. 8.7 Reported Citizen Adoption Rates for Selected GDHP Countries

delivery of discrete in-person services. Health system payers seeking to ensure that funds are spent as efficiently as possible have been reluctant to provide billing codes for online services which are harder to define and value. Newer models of primary care organizations, with innovations like team-based primary care and capitation for rostered patients have been helping to address some of these reimbursement challenges.

Question: Please indicate whether your practice offers your patients the option to communicate with your practice via email or a secure website about a medical question or concern? Request appointments online? Request refills/renewals for prescriptions online? View test results online? View patient visit summaries online?

Commonwealth Fund 2019 International Health Policy Survey of Primary Care Physicians in 11 Countries

Similar adoption rates were reported by those member countries of the GDHP (see Fig. 8.7).

8.1.7 Examples of Patient Empowering Technologies

There are many digital health examples, such as telehomecare (also know as Home Telehealth, Remote Patient Monitoring (RPM)) and patient portals. This section will provide evidence that these digital health tools can empower patients and provide tangible value for the health system as well as a compelling return on investment.

Telehomecare interventions have been used in various forms for decades. The literature includes many studies across a range of technologies that support people with chronic conditions to better manage their health at home with the support of clinical guidance and monitoring. The variability has made these hard to characterize as a whole, finding largely positive effects and great variability in efficacy and adverse effects.[13,14]

In Canada, a 2014 report, "Connecting Patients with Providers: A Pan-Canadian Study on Remote Patient Monitoring", helped Canada focus on the most promising interventions.[15] The report defined four streams of activity:

1. Enabling Information: The provision of information relating to a patient's condition through websites, patient portals and mobile applications. Enabling information may exist as a component of RPM programs, but is limited to the provision of information about a patient's condition, such as their care plan and medication regime.
2. Self-Monitoring: Programs in which patients report their health information through an enabling technology at regular intervals to a care provider. Interventions are triggered when thresholds aligned to a patient's health status are surpassed.
3. Assisted Monitoring: Programs involving patient monitoring or coaching at prescribed intervals, through the direct use of community care professionals, when complex patients are discharged into the community.
4. Environmental Monitoring: Programs designed for highly complex patients (e.g., those with a functional disability and/or multiple, complex comorbidities) involving the use of installed devices that monitor their ability to live independently. Self-monitoring is not typically a component of these programs.

With costs and health system complexity increasing dramatically across these streams, the report included a framework to help system planners consider the most appropriate interventions for different patient groups (see Fig. 8.8).

In Canada, the results of early pilots in telehomecare demonstrated strong efficacy and patient satisfaction for moderately complex patients with Congestive Heart Failure (CHF) and Chronic Obstructive Pulmonary Disease (COPD). This led to accelerated deployment in many provinces, reaching over 50,000 Canadians by 2020. Evaluations from these projects demonstrated significant reductions in utilization of health system resources consistently across the country, and despite the high cost of these intensive interventions represented a return on investment of $4 in worth of system capacity for every 1$ invested.[16]

As the expansion of telehomecare and the vast range of other monitoring technology continues to expand, the critical success factors identified in "Connecting Patients with Providers" offers guidance for system planners trying to ensure the best outcomes and value for money:

[13] https://onlinelibrary.wiley.com/doi/abs/10.1111/j.1365-2753.2010.01536.x.

[14] https://journals.sagepub.com/doi/abs/10.1258/jtt.2009.090812.

[15] https://www.infoway-inforoute.ca/en/component/edocman/1918-rpm-benefits-evaluation-study-full-report-final/view-document?Itemid=0.

[16] https://www.infoway-inforoute.ca/en/what-we-do/blog/telehomecare/7846-telehomecare-receiving-high-marks-from-patients-while-providing-significant-value-for-the-health-care-system.

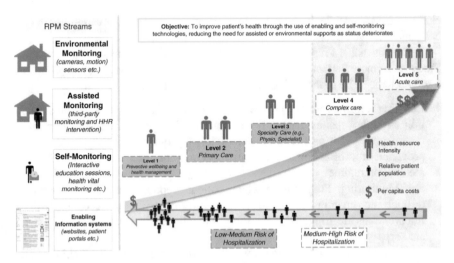

Fig. 8.8 Framework to illustrate the relationship between technological complexity and patient acuity

1. Engagement and collaboration. As clinicians are at the forefront of understanding the clinical complexity of patients, they should assist in designing an RPM program, along with the patient and/or caregiver, including the selection of appropriate technology that aligns with a patient's acuity and health care requirements. Clinicians are uniquely positioned to describe and deliver a compelling value proposition to potential patients, facilitating greater recruitment and retention.

2. Patient recruitment and retention. This is to ensure that providers identify patients that can benefit from the RPM program based on the complexity of the patient's condition, potential benefit from using the supporting technology and the actual technology involved. Appropriate recruitment and retention of patients relies on a consistent level of communication with patients regarding both the benefits of the program and the potential to track progress towards improving their health status throughout the duration of the program. The analysis also found that achieving a critical mass of patients is necessary to maximize benefits, recover program costs and return savings to the health system for reinvestment. This minimum number of patients was found to be highly variable and dependent on the scope and design of the program.

3. Benefits measurement. As RPM programs remain a relatively new care delivery enabler in Canada, determining likely benefits and consistently measuring those benefits will allow patients, clinicians and policymakers to understand the patient and system-level value RPM programs provide.

4. Integrated care and care-coordination. RPM should be integrated into a clinician's workflow through an assisted or environmental monitoring program, or coordinated across the care continuum through a self-management program to achieve the best patient benefit.

These programs, that are better for the health system as well as patients and their families, all have patient engagement in common. The derived value includes staying healthy and out of hospital and making judicious use of the health system, preserving capacity in stretched systems.

A Life Transformed

Since its launch, Eastern Health's Remote Patient Monitoring (RPM) program has been transforming patients' lives. It's been helping them stay at home instead of the hospital and it's helping them avoid trips to the emergency room. Joy Williams is one such patient. Since enrolling in the program, Joy has stopped using her blood pressure medication, left behind her walking stick and, best of all, is now able to spend more time with her energetic granddaughter.

That's because the program enabled Joy, who has diabetes, to monitor her condition using digital health tools and share the information electronically with a registered nurse in another community. Through the RPM (which is also known as telehomecare) program, she can access round-the-clock coaching, education and support that has enabled her to improve her condition.

Life was very different for Joy before enrolling in the program. She had been living with diabetes for two decades, and as a result, went on to develop hypertension and became insulin-dependent. "It seemed like no matter what I did, I just couldn't wrestle my diabetes symptoms under control," she says. "I was taking massive amounts of insulin and still not accomplishing the target levels that were suggested by my health care providers."

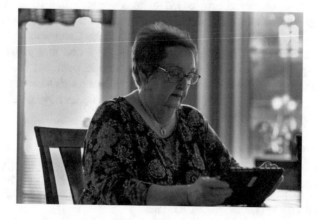

Joy's struggle with diabetes eventually led to osteoarthritis, forcing her to walk with a cane and rely on her two adult children to help complete everyday tasks. "It felt like my entire world was shrinking and I was really helpless," she says. "It was a really awful feeling." Things changed when a friend handed Joy a brochure for the RPM program which she had come across at an Eastern Health fair.

Within a week of reaching out to the RPM team, Joy received a tablet, which she used to connect to a registered nurse who remotely monitored and coached her. "It was all really instrumental in teaching me how to recognize and treat my condition, and better yet, how to avoid having symptoms altogether," she says. "That was invaluable to me because I didn't know how to do that before." Just seven months later, Joy was able to get her diabetes under control, lose weight, decrease her medication consumption, lower her blood pressure and start walking without a cane.

Patient portals often offer patients access to their own personal health information in a secure setting, and can include other information resources and e-services. "Citizen Access to Data: An international review of country approaches to citizen access to health data", a white paper by the Global Digital Health Partnership explored the value of citizen access. The primary drivers identified by most countries was citizen demand and the belief that citizens should be more engaged and empowered. However, many also identified tangible benefits they expected, including health system efficiencies, improved health outcomes, better health promotion and disease prevention and avoided visits or calls by patients. Some countries who are further ahead in the journey report experiencing many of these benefits.

The peer-reviewed literature around patient access to information is still thin, as these technologies have rapidly expanded only in recent years. One recent systematic review found "Patient portals are increasingly available, but their impact on health outcomes has yet to be established. Previous systematic reviews found positive effects on patient engagement and satisfaction, but evidence on the effect of patient portal use on care processes and health outcomes is conflicting."[17]

Evidence from Canadian project evaluations suggests that impacts of patient access to information can vary substantially based upon the functionality, ease of use, complementary educational resources, etc. "Valuing Canadians' Access to their Health Information and Digital Health e-Services"[18] found that patient access to their own information has some significant value on its own, but when combined with the ability to visit with care providers virtually through video or messaging, and the ability to renew prescriptions electronically unlocks huge potential for citizens (Fig. 8.9) and the health system (Fig. 8.10).

---

[17] Fraccaroa P, Vigoc M, Balatsoukasb P, Buchana IE, Peeka N, van der Veerb SN. Patient portal adoption rates: a systematic literature review and meta-analysis. In MEDINFO 2017: Precision healthcare through informatics: proceedings of the 16th World Congress on Medical and Health Informatics 2018 Jan 31 (Vol. 245, p. 79). IOS Press.

[18] https://infoway-inforoute.ca/en/component/edocman/3552-valuing-canadians-secure-access-to-their-health-information-and-digital-health-eservices/view-document?Itemid=0.

	Current Benefit Adoption (2016–2017)	25% Adoption	Potential Value 35% Adoption	50% Adoption
e-view Viewing of digital medical records	7% - 8% $36M – $39M	$122M	$171M	$244M
e-visit Secure e-communications (Outpatient care)	5% - 8% $26M – $42M	$132M	$185M	$265M
virtual visit Face-to-ace Videoconference	3% - 4% $14M – $18M	$110M	$154M	$221M
e-RX renew Digital prescription renewal	10% - 12% $42M – $50M	$105M	$147M	$210M
Total	$119M – $150M	$470M	$658M	$940M

Fig. 8.9 Estimated Potential Value for Canadian **Citizens:** "Valuing Canadians' Access to their Health Information and Digital Health e-Services"

	Current Benefit Adoption (2016–2017)	25% Adoption	Potential Value 35% Adoption	50% Adoption
e-view Viewing of digital medical records	7% - 8% $81– 96M	$272-293M	$381-409M	$543-583M
e-visit Secure e-communications (Outpatient care)	5% - 8% $6-15M	$19-27M	$26-35M	$36-46M
virtual visit Face-to-Face Videoconference	3% - 4% $1.8-2.3M ($27-54M)*	$14M ($927M-5B)	$20M ($1.3-7B)	$28M ($1.9-10B)
e-RX renew Digital prescription renewal	10% - 12% $18M – $20M	$57M	$79M	$113M
Total	$106–134M $13– 85M	$362–391M ($1.3-5.4B)	$505–543M ($1.8-7.5B)	$720–769M $(2.6-10.7B)

Fig. 8.10 Estimated Potential Value for Canadian **Health Systems:** "Valuing Canadians' Access to their Health Information and Digital Health e-Services"

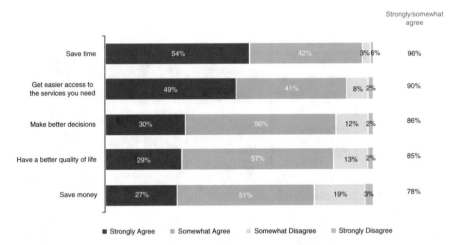

Fig. 8.11 Impacts of Digital Tools when Accessing for Common Services in Canada

This broad range of value is also evident from the feedback of citizen users of digital health tools, with saving time and improving access as leading benefits (Fig. 8.11).

Question: To what extent do you agree or disagree that these types of technology have helped you?

Mobile health apps and smart connected devices are also gaining popularity as mechanisms by which Canadians are empowering themselves to monitor their health. In 2017, researchers in Quebec published the first national study "The Diffusion of mobile health apps and smart connected devices in Canada", a study that examined Canadians' use and intentions for using mobile apps and smart devices to monitor health and well-being. It was the first national study of its kind in Canada, and the largest ever, worldwide.[19] The study found that two thirds (66%) of respondents regularly self-track one or more aspects of their health and one in four (25%) owned a wearable or smart medical device. Fitness trackers and smartwatches device made up the majority of these devices. Mobile apps and digital self-tracking devices were most commonly used for physical activity (51%), diet and nutrition (33%) and sleep (29%). Clinical tools were less common with some reporting functionality like monitoring cardiovascular and pulmonary biomarkers (13%), medication management (8%), and glucose monitoring (5%). Most users of connected care technologies are highly satisfied (83%) and many said they were able to maintain or improve their health condition (69%).

The results of the study show an opportunity to advance the health of Canadians through mobile apps and smart devices; and highlight important nuances to better understand key market segments and opportunities.

---

[19] Paré G, Leaver C, Bourget C, Diffusion of the Digital Health Self-Tracking Movement in Canada: Results of a National Survey, J Med Internet Res 2018;20(5):e177.

8.2 Health Information Technology and the Clinician

A discussion of the connected patient is not complete without a discussion of the evolution of health information technology for clinicians and for the system as a whole because citizens' experiences and relationships with the health system contribute to the development of their attitudes.[20]

In terms of medical technology in general, imaging, monitoring and interventional tools have always been a visible part of the healthcare landscape but health information technology has lagged. Many are familiar with the image of large paper charts unreliably following patients around institutions and the system.

To address this lag, the federal government funded the creation of Canada Health Infoway in 2001. Infoway is an independent, not-for-profit organization that works with its jurisdictional partners (provincial/territorial ministries/departments of health) and other stakeholders to improve the health of Canadians through digital health solutions. In the early years, the focus of Infoway investment was on the creation of electronic health records (EHRs). Moving information from paper to electronic/digital form greatly facilitated information sharing. Efforts in this regard were focused on lab information systems, drug information systems, diagnostic imaging and provider and patient registries. By 2019, much of this work was complete and approximately $30 Billion CAD in benefits with respect to improved quality (e.g. fewer drug interactions, better access to information for decision making), improved access to care (e.g. through telehealth initiatives) and greater system efficiency (e.g. fewer repeat lab tests) were generated.

Once the foundational building blocks were largely in place, focus shifted away from the infrastructure and to the clinician. Specifically, to the adoption of electronic medical records (EMRs). An EMR is a computer-based patient record specific to a single clinical practice, such as a family health team or group practice. In clinical settings where there are doctors, nurses, dietitians, pharmacists, and other health care professionals, EMRs improve communication between them and support productivity.

The adoption of EMRs in Canada, and internationally, was significant. The Commonwealth Fund, has conducted an international survey of primary care physicians on a roughly 3-year cycle since 2006.[21] In 2006, the average adoption of electronic medical records was at 64% in the relatively advanced group of countries included in the survey. By 2019, that number had risen to 93% and many other aspects of healthcare delivery had made similar gains, including a growing number of hospitals and health systems with advanced patient record systems which make possible analytics and other important opportunities for health system improvement (Fig. 8.12).

---

[20] CARTER-LANGFORD, Abigail, and David WILJER. "The eHealth trust model: a patient privacy research framework." Improving Usability, Safety and Patient Outcomes with Health Information Technology: From Research to Practice 257 (2019): 382.

[21] Reference most recent.

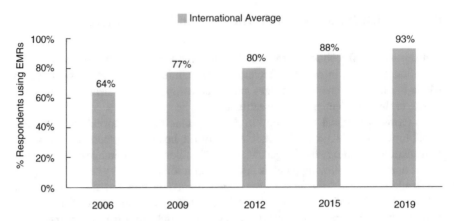

Fig. 8.12 Average Electronic Medical Record Adoption Rate for Countries Participating in the Commonwealth Fund International Survey of Primary Care Physicians

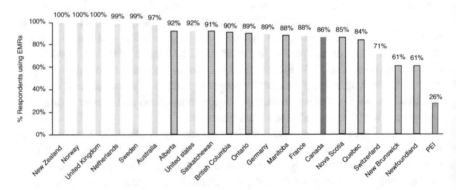

Fig. 8.13 2019 International and Canadian Provincial EMR Use Comparison

Question: Do you use electronic patient medical records in your practice (not including billing systems)?

In Canada, 86% of primary care physicians were using an EMR by 2019. It is worth noting, however, that there was substantial variability of adoption rates by jurisdiction (Fig. 8.13) and that growth in EMR use continues.

Question: Do you use electronic patient medical records in your practice (not including billing systems)?

8.3 Impact of Information Technology on Clinicians

For clinicians, the shift to EMRs has included a mix of improvements and positive impacts, as well as additional issues and stresses. In Canada, nurses, pharmacists and physicians were asked about impacts on productivity (see Table 8.1) and quality (see Table 8.2) revealing stories that are similar.

Table 8.1 Reported impact on productivity by Canadian clinicians

	Increased (%)	No change/Don't know (%)	Decreased (%)
Nurses with electronic records (2017)	50	27	23
Pharmacists with access to lab results (2016)	54	36	10
Physicians with electronic records (2013)	47	35	18

Table 8.2 Impact of electronic record keeping on quality of care

	Increased (%)	No change/Don't know (%)	Decreased (%)
Nurses with electronic records (2017)	56	34	10
Pharmacists with access to lab results (2016)	85	15	–
Physicians with electronic records (2013)	62	33	6

Productivity increases were experienced by about half in each group of respondents. Those experiencing increased productivity were more likely to be long term users of the solutions in question and more likely to work in a paperless environment. Some reported decreases in productivity by 10–23%, which is a substantive issue. Evidence points to the importance for change management, including workflow redesign to optimize productivity.

Quality increases were more commonly reported than productivity and reported decreases in quality were much rarer. These findings suggest that while the change introduces new risks overall, there are important gains increasingly being generated from digital health. More experience with digital health or use of more functionalities increases the likelihood of clinicians reporting quality of care improvements.

With such rapid change in digital health over the last decade, the peer-reviewed literature lags and many important research questions about the relationship between digital health and quality of care remain outstanding. However, findings are generally consistent with the sentiments identified in the clinician surveys. One systematic review from 2016 found that electronic health records "when properly implemented, can improve the quality of care, increasing time efficiency and guideline adherence and reducing medication errors and adverse drug events. Strategies for implementation should be therefore recommended and promoted."[22] Importantly, this study emphasized the potential value, but recognized that context and specifics of digital health initiatives can create a range of positive and negative outcomes.

Considering the variability of experiences with digital health, understanding the barriers or considerations for achieving value is important. While this topic is a

---

[22] https://academic.oup.com/eurpub/article/26/1/60/2467302.

complex one and increasingly a focus of study, clinician surveys again provide an early indication of where to focus.

Canadian nurses report a set of interconnected issues that generally relate to the range of disparate systems and processes they need to work with. Working across multiple systems, specifically having a mix of paper and electronic information is top of the list. For electronic solutions, login challenges are prevalent and closely relate to other concerns around workflows, equipment, etc. The multiple systems also create issues with fragmented patient information within healthcare organizations but more importantly when patients move between different parts of the health system.

It is important to recognize that patients will have different experiences, attitudes and perceptions about health information technology. It is equally important to understand that the same is true for clinicians. The availability of digital health solutions in different work settings, personal experiences with the technology and other factors all contribute to the clinicians' ability and desire to empower patients and help them use the available technology to better manage their health.

8.4 Considerations

There is no question that technology has had a positive impact on the way care is delivered. It has given clinicians access to more information upon which to base care decisions and has facilitated the sharing of information among the entire care team, including the patient. The use of wearable technology, sensors and other devices has provided us with more data upon which to make decisions, predict outcomes and effect change. In fact, 82% of Canadians surveyed in 2019 reported feeling that technology can help solve many of the issues within the health system.

It would be naive, however, to believe that technology is not without its challenges and that there are no important considerations that must be acknowledged and discussed if we are to ensure that the five tenets of the Canada Health Act are to be maintained and that all Canadians benefit from Canada's universal health system.

According to a 2019 Environics survey, concern about the privacy and security of their health data was the primary concern for Canadians with 78% stating that it was a significant barrier (39%) or somewhat of a barrier (39%). As per Fig. 8.14 below, other areas of concern included the cost of technology, health and technology literacy issues, perceived inability to navigate the system and lack of internet access.

Question: How much of a barrier, if at all, are the following to your own use digital health technology?

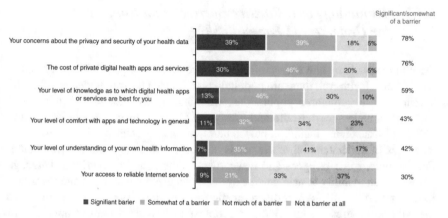

Fig. 8.14 Barriers to the Use of Digital Health Technology reported by Canadian Citizens

8.4.1   Privacy and Security

Concerns about privacy and security of their health information is consistently the most commonly cited barrier to digital health technology by Canadians. High profile data privacy breaches are a regular occurrence in Canada and while Canadians accept that technology associated with the financial sector has methods to help victims of privacy breaches when their data is compromised, they don't see how government and health care providers can offer similar protections and assurances about health information.

It is also important to note that Canadians have different thresholds of concerns, depending on the situation. For example, there is considerably less concern about sharing personal health information with a care provider. Approximately 75% of Canadians are willing to have their personal health data regularly observed by their doctor so they can be alerted if at risk for a serious health condition or share genetic information with their doctor so they can be informed about health risks. Willingness to share personal health data with private organizations decreases significantly, to 28%.

Similarly, Canadians are willing to share their anonymized health data to contribute to the 'greater good'. Most will share their data to help diagnose and treat other Canadians with conditions like theirs (82%), improve the performance of the health system (81%) and help advance scientific research (82%).

Furthermore, privacy and security concerns are more prevalent among different segments of the population. Older respondents, women, people born in Canada (rather than newcomers), and Indigenous peoples were more likely to report that "concerns about the privacy and security of your health data" is a barrier to use of digital health technology.

8.4.2 Technology as a Further Barrier or an Enabler for Underserved Populations?

Despite *accessibility* and *universality* being two of the five principles enshrined in the Canada Health Act, there are populations in Canada that are underserved in the system. These vulnerable populations, who include low socio-economic status (poverty, homelessness), health and lifestyle (LGBTQ+, mental health issues) and racialized Canadians (including newcomers), often encounter barriers to access to care, lack of understanding of the needs of their communities and discrimination. For example, some refugees and newcomers to the country experience language barriers or an inability to navigate the system; racialized populations and marginalized communities also report discrimination in a health system that does not have the cultural or lifestyle knowledge or context to provide a holistic approach to their care.

So, will technology enhance the access and quality of care for these populations or will it further marginalize them? When asked, 61% of Canadians felt confident that all Canadians will have equal access to health care technologies as they become available. A survey of underserved populations was also optimistic about the potential for technology to solve many of the challenges facing health care in Canada. They were especially interested in the role of technology to reduce problems of bias and discrimination and to include social determinants of health in the context of care provision. Overall, they identified the greatest benefit of incorporating more technology into the health system as its ability to empower underserved communities with more information and access to personal health information, allowing them to make informed health decisions.

8.4.3 The Digital Divide

Clearly, reliable internet access and availability to mobile phones and other technology will be imperative to ensure that the benefits of digital health are experienced by all. A single mother with three children, two part-time jobs and who relies on public transit, will benefit greatly from the ability to email or otherwise communicate with a clinician from her home after the children are asleep (no longer needing to take time off work, arrange for child care, pay for public transit etc....) as long as she has the technical means to do so.

While Canadians are increasingly connected and most have mobile phones, access to data plans or other technology must always be a consideration when talking about technology in health care so that we ensure our most vulnerable populations are helped by it and not further marginalized.[23] In 2019, 31% of Canadians

---

[23] Paré G, Leaver C, Bourget C, Diffusion of the Digital Health Self-Tracking Movement in Canada: Results of a National Survey, J Med Internet Res 2018;20(5):e177.

listed access to reliable internet as a barrier to the use of digital health technology. Most of these individuals lived in Canada's northern territories and rural regions. Similarly, older Canadians and low-income households were more inclined to identify this as a barrier.

8.4.4 Unconscious Bias

Technology can address issues of bias in health care, as machines are 'blind' to colour, ethnicity and other potential forms of bias. However, there is increasing evidence to suggest that biases may be programmed into the technology that sought to solve the problem. This is unconscious bias—prejudice or unsupported judgements in favour of or against one thing, person, or group compared to another, in a way that is usually considered unfair. Artificial intelligence (AI) is a good example to use to illustrate this point.

In many cases, AI can reduce the subjective interpretation of data, because machine learning algorithms learn to consider only the variables that improve their predictive accuracy, based on the training data used. At the same time, evidence suggests that AI models can embed human and societal biases and deploy them at scale. Often the data upon which algorithms are based are the issue. If AI models are trained on data containing human bias, then those biases remain. Bias can also be introduced into the data through how they are collected or selected for use. The introduction of AI must consider the nuances of social contexts and consider where and when human judgement is required.

8.4.5 Digital Health Literacy

As stated earlier, if a citizen is engaged in managing their health and they have the digital tools and information to do so, they are more inclined to have positive health outcomes. Their ability to use technology to be involved in their care will be influenced by their level of digital health literacy. Digital health literacy is defined as the ability to seek, find, understand, and appraise health information from electronic sources and apply the knowledge gained to addressing or solving a health problem.[24] Clearly, if a patient does not have the capacity or the ability to understand or navigate a digital health system, they will not be able to reap the related benefits. Many factors influence digital health literacy including age, socio-economic status and health status. Usually those who are elderly, have lower incomes and are less healthy, have the highest levels of digital health illiteracy. Those who are digitally

---

[24] Source: Norman CD, Skinner HA. eHealth Literacy: Essential Skills for Consumer Health in a Networked World. J Med Internet Res 2006;8(2):e9. https://doi.org/10.2196/jmir.8.2.e9.

illiterate are usually impaired in two ways; they are not comfortable with technology in general and they have a low level of understanding of their health information.

As digital health solutions become more common it will be imperative to ensure that issues of digital literacy are addressed. Co-design of solutions with patients may help overcome some of the barriers by building solutions that are user-friendly, use video, infographics and plain language (and multiple languages) so they are less intimidating. It is also important to understand that the introduction of digital health solutions may change the clinician-patient relationship in that clinicians may be asked to take on a role of digital health educator/advisor to some of their patients. It is important that they are comfortable in this role.

For clinicians, like patients, there are different levels of digital health literacy. While the next generation of clinicians will likely be the most digitally savvy to date, tailored education resources and tools can support them in using technology optimally and safely and in educating their patients to do the same. Since 2011, Canada Health Infoway has been working with three national organizations—the Canadian Association of Schools of Nursing (CASN), the Association of Faculties of Medicine (AFMC) and the Association of Faculties of Pharmacy of Canada (AFPC)—to encourage digital health education for clinicians in training. The broader work with all three organizations morphed into a faculty peer network program, the Digital Health Faculty Associations Content and Training Solutions program, which strove to provide faculty in these programs with the tools and resources to integrate health informatics into their teachings. This program received the 2017 Ted Freeman Award for Innovation in Education.

8.5 Nurses Play a Key Role

The healthcare landscape in which nurses are working has never been more complex. The patient demographic is changing such that there is an increased burden of disease on patients who are living longer. Mental health issues are becoming increasingly prevalent and the lines between health and social care are becoming more blurred. In this context, technology solutions can improve patient safety by facilitating access and exchange of information. They can empower patients with information to better manage their health.

Nurses play a pivotal role. As health professionals that are most accessible to patients, nurses can ensure that patients can effectively navigate the system, are aware of the digital options available to them and that they have the skills and confidence to use them. Likewise, nurses can advocate to ensure that technology is being used to support vulnerable and underserved populations and ensure that the benefits of digital health are enjoyed by all.

Review Questions
1. We know that technology has had a significant impact on our lives by giving us, as consumers, more control. Give one or two examples of how empowered con-

sumers have become empowered patients and describe the benefits in terms of the Triple Aim.

2. You have been asked to participate on a team that is looking to develop digital tools and strategies to improve the ability of patients and families to participate in their care. What are some strategies/tactics you might deploy throughout the project to ensure its success?

Answers

1. Technology has given consumers more choice of product, made it more convenient to shop, and given us more information about the product and the buying experience—all these changes have resulted in consumers having more control. The same benefits can accrue when these attributes are available in the health context. For example, a patient with more information about their health condition and the treatment options, can have a more informed discussion with their care team and make a decision that is best for them. A patient who can access digital tools and services at their convenience (e.g. have a virtual visit, renew prescriptions online) can save time and money and not need to take time off work or school to attend an appointment. Answers to this question should speak to the value to the patient (as per above), the value to the health of the (e.g. employing digital solutions to keep vulnerable populations from being exposed) and the cost of care (e.g. telehomecare as a mechanism to keep people at home rather than in the hospital).

2. There are many ways to ensure the success of a project designed to empower patients through technology. First and foremost, patients and their families should co-lead the design of the tools. As per the 'nothing about me, without me' principle outlined in the chapter, including patients from the outset will ensure that their views, experiences, expertise and expectations are incorporated from the beginning. Understanding and addressing some of the barriers to digital health will also be important. The chapter outlined several considerations for digital health solutions. The project team should ensure that these issues have been considered and addressed in the design and implementation plan. For example, is the solution private and secure? Will it be easy to understand by those who are not comfortable with technology and/or don't understand complex health terminology? Does the solution address the needs of vulnerable populations? Is there a way to support users post-implementation? How have patients and clinicians been engaged to help promote the solution?

Glossary

AI Artificial Intelligence

Ambient assistant living The term ambient relates to the use of unobtrusive, or non-invasive sensors, such as motion detectors, which help us understand how people live their lives and to detect when things change—a possible indicator of health decline. The goal of AAL is to enhance the quality of life of older people through the use of ICT.

CIHR Canadian Institute for Health Research

Digital consumer A trend of escalating consumer use of digital technology

GDHP Global Digital Health Partnership

ICT Information and Communication Technologies.

Independent Able to exist without dependency on another concept, variable, person

Independent living Independent living refers to a person's ability to go about their daily lives and carry out activities of daily living, without the need of help or support from others.

Older adults Typically the target group of many independent living and ICT products and services. There is no wide agreement on what age 'old' age begins. For the purposes of this chapter we will take the term older adults to refer to anyone of or over the age of 60.

Patient engagement A term used to describe patients' ability and desire to being active participants in their health journey and being equipped, enabled, and empowered to do so

Patient portal A website where patients can securely access their own medical and healthcare information

RPM Remote Patient Monitoring

Smart Home Smart Homes are domestic residences, augmented with AAL technologies and ICT-based services, that provide support to facilitate ageing-in-place

SPOR Strategy for Patient-Oriented Research

Telecare *Telecare*—the umbrella term of healthcare services planned, facilitated and delivered using technology

Telehealth Telehealth is the remote exchange of data between a patient and a healthcare professional to assist in the diagnosis and management of a health condition. Examples include blood pressure and blood glucose monitoring. These technologies are generally provided to patients with long-term health conditions such as diabetes

Telehomecare Homecare services delivered or facilitated by digital/telehealth technologies

References

Carter-Langford A, Wiljer D. The eHealth trust model: a patient privacy research framework. Stud Health Technol Inform. 2019;257:382–7.

Doty MM, et al. Primary care physicians' role in coordinating medical and health-related social needs in eleven countries: results from a 2019 survey of primary care physicians in eleven high-income countries about their ability to coordinate patients' medical care and with social service providers. Health Aff. 2020;39(1):115–23.

Ferguson T. E-patients: how they can help us heal healthcare. 2007. http://e-patients.net/e-Patients_White_Paper.pdf. Accessed 15 March 2015.

Fraccaroa P, Vigoc M, Balatsoukasb P, Buchana IE, Peeka N, van der Veerb SN. Patient portal adoption rates: a systematic literature review and meta-analysis. In: MEDINFO 2017: precision healthcare through informatics: proceedings of the 16th World Congress on Medical and Health Informatics, vol. 245. Amsterdam: IOS Press; 2018. p. 79.

https://academic.oup.com/eurpub/article/26/1/60/2467302.

https://changefoundation.ca/wp-content/uploads/2016/05/PFAC-Part3-FINAL-web.pdf.

https://cihr-irsc.gc.ca/e/41204.html.

https://imaginecitizens.ca.

https://infoway-inforoute.ca.

https://journals.sagepub.com.

https://onlinelibrary.wiley.com.

https://www.cihi.ca/en/commonwealth-fund-survey-2019.

https://www.longwoods.com.

Paré G, Leaver C, Bourget C. Diffusion of the digital health self-tracking movement in Canada: results of a National Survey. J Med Internet Res. 2018;20(5):e177.

Norman CD, Skinner HA. eHealth literacy: essential skills for consumer health in a networked world. J Med Internet Res. 2006;8(2):e9. https://doi.org/10.2196/jmir.8.2.e9.

Survey of Canadian Citizens, Environics, March 2020, Commissioned by Canada Health Infoway.

Chapter 9
Administrative Applications

Gemma Doleman and Christine Duffield

Abstract Nurse managers play a critical role in ensuring an appropriate number and mix of staff are available to ensure safe patient care is provided. When leadership decisions are effective, we see improved patient care outcomes, better staff performance, increased job satisfaction and staff retention. However, when decision making is less effective both patients and staff can be negatively impacted. The impact is particularly noticeable for patients who may experience increased adverse events, including greater risk of dying. Making evidence-based staffing decisions can be challenging for nurse managers given the complexity of today's workplace and importantly, a lack of access to real-time data. Many factors impact on their decisions including nursing shortages; challenges to skills mix (human capital such as experience and qualifications); staff stress, burnout and fatigue; changes to the complexity of patient care needs; an aging workforce and communication inefficiencies. There are many workload measurement tools used internationally, but most are not based on real-time data showing patient acuity, bed occupancy rates and the quality and availability of staffing resources, all factors which are necessary to make cost-effective staffing decisions. Instead, nurse managers are left with many static and disparate reporting systems that do not meet managerial requirements for decision-making. This can result in increased workloads and stress for nurse managers, which also ultimately impact clinical staff. Hospitals need to develop and use software systems which will harness existing data, allowing nurse managers to

Electronic Supplementary Material The online version of this chapter (https://doi.org/10.1007/978-3-030-58740-6_9) contains supplementary material, which is available to authorized users.

G. Doleman (✉)
School of Nursing and Midwifery, Edith Cowan University, Perth, WA, Australia
e-mail: g.doleman@ecu.edu.au

C. Duffield
School of Nursing and Midwifery, Edith Cowan University, Perth, WA, Australia

Faculty of Health, University of Technology Sydney, Sydney, NSW, Australia
e-mail: christine.duffield@uts.edu.au

extract, analyze and interpret data in a timely manner to support appropriate and safe nurse staffing decisions.

Keywords Nurse manager · Nursing workloads · Nurse staffing · Software systems · Dashboards · Patient outcomes

Learning Objectives for the Chapter
1. Discuss the role of the nurse manager in the deployment and allocation of nursing resources to meet patient care needs.
2. Examine the factors which impact nursing workload and analyze the advantages and disadvantages of current workload measurement tools used.
3. Explain nursing sensitive outcomes and how these are measured in the healthcare system.
4. Describe the complex factors that impact on managerial decision making and nursing workloads.
5. Discuss the implications of staffing a ward with an insufficient number of nurses or poor skill mix.
6. Discuss some of the administrative data which could be useful in nurse staffing decisions.

9.1 Introduction

Over the last decade there have been many changes impacting on nursing work including changes to patient mix and acuity, restructuring of services, bed shortages, cost containment measures and staff shortages (Kutney-Lee et al. 2013; Boudrias et al. 2019). These factors increase complexity in the workplace and are expected to have an impact on the workload of nurses, stress levels and overall job satisfaction. In addition, more sophisticated technologies are now used in health and there are ever-increasing consumer expectations (Duffield et al. 2019a). It has been the responsibility of nurse managers, as part of the administrative team leading the largest workforce in most health facilities, to guide their staff through these changes by maintaining adequate communication (Doleman 2017), appropriate staff allocation and skills mix (human capital), and to offer staff support and guidance as needed. The use of informatics by nursing management has been identified as an important part of the future of nursing, propelling the profession towards health systems transformation. This shift is expected to create a whole of systems approach that focuses on patient safety, use of evidence-based practice, collaboration amongst and between health professionals and improvement of patient health (Remus and Kennedy 2012; Barron McBride 2005). This chapter is focused on the administrative application of informatics in nursing. Current workforce trends, skills mix, workloads, patient outcomes, and current data limitations will be outlined.

9.2   The Nurse Manager Role

Nurse managers play a critical role in the delivery of health care services, by creating positive work environments and ensuring organizational obligations are met (Labrague et al. 2018). While managerial responsibilities may vary slightly across healthcare organizations, the nurse manager has one of the most demanding roles, ensuring standards of care are being met, ensuring successful deployment of a skilled and trained workforce and overseeing patient care (Scott and Timmons 2017). When leadership decision-making is effective, staff performance improves and this has been linked to quality of care, increased job satisfaction (Scott and Timmons 2017), and retention of the workforce. However, when nurse leaders fail or are unable to make appropriate staffing decisions, patient outcomes are negatively affected, reducing patient safety and in some cases, death can result (Department of Health 2010).

In recent times, there has been much debate about using generic non-clinical business managers rather than nurses with knowledge and expertise from both the clinical and management disciplines. There is a view that managing the complexity of the current healthcare environment, including the changes in patient demand, acuity and occupancy as well as unplanned admissions and staffing, and the impact these factors have on staffing decisions, can only be undertaken with knowledge and experience in the clinical setting (Duffield et al. 2019a). However, another view is that nurse managers cannot successfully reconcile the values and skills required of being a manager with those of a clinician, arguing that lay managers are necessary for effective decision-making, particularly where resources are concerned (Stanley 2016).

New Zealand adopted this latter view, introducing non-clinical managers in the 1990s. These managers had a background in business and managed finances, staffing and logistics of hospital wards. However, following implementation of these changes to nurse manager roles, there was an associated increase in adverse patient outcomes, including an increase in urinary tract infections, hospital-acquired pneumonia, deep venous thrombosis and sepsis (Carryer et al. 2010). The authors stated that managers with no nursing background were less likely to identify and understand the often-conflicting demands between hospital policies and patient outcomes. Clinical knowledge arising from having worked at the front line as a clinician was essential for ensuring services were aligned with patients' care needs.

This view is supported by Duffield and colleagues (Duffield et al. 2019b) who recently identified that nurse managers believe they are engaged in clinically related activities despite not providing direct patient care. Using a self-report tool, they found that clinically focused activities, albeit undertaken in a different manner than a front-line clinical nurse, were not entirely lost from middle management roles.

Examples of clinical activities in which nurse managers were involved included interdisciplinary collaboration and facilitating the patients' journey through the health system, to name two. They concluded that this link to clinical knowledge and skills, as well as managerial expertise, are critical for ensuring safe and effective care is provided (Duffield et al. 2019b). This research supports the findings of the Francis inquiry conducted in the United Kingdom (Francis 2013), which found that when senior managers were more concerned with administrative tasks and meeting targets than addressing patient care issues, there were higher rates of errors in care, higher patient mortality rates and shortages of skilled nurses. Following this Inquiry it was suggested that nurse managers have greater involvement in the supervision of clinical staff and oversight of clinical care to minimize errors and adverse patient events.

Many managers however struggle to achieve this degree of involvement due to increased monitoring and reporting requirements by the organization (Scott and Timmons 2017; Rankin et al. 2016; Smiley et al. 2018). Hewko and colleagues (2015) identified that nurses managers intended to leave their job due to work overload, inability to ensure quality patient care, insufficient resources and a lack of recognition and empowerment. In addition, the rise in administrative demands has resulted in an increase in nurse managers' stress levels, which has reduced their ability to lead front-line nurses effectively, also making these roles unattractive to the next generation of nurse leaders. Most importantly, nurse managers often have minimal data to be able to proactively match the demand for patients with the appropriate level of nurse staffing (Scott and Timmons 2017), and instead are left with many static and disparate reporting systems that do not meet managerial requirements for decision making (Rosow et al. 2003; Ghazisaeidi et al. 2015). This can result in increased workload and stress for managers and as a consequence, clinical staff.

9.2.1 Nursing Sensitive Outcomes

Over the last two decades a great deal of research has been undertaken in many countries to examine the link between nursing workload, staffing numbers, the mix of staff and the quality of nursing care (Ball et al. 2018; Aiken et al. 2014; Duffield et al. 2011a; Needleman et al. 2011). This work has been facilitated following the development, refinement and adoption of Nursing Sensitive Outcomes (NSOs), a measure of nursing's contribution to patient safety.

Nursing Sensitive Outcomes are defined as adverse events which are considered sensitive to changes in nurse staffing (Kane et al. 2007a; Needleman et al. 2002). These NSOs include CNS complications, deep vein thrombosis (DVT), pressure injury, Gastro-intestinal (GI) bleeding, pneumonia, sepsis, shock/cardiac arrest, Urinary tract infection (UTI), failure to rescue, mortality, length of stay, physiologic/metabolic derangement, pulmonary failure and surgical wound infection (Needleman et al. 2001). Needleman et al. (2002) developed an algorithm to identify each of these outcomes from the hospital discharge database using coded medical records. Each algorithm specified inclusion and exclusion criteria for the specific adverse outcome so that only those patients who experienced a preventable adverse outcome, rather than one associated with the disease process, were identified. Algorithms were based on variables, such as diagnosis related groups (DRG) and major diagnostic categories (MDC), presence of a surgical procedure and age. They also developed an estimate of nursing care hours needed based on the diagnostic related group (nursing cost-weights).

Research shows that when there are not enough staff there are higher rates of negative outcomes for patients associated with insufficient nursing care being provided (Duffield et al. 2006). In the United States for example, patient death increased by 2% on a shift where a patient was exposed to staffing levels which were eight or more hours below the defined target staffing (Needleman et al. 2011). In seminal work, Aiken and colleagues conducted a study over 168 non-federal adult general hospitals and identified that with an additional patient per nurse, there was an increase of 7% in the rate of mortality within 30 days of admission and a likelihood of failure to rescue (Aiken et al. 2002). Lower levels of staffing are also associated with higher rates of drug administration errors, episodes of care left undone or missed nursing care (Ball et al. 2018; Griffiths et al. 2018).

Perhaps more important than the number of staff is the proportion of hours of care provided by registered nurses, as opposed to unregulated care givers. For example, Needleman and colleagues noted that when there is a higher number of hours of care provided by registered nurses there was a reduction in the rate of failure to rescue (Needleman et al. 2002). Australian work has found that increasing RN hours by 10% decreases the following adverse event rates by:

- Central nervous system complications 45%
- GI bleed 37%
- UTI 34%
- Failure to rescue 27%
- Decubitus ulcers 19%
- Sepsis 15% and
- Pneumonia 11% (Roche et al. 2012).

These studies highlight the importance of understanding the elements which comprise nursing workload in order to determine an appropriate mix and number of staff to ensure the best outcomes for patients possible.

9.3   Workloads

One of the most important tasks of a first-line nurse manger (the manager at the ward or unit level) is to assign patients to nurses for care. This allocation determines a significant portion, but not all, of a nurse's workload. Nursing workload is usually described in terms of direct care activities (e.g. bathing, medication administration, patient interaction) and indirect nursing care (e.g. clerical work, interaction with team members), and these activities can be different depending on the specialty, ward area and patient acuity level. However, the nature and breadth of activities that comprise nursing has resulted in difficulties with defining the contribution that nursing makes to patients' care and more importantly, the measurement of nursing workload. Much of what nurses do is invisible and difficult to quantify and allocate as workload (Lawler 1991). As discussed in Chaps. 2 and 3, now more than ever with shifting models of care delivery, nursing informatics needs to not only facilitate the measurement of nursing workload, but more importantly, make visible and measurable the nursing contribution. For example, it is hard to define and measure empathy and support towards patients and families, but perhaps more importantly, in a time frame that measures effectiveness and completion of the activity or intervention. This is in contrast to the production of goods, in which a set amount of time for task completion can be allocated.

Due to the lack of definition and difficulties in the measurement of workloads, it is currently impossible to determine whether a nurse is working harder than they need to or whether they could be more productive. This is important to note as excessive workloads are a major cause of stress for nurses and a cause of job dissatisfaction (Duffield et al. 2006; Lu et al. 2019), which contribute to a nurse deciding whether to remain in the job and/or the profession (Duffield et al. 2006). Additional negative effects of high workloads include:

- Increased absenteeism,
- Increased overtime,
- Burnout,
- Work related musculoskeletal disorders (MSD) and
- An increased rate of injuries (Qureshi et al. 2018).

Research has shown that these negative impacts continue to fuel the turnover intentions of nurses (Lu et al. 2019). Unfortunately, as nurses continue to exit the workforce and workforce shortages persist, there is an increase in workload for those nurses remaining (MSSS and AAA 2015).

Nurses facilitate the provision of safe quality patient care through the use of observational skills, knowledge and understanding of interventions (Sensmeier 2016; Snavely 2016) that allows for early recognition and management of patient deterioration (Dalton et al. 2018) . Factors which increase nursing workload can impact on a nurse's ability to provide the necessary oversight of patients. There is now a substantial body of research internationally, which demonstrates the strong link between nursing workload and patient mortality and morbidity.

9.4 Workload Measurement Tools

Since the early 1920s, the development of tools to measure nursing workload has been extensively researched. Determining workload is critical as it informs the decisions about allocation of patients to staff. Determining optimal staffing levels is difficult for managers due to limitations in data collection specifically related to staffing levels and the skills mix of nursing teams (National Quality Board 2016; Hurst 2003). Health care organizations across many countries have adopted different methods of managing and assigning nursing workloads. Mandated nurse to patient ratios are used for example in California (USA), and Victoria and Queensland in Australia. The United Kingdom uses a recommended national nurse staffing level; however these are not mandated (National Quality Board 2016; Ball 2010; Health Do 2018). In 2016, Wales introduced a Nurse Staffing Levels Act that recommends the nurse to patient ratio based on decisions of staffing (Welsh Government 2016). Ireland has introduced the Nursing Hours per Patient Day (NHPPD) model based on the Western Australia staffing model (Drennan et al. 2018).

There are many methods used around the world to measure staffing requirements. The most popular methods will be explained in greater detail below.

9.4.1   Patient Assessment and Information System (PAIS)

One of the earliest tools used to determine nursing workload in Australia was the Patient Assessment and Information System (PAIS). Designed in the United States, this method was introduced into the health system in Victoria (Australia) in the early 1980s. Patients are assessed and classified into one of six groups depending on their level of dependency, that is, their need for nursing care, which in part determines nursing workload. An amount of time is then allocated for each dependency indicator, for example, how independent/dependent the patient is in being able to shower themselves. These numbers are added together to provide a total number of care hours required for each patient. The greater the number of indicators for each patient, the greater the workload and resources (nursing hours) required to care for that patient (Hovenga 1996).

Use of this measurement tool required nurses to enter data following their assessment/reassessment of patients. PAIS was sensitive to patients' conditions and could be adjusted for each shift and indeed, on an *as required* basis, which accounted for patient variability and deterioration. This system is no longer in use, in part because there was a belief that nursing staff could 'play the system' and inflate patient scores. This resulted in an increase in care hours and as a result, increased staff numbers (Hovenga 1996).

9.4.2   Diagnostic Related Groups (DRG) Nurse Costing Models

Diagnostic Related Groups (DRGs) were developed as a method to determine resource allocation (all resources not just human resources) by categorizing patients based on their diagnosis and characteristics such as age and the presence of other illnesses which might increase resource requirements, for example diabetes

(Queensland University of Technology 2001). The argument is that if patients can be categorized into clinically meaningful and homogenous groups, then resource allocation can be determined for each hospital based on the institution's patient mix (casemix). Developed in the United States, this system is used extensively now throughout the world for example in Canada and in many European countries. In Australia there is agreement that all jurisdictions move to casemix-based activity funding in all hospitals (Heslop 2012).

The DRG classification is determined on discharge but its advantage is that it is derived from administrative data, the patient's chart, and can be linked to other administrative data sets such as finance and payroll. The nursing resources required for each DRG, defined as nursing service weights, have been incorporated into each DRG (Diers and Bozzo 1997) and these are used to determine the number of nurses needed for a particular ward. However, the resources are determined across the DRG grouping post-discharge and so are not sensitive to an individual patient's condition or changes to that condition during a shift or day. Nursing care is averaged out for a patient's entire length of stay, which does not allow for days when these requirements may be greater or lesser than those estimated (Duffield et al. 2006). The nursing service weights have been criticized as underestimating the requirements for nursing care (Heslop 2012), but perhaps a more important criticism is that DRG determinations are derived from medical diagnoses and are not sensitive enough to variations, which can affect nursing care (O'Brien-Pallas et al. 1997).

9.4.3   Nursing Hours of Care per Patient Day (NHpPD)

Collecting data for the number of Nursing Hours per Patient Day (NHpPD) is easily achieved using administrative data sets. It is a simple calculation which divides the number of nursing hours allocated to each ward by the average number of patients on the ward (usually calculated at the midnight census) to determine the average number of hours of care each patient could potentially receive (Twigg and Duffield 2009).

There are several issues with this method. First of all, the basis on which the determination of hours of care patients required is not clear. Secondly, it isn't really a method for determining workload but rather, a method of allocating paid nursing hours to a certain number of patients. It does not take into account patient complexity or specific care needs or changes to these over a shift or day (Twigg and Duffield 2009; Hodge et al. 2004). Nor does it take into account the 'indirect' aspects of nursing care—documentation, education of patients and their families to name just two (Hodge et al. 2004).

The exception to this is the model introduced in Western Australia (WA) in 2002 and currently being implemented in Ireland (Drennan et al. 2018). This method of staffing uses a 'bottom up' approach to classify wards into seven categories based on characteristics, such as patient complexity, patient turnover, emergency vs elective admissions and presence of a high dependency unit (Twigg et al. 2011). All wards in WA (emergency departments, ICU and CCU, high dependency and renal units have separate allocations) are then be classified according to these characteristics into one of seven bands of staffing (Department of Health 2019). These then prescribe the NHpPD allocated to the ward ranging from 3.0 (day surgery) to 7.5 h (high complexity, high intervention levels, tertiary pediatrics). Table 9.1 shows the ward categorization and the number of hours of nursing care required to care for

Table 9.1 Western Australian model showing ward categorization and the number of nursing hours required (Department of Health 2019)

Ward Category	NHPPD	Criteria for measuring diversity, complexity and nursing tasks required

A	7.5	• High Complexity
		• High Dependency Unit @ 6 beds within a ward
		• Tertiary Step Down ICU
		• High Intervention Level
		• Specialist Unit/Ward Tertiary Level 1:2 staffing
		• Tertiary Paediatrics
		• Mental Health Secure Beds
		   – Seclusion used as per the Mental Health Act 1996 (WA)
		   – High risk of self-harm and aggression
		   – Intermittent 1:1/2 Nursing
		   – Patients frequently on 15 minutely observations

B	6.0	• High Complexity,
		• No High Dependency Unit
		• Tertiary Step Down CCU/ICU
		• Moderate/High Intervention Level
		• Special Unit/Ward including Mental Health Unit
		• High Patient Turnover (Kutney-Lee et al. 2013) >50%
		• FHHS Paediatrics (Boudrias et al. 2019)
		• Secondary Paediatrics
		• Tertiary Maternity
		• Mental Health—High risk of self-harm and aggression
		   – Patients frequently on 30-minute observations
		   – Occasional 1:1 nursing
		   – Mixture of open and closed beds
		   – Seclusion used as per the Mental Health Act 1996 (WA)

C	5.75	• High Complexity Acute
		• Care Unit/Ward
		• Moderate Patient Turnover >35%, OR
		• Emergency Patient Admissions >50%
		• Mental Health—moderate risk of self-harm and aggression
		   – Psycho geriatric Mental Health Unit
		   – Mental health unit incorporating ECT facility

(continued)

Table 9.1 (continued)

Ward Category	NHPPD	Criteria for measuring diversity, complexity and nursing tasks required
D	5.0	• Moderate Complexity • Acute Rehabilitation Secondary Level • Acute Unit/Ward • Emergency Patients Admissions >40% OR • Moderate Patient Turnover >35% • Secondary Maternity • Mental Health—medium to low risk of self-harm and aggression – Mental Health Forensic Patients in open beds
E	4.5	• Moderate Complexity • Moderate Patient Turnover >35% • Sub-Acute Unit/Ward • Rural Paediatrics • Rural Maternity
F	4.0	• Moderate/Low Complexity • Low Patient Turnover <35% • Care Awaiting Placement/Aged Care • Sub-Acute Unit/Ward • Mental Health Slow stream rehabilitation
G	3.0	• Ambulatory Care including: • Day Surgery Unit
Emergency Department		• ED Nursing Hours per Patient Day are worked out using the following formula NHpPD = B + (CxD) + E
Intensive care (ICU)	31.60	• Tertiary designated ICU
Coronary Care Unit (CCU)	14.16	• Designated stand alone CCU
High Dependency Unit	12.00	• Designated stand alone HDU • High Dependency Unit at >6 beds
Renal (T)	3.02	• Stand alone Tertiary Renal unit
Renal (S)	2.18	• Stand alone Satellite renal unit

Note: Turnover = Admissions + Transfers + Discharges divided by Bed Number

patients on each ward in Western Australia and the characteristics which are considered. From this allocation of hours/patient the staffing numbers are determined for each ward. The nurse in charge of the ward can then determine how to allocate those hours of care by shift and day of the week to determine the number of nurses rostered on. Wards can apply to have their classification changed based on changes to the characteristics for example, an increase in emergency rather than elective patients over time (Department of Health 2019).

In 2016, the Department of Health in Ireland issued the *Framework for Safe Nurse Staffing and Skill Mix in General and Specialist Medical and Surgical Care Settings in Adult Hospitals*. Following publication of this document the WA NHpPD model of nurse staffing was introduced to three hospitals as pilot sites to test the impact that planned changes in nurse staffing and skill-mix have on patient, staff and organizational outcomes (Drennan et al. 2018). Administrative data were used to measure the association between the introduction of the staffing recommendations from the *Framework* and nursing sensitive outcome indicators related to patient care (Needleman et al. 2002). These included

- mortality,
- urinary tract infections,
- pressure ulcers,
- hospital acquired pneumonia,
- deep vein thrombosis/pulmonary embolism,
- upper gastro-intestinal bleeding,
- central nervous system complications,
- sepsis and shock/cardiac arrest,
- wound infection,
- pulmonary failure,
- metabolic derangement and
- length of stay (Needleman et al. 2002).

Cross-sectional data were used to measure staff outcomes including nurses' perceptions of the working environment, job satisfaction, burnout, and missed care. At an organisational level, data were used to measure levels of staff turnover, absenteeism, agency and bank use by wards, and the extent to which actual and required staffing was in place on a day-to-day basis. The economic costs of implementing the NHpPD model were also examined and these included: the costs of changes to levels of staffing, agency and bank costs and the costs associated with nursing sensitive outcomes. The overall aim of the research was to measure the impact of the introduction of the *Framework* and to identify the extent to which key patient, staff and organisational outcomes changed as a consequence of the introduction of the NHpPD model of nurse staffing. At the time of writing this work is ongoing in the Emergency Departments.

9.4.4   Nurse to Patient Ratios (Ratios)

This method of determining the number of staff needed per ward/unit has gained wide-spread acceptance internationally, in part because of its simplicity. Wards are allocated staffing on the basis of a ratio, the number of patients nurses are to care for such as 1:3 = 1 nurse to 3 patients. California was the first state in the USA to mandate nurse to patient ratios across their hospitals and many other states and countries have since followed. Two States in Australia, Victoria and Queensland, have adopted this method of staffing. Ratios are established at the unit level and are meant to reflect patient acuity. The more acutely ill patients on the ward are, the fewer patients each nurse would be assigned. The issue with this method of determining staff numbers is that is it hard to determine the optimal ratio for each ward based on patient and staffing characteristics (Duffield et al. 2006).

9.4.5 Commercial Software Packages

There are several software packages which have been developed to plan care and the number of nurses needed. This involves nurses completing a care plan for each patient, which then forms the basis for the determination of their individual care hours. Each nursing activity is added to the system, which then calculates the staffing requirements. Patient acuity is indirectly measured on the basis of clinical hours required for care. However, consideration needs to be taken of patient co-morbidities, skills mix, complications, support staff and other specialty variations. In addition, some packages do not account for time nurses are undertaking indirect nursing duties (Duffield et al. 2006).

In summary, the methods of determining the number of nurses required to provide care for the patients on any given ward, and thus nursing workload, are varied. Some methods are based on the use of administrative data while others rely on nursing staff to provide additional documentation. None of the methods described take account of the mix of staff (registered nurses or unregulated workers) or skills mix (human capital—qualifications and experience of the staff member). While some methods endeavor to take account of the time nurses spend in indirect nursing activities (e.g. patient transfers in the WA NHpPD model) none adequately account for patient variability or patient deterioration, nor are they flexible enough to adjust staffing in the course of a shift or even a day (Duffield et al. 2006).

Probably the most critical skill for nurse managers, particularly first-line nurse managers, is to staff their wards with the appropriate number and mix of staff to ensure patients are safe and receive quality care and their nursing staff are not overworked (Scott and Timmons 2017). To do so requires real-time data to identify bed occupancy levels, patient care needs and resource allocation.

9.5 Challenges for Nurse Managers

Research has identified several complex factors that can impact on managerial decision-making regarding nurse staffing. These factors include nursing shortages, skills mix, stress, burnout and fatigue, changes to patient care needs, an aging workforce, decreased job satisfaction, and poor organizational communication. These areas will be discussed in the following sections.

9.5.1 Nursing Shortages and Workforce Trends

For many years research has documented insufficiencies in the supply and demand of nursing professionals (Marć et al. 2019). These shortages are set to impact countries across all levels of socioeconomic development. The World Health Organization estimates 9 million additional nurses and midwives will be needed by 2030 to ensure sustainability in the workforce. Shortages result from challenges with educational preparation, employment, retention, and workforce performance (World Health Organization 2018). As a consequence of these shortages many researchers and healthcare organizations are now focusing on retention of staff as a priority to ensure patient safety (Sermeus et al. 2011). As indicated earlier, ensuring patients receive safe quality care requires an adequate supply of nurses, particularly registered nurses. An imbalance between supply and demand of these human resources challenges nurse managers. As one of their main functions is to allocate enough nursing resources to meet patient care needs, doing so means they often have to rely on temporary nursing staff or less skilled workers to meet demands (Duffield et al. 2019a). The strain of staff allocation is further exacerbated by lack of real time data showing bed configuration, patient acuity and nursing resource requirements.

Nursing shortages also impact on the economic health of a country by increasing the costs associated with the provision of care (Snavely 2016). These costs are associated with the following:

1. Higher patient re-admission rates (McHugh et al. 2013),
2. Increase in infections including pneumonia, urinary tract infections (Scott 2009), surgical site infections (Cimiotti et al. 2012) and longer length of stay (Kane et al. 2007b), and
3. High turnover of nurses (Snavely 2016).

9.5.2 Skills Mix

Skills mix on a ward or unit can also contribute to the individual nurses' workload but also impacts on patient outcomes. Skills mix refers to the different levels of qualifications, level of nurse (registered or enrolled), experience levels and expertise of staff (Buchan and Dal Poz 2002). In recent times the healthcare system has seen the increased use of unregulated nursing support workers, also known as unlicensed assistive personnel in the USA, health care assistants in the UK, and assistants in nursing in Australia (Duffield et al. 2014). These roles account for approximately 25% of the health workforce in each of these three countries (Australian Bureau of Statistics 2013; Cavendish 2013; Squillace et al. 2007). Support workers usually undertake a range of activities including bathing, feeding, mobilizing and monitoring of patient vital signs (U.S Bureau of Labour Statistics 2013; National Health Service 2015; Blay and Roche 2020) usually under the direct supervision of an enrolled or registered nurse (Blay and Roche 2020). Support workers can be utilized in one of two ways, either a complementary or substitution model.

The complementary model involves the addition of nursing support workers to ward/unit staffing. This model has been identified as a potential strategy to decrease nursing workloads by increasing hours of care available resulting in increased patient contact, fewer tasks being delayed or not completed, better quality of patient care and improvements in nursing job satisfaction (Duffield et al. 2018). Australian research suggests that effective integration of support workers into ward staffing is associated with a higher rate of task completion for RNs (Roche et al. 2016). However, there is evidence that despite the addition of nursing support workers to the nursing team there is a negative impact on patients' outcomes. Twigg and colleagues (Twigg et al. 2016) identified that for every 10% of time a patient spent on a ward with nursing support workers added to nurse staffing, there was a 1% increased chance of developing a hospital acquired urinary tract infection and a 2% chance of acquiring pneumonia. Likewise, Aiken and colleagues (2017) identified that increasing the percentage of assistive personnel resulted in an 11% increase in the chance of a preventable death and a decrease in the quality and safety of hospital care.

In contrast to this is the substitution model, whereby registered nurses are replaced with unregulated workers. While this maintains the number of hours of care available, it reduces the hours of care provided by registered nurses, which has been shown to have a negative impact on patient outcomes (Needleman et al. 2002, 2011; Twigg et al. 2011). In addition, some unregulated workers feel powerless in refusing to perform delegated activities, resulting in them undertaking activities outside of their scope of practice that they are not competent or trained to undertake. This may also result in an increase in negative patient outcomes (Blay and Roche 2020).

These negative patient outcomes identified with lower regulated nursing levels include:

- shock and cardiac arrest,
- upper gastrointestinal bleeding
- failure to rescue
- length of stay (Needleman et al. 2001, 2002).

Through the substitution model there is also likely to be a greater burden on the remaining regulated nurses in terms of delegation to and supervision of unregulated staff (Butler et al. 2011). Hegney and colleagues (2019) identified that nurses were very dissatisfied with a poor mix of staff, which negatively impacted on their workloads. Nurses indicated they were working with too many inexperienced staff without the necessary skills, thereby increasing their workload.

Unfortunately, as nurses are the largest workforce in most if not all health care facilities, many hospitals and health care organizations try to contain costs by reducing the number of registered nurses or substituting professional nursing staff with less skilled nursing aids, licensed practical nurses and other assistive personal (Needleman 2017). Budgetary constraints can be challenging for nurse managers as they try to provide optimal staffing to meet patient needs, while trying to remain within budget (Hughes et al. 2015). Staffing decisions are made more difficult because of limited access to timely and accurate data showing bed occupancy and resource needs.

9.5.3   Stress, Burnout and Fatigue

Stress, burnout and fatigue have been identified as factors that impact on nurses' workloads and their turnover intentions, resulting in some nurses leaving after only a few years in the profession (Snavely 2016). An estimated 30–50% of nurses leave their position in nursing or leave the profession altogether after the first three years (MacKusick and Minick 2010). It is estimated that in the twenty-first century a nurse's career is five years or less with an estimated 2.5 million nurses not practicing (Goodare 2017).

Nurses experience one of the highest levels of occupational stress as a result of high workload demands, emotional strain, long working days, overtime, staff shortages, a lack of support and conflict between healthcare teams (Williams and Smith 2013; Rothmann et al. 2006). In recent years increased stress has also been associated with the advancement in technologies, increasing financial constraints on the health system and changes in workplace environments (Jennings 2007). The National Health Service conducted a review of the health and wellbeing of its staff and identified that one quarter of staff absences were due to stress, depression and anxiety (Fearon and Nicol 2011). This impacts on job satisfaction, productivity and performance and can compromise wellbeing, leading to nurses feeling inadequate and burned out (Najimi et al. 2012). Nurses who show changes in their psychological wellbeing are more inclined to resign from their position and leave the nursing profession (Drury et al. 2014). In addition, high levels of stress among nurses can result in a failure to recognize patient deterioration, leading to negative outcomes for patients including mortality (Stewart and Terry 2014).

Burnout is a psychological concept defined as complete emotional, physical and mental exhaustion caused from continual physical and psychological stress (Okwaraji and En 2014). Symptoms can also include depersonalization and a reduction in perceived accomplishments (Goodare 2017). Nurses are considered to be at high risk of burnout due to unpredictable and stressful working environments resulting from financial and managerial constraints, which impact on nurses' ability to provide the quality of care they expect to deliver (Macken and Hyrkas 2014; Manzano García and Ayala Calvo 2012). Associated with burnout are the increased financial costs related to absenteeism, lost productivity, staff turnover and poor quality of care resulting in potential adverse events for patients. For example, in 2014 the average cost, in American dollars, of turnover per Full Time Equivalent (FTE) nurse is estimated at $48,790 in Australia, $20,561 in the USA, $26,652 in Canada and $23,71 in New Zealand. Akman and colleagues (2016) identified a direct link between job satisfaction and burnout. When job satisfaction was high burnout was low, and when job satisfaction was low burnout was high. High burnout negatively effects employees and impacts on the quality of care provided to patients (Gosseries et al. 2012). Interestingly, satisfaction with care is also lower in hospitals where nurses are dissatisfied and experience burnout. Research suggests that there is a link between nursing burnout and compassion fatigue (Foureur et al. 2013).

All nurses are at risk of developing compassion fatigue due to prolonged stressful situations and their inability to remove themselves from direct patient care. Compassion fatigue is noticed when a nurse shows declining empathy towards patients related to continual exposure to another's suffering, both physical and emotional, as well as a lack of support from the workplace (Hegney et al. 2014). Unfortunately, research shows that when one reaches compassion fatigue it is hard to recover as the person is completely drained of all compassionate energy (Jenkins and Warren 2012; Coetzee and Klopper 2010). Compassion fatigue has been identified worldwide as a contributor to nursing shortages (Nolte et al. 2017; Harris and Griffin 2015; World Health Organization 2016). The symptoms of compassion fatigue include;

- Sadness
- Depression
- Anxiety
- Intrusive images
- Flashbacks
- Numbness
- Avoidance and
- Poor self-esteem (Hooper et al. 2010).

When nurses feel compassion fatigue the desire to leave the profession increases as does turnover intentions (Coetzee and Klopper 2010; Nolte et al. 2017; Harris and Griffin 2015; Sheppard 2016; Bohnenkamp 2016). Compassion fatigue also impacts patient care and safety resulting in an increase in patient dissatisfaction, and financial strain for the institution resulting from increased costly negative patient outcomes. It has been suggested that if organizations empower their nurses, they may potentially protect them from the development of compassion fatigue (Berger et al. 2015). In addition, workplaces that are supportive, nurturing, caring and compassionate towards staff are seen to combat compassion fatigue (Harris and Griffin 2015). Nurse managers need to consider the risk of stress, burnout and compassion fatigue when scheduling staff and allocating workloads in order to maintain staff health and wellbeing. This can be challenging due to the lack of real-time data available to assist with workload allocation, determination of patient care requirements and the number of nursing staff needed.

9.5.4 Changes to Patient Care Needs

In recent times, a variety of changes in patient characteristics has impacted nursing workload. One of the most significant is aging of the population, noticed in most developed countries. The United Nations reported that the world's population aged 60 years and older will double over the next 30 years accounting for between 20–30% of the population in some countries (Giacalone et al. 2016; Vespa et al. 2018; McPake and Mahal 2017; Department of Economic and Social Affairs

Population Division 2017). Patients above the age of 60 years usually have more than one diagnosis and multiple comorbidities. This increases the complexity of care required and results in greater consumption of resources, that is more nursing hours required to care for the patient (Snavely 2016; Duffield et al. 2015; Anderson 2014). In addition, many diseases that once resulted in death are now treatable, leading to an increased number of people living for many years with a chronic condition, increasing demands for care over time and as a consequence, more staff to meet those needs (Haddad and Toney-Butler 2019).

Patient churn is a factor which can significantly impact workloads at the unit level in hospitals (Duffield et al. 2019a). Patient churn is the excessive movement of patients due to admissions, transfers and discharges (Hughes et al. 2015; Blay et al. 2017). During times of churn a nurse's workload increases beyond the work demands of direct patient care (Hughes et al. 2015). Blay et al. (2017) found that as a result of poor bed management policies resulting in patient churn, the amount of time needed to move medical-surgical patients between and within wards in one hospital site was equivalent to 11.3 Full-time Equivalent (FTE) nurses. These extra ward requirements are difficult for managers to plan for, as churn is unpredictable, resulting from a fluctuation occurring during a shift (Hughes et al. 2015). In addition, some hospitals still manage patient flow on paper, white boards and via phone calls, which does not allow precise and timely information to match bed availability and human resource requirements (nurses).

A study conducted by Duffield and colleagues (2019a) explored the impact of bed configuration changes on nursing workload. The study identified that there was a noticeable increase across most ward activities following planned changes to patient mix. Specifically, nurses noticed a substantial increase in workloads associated with transfers in and out of the ward, noting lengthy and repetitive contacts with bed management staff and staff on other wards or in different facilities. The addition of temporary staff also meant that many permanent nurses were left performing indirect care for patients that required knowledge of the ward, including discharge, liaison with doctors and communication with families. The ward had mandated nurse-to-patient ratios of 4 patients to 1 nurse. However, nurses stated that this ratio did not reflect the acuity of patients and resulted in some nurses being assigned four very sick patients. Nurses felt that the ward had become a difficult place in which to work. Further, the nurse staffing figures indicated that the planned staffing numbers did not accurately predict the impact of increased patient churn and changes to patient casemix (Duffield et al. 2019a).

Unfortunately, when patients are not discharged in a timely manner the result is system wide congestion. This results in poor quality of care including higher patient mortality rates, higher rates of readmission, greater exposure to error, decreased patient satisfaction, emergency blockage due to a lack of beds, increased length of stay, understaffing or overstaffing and strain on nursing and ancillary staff (Morley et al. 2018). As a consequence nurses increase their focus on improving bed capacity by speeding up discharges thereby increasing their workload, instead of focusing on their primary role of caring for patients (Ward et al. 2010). Interestingly, patients who are discharged early have a higher risk of being readmitted within 72 h of discharge, especially if they are discharged before they have adequately recovered (Anderson et al. 2011).

When workloads are high a nurse may ration care according to patient needs. Care rationing is used when a nurse needs to prioritize care according to resources and their capacity to undertake the work (Kalisch et al. 2009). In times of patient deterioration a nurse will assess, respond and intervene in a timely manner to prevent adverse events (Dalton et al. 2018). Patient deterioration may necessitate one-to-one patient care and at times, more than one nurse per patient, such as in a cardiac arrest. Unfortunately, this can also limit the time a nurse has with other patients allocated to them for the shift, resulting in missed or delayed nursing care (Kalisch et al. 2009; Duffield et al. 2011b). It is hard for nurse managers to anticipate staff workloads and staffing levels in the absence of timely and accurate data and this situation is compounded by ward instability (Duffield et al. 2015), difficult practice environments (Halpin et al. 2017), low staffing levels, inadequate time (Schubert et al. 2008) and violence towards healthcare professionals (Phillips 2016). Any of these factors can result in episodes of missed or delayed patient care, and it is unlikely that any staffing method could take account of these issues. This is where the role of experienced nurse managers becomes critical. Their expertise is essential in making effective staffing decisions, which can have life or death consequences for those in their care.

The ever-increasing expectations of patients and family members about treatment options and care they expect to receive while in hospital is also adding to the workload and stress levels of nurses. More than ever before nurses are being exposed to google doctor, terms like cyberchondriacs and the development of the e-patient. Many nurses have witnessed the increasing emphasis and influence that cyber reality has on healthcare, patients and their families (Holyoake and Searle 2015). There are benefits for patients searching the internet for healthcare related information including increased empowerment, knowledge, support, alleviation of anxiety (Power and Kirwan 2013) and taking more responsibility for their own health and wellbeing (Gee et al. 2012). The use of digital technologies by an older person may also have the added benefit of allowing them to remain in the community longer by supporting their own care needs (Georgsson 2018). However, the negative consequences of cyber reality can include misinformation, loss of professional authority and search anxiety. The loss of professional authority includes reduced confidence by the community in health professionals' knowledge, and reduced effectiveness of health professionals' intervention (Holyoake and Searle 2015), which can increase nursing workloads. This can also have a direct impact on patients as they may follow inaccurate and dangerous practices from untrustworthy sources (McMullan 2006), which can result in negative outcomes and even death.

Managers are meant to adjust nursing resources by reviewing shift-by-shift fluctuations in the number of patients but as the midnight census is used, it is difficult to take account of patient flow throughout shifts (Kane et al. 2007b; Unruh and Fottler 2006; Clements et al. 2008). This is critical as research shows that if managers allocate resources effectively the quality of care is improved and the consequences of nurse overload are reduced (Hughes et al. 2015). In contrast to this, when successful deployment of nursing personnel is not achieved, an increase in patient adverse events is noted, including an increase in mortality and morbidity and poor nursing outcomes such as job dissatisfaction, stress and burnout (Aiken et al. 2012, 2013), and increased turnover intentions. The difficulties with successful deployment of resources needs to be noted in terms of the limited data available for managers showing bed occupancy and patient acuity. Timeliness of data availability is also an issue.

9.5.5   Aging Workforce

As the generation of baby boomers is now reaching retirement age (Graham and Duffield 2010), the number of nurses leaving the profession in the next 15–20 years is set to increase (Snavely 2016). This has a direct impact on nursing care and patient outcomes due to the increase in less experienced and skilled nurses within the workforce (Collins-McNeil et al. 2012). Unfortunately, in the twenty-first century the ageing nursing workforce is a problem for most developed countries, as shown below;

- The average age of nurses in Australia is 44 years of age with 2 in 5 nurses being over 50 (Australian Insitute of Health and Welfare 2016).
- In the United States the average of nurses is higher, at 51 years of age (Smiley et al. 2018).
- The labor force survey in the United Kingdom shows that 48.9% of registered nurses are 45 years or older (Royal College of Nursing 2017).

The greatest loss associated with the aging workforce is the loss of clinical expertise and intellectual capital that these nurses possess. These attributes are central to the education of new nurses, improvement in patient outcomes and the identification of improvements needed (Kirgan and Golembeski 2010; Glasper 2011). Unfortunately, as workloads increase this also has an impact on older nurses resulting in increased stress, poor health and injury (Gabrielle et al. 2008). Research suggests that nurse managers need to identify ways to retain older, more experienced and knowledgeable nurses, while trying to recruit younger nurses into the profession (Collins-McNeil et al. 2012; Kirgan and Golembeski 2010; Glasper 2011). One such strategy is for nurse managers to decrease workloads of older nurses to prevent stress and injury (Graham and Duffield 2010). This can be challenging for nurse managers due to the lack of real-time data showing bed occupancy, patient acuity and availability of nursing resources.

9.5.6   Communication

Poor communication within a healthcare organization has also been identified as a source of errors, job dissatisfaction and a contributor to nurse turnover intentions (Doleman 2017). Specifically, nurses have rated communication with supervisors, communication climate and media quality as the factors that most impact on job satisfaction and turnover intentions (Doleman 2017). Poor communication has been implicated in negative patient events leading to death or serious injury in patients. It is also the cause of patient dissatisfaction, lack of continuity of care and ineffective use of resources and worktime, all of which impact on the economics of a healthcare organization (Vermeir et al. 2015). Nurses often feel frustrated with information accessibility, hierarchical filtration, distortion and ease of access, all features of inefficient work environments (Yazici 2002). Agarwal and colleagues (2010) identified that communication inefficiencies cost the U.S healthcare system over $ 12 billion annually with a 500 bed hospital costing on average $4 million per year.

Effective organizational communication is needed for quality and safety for patient care and also, operational effectiveness (Agarwal et al. 2010). Effective communication relies on management's ability to maintain the communication flow within an organization. Research suggests that by restructuring and improving communication systems, distortion of information will reduce (Doleman 2017; Duffield et al. 2011b), which may also have the benefit of reducing the mean length of stay, maintaining high patient satisfaction levels (Friedman and Berger 2004) and supporting the sustainability of the workforce.

9.6   Implications of Incorrect Staffing

Nurse managers are challenged in their attempts to allocate staff resources successfully by a variety of factors that impact on nursing workloads. They often struggle to make evidence-based decisions due to limited access to critical real-time data at the point of delivery. These limitations can impact on nursing resource allocations, workloads and the optimization of patient outcomes (Hussey et al. 2015).

The current workload models show limited evidence for the reliability of measuring workloads and staffing requirements. Fasoli and colleagues (2011) and Fasoli and Haddock (2010) concluded that many systems are not accurate enough for resource allocation or decision-making. The problem in Australia lies in the limited information collected by government funded agencies about nursing in the hospital and the characteristics of patients that create the demand for nursing resources. In the United States of America, the utilization of patient data for quality assurance has been undertaken since the early 1990s (Rosser and Kleiner 1995). However, the data and the outcomes measured are linked to medical management rather than nursing care. Unfortunately, data available on the patient, nurse, organization and outcomes are not routinely extracted to quantify their effect on costs, patient safety and quality of care (Duffield et al. 2006).

In addition, most workload measurement tools use some degree of professional judgement to measure the demand for nursing care and each makes an underlying assumption about what constitutes adequate safe care or quality staffing (Griffiths et al. 2020). Further, each method provides a basis for nurse staffing, but fails to provide insight into the most appropriate mix of staff, and fails to take into consideration casemix variability (patient mix); all aspects which are required for the provision of adequate and safe care. There are also implications for full time nurses that are often left working hours around those that are part time and casual. This loss of control over practice and work life has been identified internationally as a key issue for nurses and a challenge for nurse managers when making decisions about the allocation of nursing resources (Duffield et al. 2006; Aiken et al. 2001; Duffield and O'Brien-Pallas 2002).

The current method of measuring and allocating nursing resources can also have an impact on the quality of patient care if insufficient or inadequate information is available on which to base decision-making. For example, current workload measures assume that patient volume is static and due to the lack of real time data on patient movement, renders workload associated with patient churn invisible. As a result, shifts that have high patient turnover or churn show an increase in patient mortality related to an increase in nursing workloads (Hughes et al. 2015; Blay et al. 2017). Similar results were identified In the United Kingdom, where a 9% increase in the risk of death in one trust hospital was noted due to inadequate staffing levels (Griffiths et al. 2018). They also identified that the relationship between registered nurse staffing and mortality appeared to be linear with no clear threshold effect, highlighting the difficulties for managers assessing optimal staffing levels to meet patient care needs. Further, in a study conducted in Finland, an increase in negative patient outcomes including mortality was noted when workloads were above optimal levels (Fagerström et al. 2018; Junttila et al. 2016).

In addition, the costs of negative outcomes due to increased hospital stay and additional resource demands need to be considered as the average cost of a patient stay in 2013–2014 in an acute care setting was $1839 per day in Australia (Independent Hosptial Pricing Authority n.d.). These costs increase pressure on the already tight healthcare budget in most countries. Based on data limitations, fragmentation of services, poor coordination of care and a lack of real time information at the point of care continue to impede the provision of quality and safe patient care (Agency Healthcare Research and Quality 2014).

9.7 The Future

Over the years, safety concerns linked to staffing, nurses' workloads and patient outcomes have been noted, in part due to the lack of real time data available on which nurse managers can make decisions. These limitations in data availability provide a continual challenge for nurse managers in measuring the complex and dynamic workload of nurses. They need access to real-time data on aspects such as bed occupancy, patient acuity and the characteristics and availability of nursing resources (Duffield et al. 2019a).

Unfortunately, the static nature of performance reporting systems is caused by lack of consensus on key measures, lack of consistency in data sources, poor quality of available data and lack of support from IT (Ghazisaeidi et al. 2015). This results in inconsistent and poor-quality reports which are time consuming to develop, but which in many instances, do not allow managers to identify or monitor ward performance, therefore hindering decision-making. As nurse managers are in a critical position responsible for the utilization of information to ensure positive patient outcomes (Hart 2010) and nurse staffing sustainability, they require interactive tools to transmit, organize, analyze and display performance data in real time (Ghazisaeidi et al. 2015). Nurse managers should be able to advocate for appropriate systems, known more commonly as performance dashboards, to be installed (Ghazisaeidi et al. 2015), which will allow them to create an environment that will promote quality patient care (Strudwick et al. 2019a).

A performance dashboard is a layered information system that has the capacity to allow managers to measure, monitor and manage ward performance effectively (Ghazisaeidi et al. 2015). By having these systems in place managers are able to focus on other activities which promote patient safety and the corrective actions needed to improve care provision (Ghazisaeidi et al. 2015; Duffield et al. 2006). The successful implementation of a performance dashboard can support evidence-based nursing care by allowing support for clinical judgement and client values based on proven outcomes (Nursing Informatics Awareness Task Force 2007). In addition, the availability of accurate and timely data will allow nurse managers to successfully allocate nursing resources based on patient care needs. This will allow nurse managers to successfully manage and progress patients through the health facility while facilitating effective clinical leadership of front-line nurses, which drives safe and quality patient care (Wise and Duffield 2019).

A study conducted in Queensland (Australia) provides an example of the administrative data required for the creation of a successful hospital performance dashboard. In the study, administrative data were collected over a two-year period to explore the impact that bed configuration changes and patient mix have on a nurses' workload. The administrative data collected examined ward activity, acuity indicators, resource intensity and nurse staffing requirements. See Table 9.2 for a summary of some data elements which can be readily accessed from administrative datasets. Results from the study determined that the bed configuration changes resulted in an increase in patient transfers, greater variability in casemix and an increase in nursing workloads. The study concluded that nurse managers should be supported with the necessary skills to access and utilize available administrative data, allowing for expert decisions to be made regarding the complex and often hidden aspects of nursing workloads (Duffield et al. 2019a). By harnessing administrative data, organizations will have the ability to measure and act on key indicators and events in real-time.

In another example also in Queensland, a digital reporting and monitoring dashboard system was implemented into community child health services to inform service improvements, guide strategic planning and support implementation of strategic priorities. This dashboard collected information on service activity, workforce, consumer feedback and socio-demographic data, and was accessible to all child health services and programs. The data allowed for baseline establishment prior to

Table 9.2 Administrative data

Ward activity	Acuity indicators and resource intensity	Nursing staffing requirements
Occupancy	**Acuity Indicators**	**Planned Vs. Actual staffing**
• occupancy %	• Intensive care transfers in	• Planned Staffing
• Length of stay	• Medical Emergency Team (MET) Calls	• Actual Staffing
• Occupied Bed Days	**Resource Intensity Data**[a]	• *Difference (Planned-actual)*
Patient Movements	• Highest intensity	**Employment Status**
• Admissions	• Second highest	• Full-time
• Transfers In	• Third highest	• Part-time
• Transfers Out	• Fourth highest	• Internal Casual
• Deaths	• Other (intensity not categorized)	• External Agency
• Discharges		**Skillmix**
• Total Patient Movements		• Registered nurses
Emergency status		• Enrolled nurses
• Emergency		• Nursing assistants
• Elective		**Specials**
• Unassigned		• Number of Specials

[a]Determined from AR-DRG codes

interventions to improve service delivery. Each team accessing the dashboard identified areas of improvements based on information reported in the dashboard. As a result of the implementation of the dashboard child health services were able to make informed decisions about clinical service, utilization of resources and future planning (Kennedy and Tracey 2018). In addition, Rosow et al.'s (2003) seminal work identified the benefits of performance dashboards as

- Increased performance and reduced costs and time.
- Process improvement optimizing patient placement,
- Increasing staff efficiency,
- Improving bed utilization, occupancy and patient flow,
- Optimizing utilization of materials,
- Predicative capacity management which reduced overcrowding, operating delays,
- Increased staff satisfaction,
- Better treatment of patients
- On-demand historical, real-time and predicative reports,
- Alerts warning and recommendations, ability to share information throughout the hospital
- Timely data driven decision making regarding staffing levels,
- Improved crisis management

Collectively these integrated applications directly benefit health care providers, insurers, and most importantly, patients. Improvements in the workflow of service co-ordination is also noted (Hussey et al. 2015) as nurse managers will have real-time data showing patients' diagnoses, patient acuity, census data, patient rooms, admission dates and estimated discharge and requirement of specialty staff (Punnakitikashem et al. 2013).

9.7.1 Challenges

There are several requirements that must be met before dashboards can be utilized for quality improvement (Weggelaar-Jansen et al. 2018). These include the efficiency and effectiveness of information presented to the user; content needs to align with needs; there must be an ability to customize visualization and display timely and complete data for users; and the system must be capable of inter-connectivity and performance indicator development (Ghazisaeidi et al. 2015; Weggelaar-Jansen et al. 2018). Unfortunately, these issues have been identified in the literature as areas that hospitals and health care facilities fail to manage appropriately.

Regardless of the dashboard system used, the output will only be as good as the data being entered into the system. Support will need to be provided to clinicians to ensure the input of quality data. This also requires managerial and staff commitment as an essential component for successful implementation and use (Taylor et al. 2015). Staff training is also important, as is staff understanding of expected benefits and uses. Research continues to identify that nurse managers are underprepared for their roles, particularly in the use of data (Collins et al. 2017; Westra and Delaney 2008; Strudwick et al. 2019b; Moore et al. 2016). Therefore, educational institutions and employers must strengthen efforts to improve the knowledge and skills of individuals to be able to undertake these roles successfully. The importance of this cannot be underestimated as the need for health practitioners to engage and use technology successfully now and into the future escalates (Hussey et al. 2015).

Importantly, staff will become cynical if there are limited perceived benefits of system implementation. Tools must be tested for reliability in each new setting where implementation occurs (van Oostveen et al. 2016). If this is not undertaken, engagement may be impacted, especially if important aspects of care are omitted because they are deemed to be less important (Brennan and Daly 2015). While the use of dashboards has been developed to unite disparate data sources into meaningful readily available reports, the satisfaction with such deployment has been modest (Kennedy and Tracey 2018; Lachev and Price 2018; Lytvyak et al. 2018). The challenges include incomplete or out of date data, limited system access and usability. These challenges need to be addressed to facilitate successful infiltration of dashboards in the future. Despite the importance for quality patient care and staffing costs there is little available research that pays attention to the impact that these tools and systems can have in facilitating nurse staffing decisions (Griffiths et al. 2020).

9.8 Conclusion

This chapter highlights the challenges faced by nurse managers in terms of measuring nurses' complex and dynamic workload at the ward level (Duffield et al. 2015; Douglas 2010). Without the use of real time data at the point of care, the mismatch between the supply of nursing resources and patient needs will continue with consequences for patients, staff and the health care system as a whole (Douglas 2010; Tierney et al. 2013). As reported in Chaps. 2 and 14, artificial intelligence (AI) and machine learning (ML) increasingly are being considered useful for decision support in health and social care delivery. Hospitals rarely use the extensive administrative data they collect about patients and staff on each ward to make evidence-based staffing decisions. To harness existing data, software must be employed that allows data to be extracted, analyzed and interpreted for visualization in a timely manner to support staffing decision making (Leary et al. 2016). Evidence-based staffing decisions need to incorporate both comparative and longitudinal trends offered by quantitative administrative data, with the perspective of expert nurses who have the knowledge to contextualize the data and provide a full picture of nursing workload at the ward level.

9.9 Review Questions

1. Can you list some of the challenges that nurse managers face in allocating enough resources to meet patent care requirements and consider how these challenges are overcome in your practice?
2. Can you list some of the nursing sensitive outcomes mentioned in this chapter and consider how they are captured in existing healthcare systems in your practice?
3. Can you recall the different types of workload measurement systems listed in this chapter, select one of them and explain why you consider it to be your preferred choice to implement in practice?

9.9.1 Answers

1. The challenges faced by nurse managers include,
   Nursing shortages and workforce trends,
   Skills mix.
   Stress, burnout and fatigue.
   Changes to patient care needs.
   Aging workforce.
   Communication.

2. Needleman and colleagues (2001) identifies the following Nursing Sensitive Outcomes;
   Mortality,
   Failure to Rescue (FTR),
   Shock/ Cardiac Arrest,
   Deep Vein Thrombosis,
   Central Nervous System Complications,
   Decubitus Ulcer,
   Gastrointestinal Bleeding,
   Pneumonia,
   Sepsis.
   Urinary Tract Infection,
   Length of Stay,
   Physiologic/Metabolic Derangement,
   Pulmonary Failure.
   Surgical Wound Infection.
3. In this chapter, five workload measurement systems are listed
   The patient assessment and information system (PAIS),
   The Diagnostic Related Grouping (DRG) Nurse Cost Model,
   The Nurse Hours of Care per day,
   Nursing to patient ratios and mandated ratios, and
   Commercial software packages.

Glossary

CQI Continuous Quality Improvement

DRG Diagnosis Related Groups

Failure to rescue FR As a safety and quality measure, *failure to rescue* has been *defined* as the inability to prevent death after the development of a complication.

MDC Major Diagnostic Categories

MIS Management Information System

NHpPD Nursing Hours per Patient Day

NSO Nursing Sensitive Outcomes—a measure of nursing's contribution to patient safety.

NWMS Nursing Workload Management System, which measure direct, indirect, and nonclinical patient care hours by patient acuity

PAIS Patient Assessment and Information System

Patient churn The excessive movement of patients due to admissions, transfers and discharges

PCS Patient Classification System, also used interchangeably with NWMS

TQM Total Quality Improvement

References

Agarwal R, Sands DZ, Díaz Schneider J. Quantifying the economic impact of communication inefficiencies in US hospitals. J Healthc Manag. 2010;55(4):265.

Agency Healthcare Research and Quality. Care coordination measurement atlas. California 2014. Contract No.: 14-0037-EF.

Aiken LH, Clarke SP, Sloane DM, Sochalski JA, Busse R, Clarke H, et al. Nurses' reports on hospital care in five countries. Health Aff. 2001;20(3):43–53.

Aiken LH, Clarke SP, Sloane DM, Sochalski J, Silber JH. Hospital nurse staffing and patient mortality, nurse burnout, and job dissatisfaction. J Am Med Assoc. 2002;288(16):1987–93.

Aiken LH, Sermeus W, Van den Heede K, Sloane DM, Busse R, McKee M, et al. Patient safety, satisfaction, and quality of hospital care: cross sectional surveys of nurses and patients in 12 countries in Europe and the United States. Br Med J. 2012;344:20.

Aiken LH, Sloane DM, Bruyneel L, Van den Heede K, Sermeus W, Consortium Rc. Nurses' reports of working conditions and hospital quality of care in 12 countries in Europe. Int J Nurs Stud. 2013;50(2):143–53.

Aiken LH, Sloane DM, Bruyneel L, Van den Heede K, Griffiths P, Busse R, et al. Nurse staffing and education and hospital mortality in nine European countries: a retrospective observational study. Lancet. 2014;383(9931):1824–30.

Aiken LH, Sloane D, Griffiths P, Rafferty AM, Bruyneel L, McHugh M, et al. Nursing skill mix in European hospitals: cross-sectional study of the association with mortality, patient ratings, and quality of care. BMJ Qual Saf. 2017;26(7):559–68.

Akman O, Ozturk C, Bektas M, Ayar D, Armstrong MA. Job satisfaction and burnout among paediatric nurses. J Nurs Manag. 2016;24(7):923–33.

Anderson A. The impact of the Affordable Care Act on the health care workforce, vol. 2887: The Heritage Foundation; 2014. p. 1–20.

Anderson D, Price C, Golden B, Jank W, Wasil E. Examining the discharge practices of surgeons at a large medical center. Health Care Manag Sci. 2011;14(4):338–47.

Australian Bureau of Statistics. April 2013-Doctors and Nurses Canberra, Australia Australian Bureau of Statistics; 2013.

Australian Insitute of Health and Welfare. Nursing and midwifery workforce 2015: Australia Australian Insitute of Health and Welfare; 2016.

Ball J. Guidance on safe nurse staffing levels in the UK: RCN; 2010.

Ball JE, Bruyneel L, Aiken LH, Sermeus W, Sloane DM, Rafferty AM, et al. Post-operative mortality, missed care and nurse staffing in nine countries: a cross-sectional study. Int J Nurs Stud. 2018;78:10–5.

Barron McBride A. Actually achieving our preferred future. Reflect Nurs Leadersh. 2005;31(4):22–3.

Berger J, Polivka B, Smoot EA, Owens H. Compassion fatigue in pediatric nurses. J Pediatr Nurs. 2015;30(6):e11–e7.

Blay N, Roche M. A systematic review of activities undertaken by the unregulated nursing assistant. J Adv Nurs. 2020;76:1538–51.

Blay N, Roche MA, Duffield C, Gallagher R. Intrahospital transfers and the impact on nursing workload. J Clin Nurs. 2017;26(23–24):4822–9.

Bohnenkamp S. Decreasing moral distress: what do we need to do to keep our nurses at the bedside? Medsurg Nurs. 2016;25(6):378.

Boudrias V, Trépanier S-G, Foucreault A, Peterson C, Fernet C. Investigating the role of psychological need satisfaction as a moderator in the relationship between job demands and turnover intention among nurses. Empl Relat. 2019;

Brennan CW, Daly BJ. Methodological challenges of validating a clinical decision-making tool in the practice environment. West J Nurs Res. 2015;37(4):536–45.

Buchan J, Dal Poz MR. Skill mix in the health care workforce: reviewing the evidence. Bull World Health Organ. 2002;80:575–80.

Butler M, Collins R, Drennan J, Halligan P, O'Mathúna DP, Schultz TJ, et al. Hospital nurse staffing models and patient and staff-related outcomes. Cochrane Database Syst Rev. 2011;(7)

Carryer JB, Diers D, McCloskey B, Wilson D. Effects of health policy reforms on nursing resources and patient outcomes in New Zealand. Policy Polit Nurs Pract. 2010;11(4):275–85.

Cavendish C. The Cavendish review: an independent review into healthcare assistants and support workers in the NHS and social care settings. London: Department of Health; 2013.

Cimiotti JP, Aiken LH, Sloane DM, Wu ES. Nurse staffing, burnout, and health care–associated infection. Am J Infect Control. 2012;40(6):486–90.

Clements A, Halton K, Graves N, Pettitt A, Morton A, Looke D, et al. Overcrowding and understaffing in modern health-care systems: key determinants in meticillin-resistant Staphylococcus aureus transmission. Lancet Infect Dis. 2008;8(7):427–34.

Coetzee SK, Klopper HC. Compassion fatigue within nursing practice: a concept analysis. Nurs Health Sci. 2010;12(2):235–43.

Collins S, Yen P-Y, Phillips A, Kennedy MK. Nursing informatics competency assessment for the nurse leader: the Delphi study. J Nurs Adm. 2017;47(4):212–8.

Collins-McNeil J, Sharpe D, Benbow D. Aging workforce: retaining valuable nurses. Nurs Manag. 2012;43(3):50–4.

Dalton M, Harrison J, Malin A, Leavey C. Factors that influence nurses' assessment of patient acuity and response to acute deterioration. Br J Nurs. 2018;27(4):212–8.

Department of Economic and Social Affairs Population Division. World population aging 2017: New York United Nations; 2017.

Department of Health. Equity and excellence: liberating the NHS. London: Department of Health; 2010.

Department of Health. NHpPD application manual: guiding principles Western Australia: Department of Health; 2019.

Diers D, Bozzo J. Nursing resource definition in DRGs. Nurs Econ. 1997;15(3):124–32.

Doleman G. The impact of communication satisfaction on paediatric nurses' job satisfaction and intention to stay [doctoral dissertation]: Edith Cowan University; 2017.

Douglas K. Ratios – if it were only that easy. Nurs Econ. 2010;28(2):119–26.

Drennan J, Duffield C, Scott AP, Ball J, Brady NM, Murphy A, et al. A protocol to measure the impact of intentional changes to nurse staffing and skill-mix in medical and surgical wards. J Adv Nurs. 2018;74(12):2912–21.

Drury V, Craigie M, Francis K, Aoun S, Hegney DG. Compassion satisfaction, compassion fatigue, anxiety, depression and stress in registered nurses in A ustralia: Phase 2 results. J Nurs Manag. 2014;22(4):519–31.

Duffield C, O'Brien-Pallas L. The nursing workforce in Canada and Australia: two sides of the same coin. Aust Health Rev. 2002;25(2):136–44.

Duffield C, Roche M, Merrick ET. Methods of measuring nursing workload in Australia. Collegian. 2006;13(1):16–22.

Duffield C, Roche MA, Blay N, Thoms D, Stasa H. The consequences of executive turnover in Australian hospitals. J Res Nurs. 2011a;16(6):503–14.

Duffield C, Diers D, O'Brien-Pallas L, Aisbett C, Roche M, King M, et al. Nursing staffing, nursing workload, the work environment and patient outcomes. Appl Nurs Res. 2011b;24(4):244–55.

Duffield CM, Twigg DE, Pugh JD, Evans G, Dimitrelis S, Roche MA. The use of unregulated staff: time for regulation? Policy Polit Nurs Pract. 2014;15(1–2):42–8.

Duffield CM, Roche MA, Dimitrelis S, Homer C, Buchan J. Instability in patient and nurse characteristics, unit complexity and patient and system outcomes. J Adv Nurs. 2015;71(6):1288–98.

Duffield C, Roche M, Twigg D, Williams A, Rowbotham S, Clarke S. Adding unregulated nursing support workers to ward staffing: exploration of a natural experiment. J Clin Nurs. 2018;27(19–20):3768–79.

Duffield C, Roche MA, Wise S, Debono D. Harnessing ward-level administrative data and expert knowledge to improve staffing decisions: a multi-method case study. J Adv Nurs. 2019a;76(1):287–96.

Duffield C, Gardner G, Doubrovsky A, Wise S. Manager, clinician or both? Nurse managers' engagement in clinical care activities. J Nurs Manag. 2019b;27(7):1538–45.

Fagerström L, Kinnunen M, Saarela J. Nursing workload, patient safety incidents and mortality: an observational study from Finland. BMJ Open. 2018;8(4)

Fasoli DR, Haddock KS. Results of an integrative review of patient classi cation systems. Annu Rev Nurs Res. 2010;28(1):295–316.

Fasoli DR, Fincke BG, Haddock KS. Going beyond patient classification systems to create an evidence-based staffing methodology. J Nurs Adm. 2011;41(10):434–9.

Fearon C, Nicol M. Strategies to assist prevention of burnout in nursing staff. Nurs Stand. 2011;26(14)

Foureur M, Besley K, Burton G, Yu N, Crisp J. Enhancing the resilience of nurses and midwives: Pilot of a mindfulnessbased program for increased health, sense of coherence and decreased depression, anxiety and stress. Contemp Nurse. 2013;45(1):114–25.

Francis R. Report of the Mid Staffordshire NHS Foundation Trust public inquiry: executive summary: The Stationery Office; 2013.

Friedman DM, Berger DL. Improving team structure and communication: a key to hospital efficiency. Arch Surg. 2004;139(11):1194–8.

Gabrielle S, Jackson D, Mannix J. Adjusting to personal and organisational change: views and experiences of female nurses aged 40–60 years. Collegian. 2008;15(3):85–91.

Gee PM, Greenwood DA, Kim KK, Perez SL, Staggers N, DeVon HA. Exploration of the e-patient phenomenon in nursing informatics. Nurs Outlook. 2012;60(4):e9–e16.

Georgsson M. An aging population, larger chronic disease burden, and reliance on digital self-management tools require contributions from nurse informaticians. Online J Nurs Inform. 2018;22:3.

Ghazisaeidi M, Safdari R, Torabi M, Mirzaee M, Farzi J, Goodini A. Development of performance dashboards in healthcare sector: key practical issues. Acta Informatica Medica. 2015;23(5):317.

Giacalone D, Wendin K, Kremer S, Frøst MB, Bredie WL, Olsson V, et al. Health and quality of life in an aging population – food and beyond. Food Qual Prefer. 2016;47:166–70.

Glasper A. Can older nurses still provide care? Br J Nurs. 2011;20(18):1206–7.

Goodare P. Literature review: why do we continue to lose our nurses? Aust J Adv Nurs. 2017;34(4):50.

Gosseries O, Demertzi A, Ledoux D, Bruno M-A, Vanhaudenhuyse A, Thibaut A, et al. Burnout in healthcare workers managing chronic patients with disorders of consciousness. Brain Inj. 2012;26(12):1493–9.

Graham EM, Duffield C. An ageing nursing workforce. Aust Health Rev. 2010;34(1):44–8.

Griffiths P, Ball J, Bloor K, Böhning D, Briggs J, Dall'Ora C, et al. Nurse staffing levels, missed vital signs observations and mortality in hospital wards: retrospective longitudinal observational study. NIHR Journals Library. 2018;

Griffiths P, Saville C, Ball J, Jones J, Pattison N, Monks T, et al. Nursing workload, nurse staffing methodologies and tools: a systematic scoping review and discussion. Int J Nurs Stud. 2020;103:103487.

Haddad LM, Toney-Butler TJ. Nursing shortage. StatPearls [Internet]: StatPearls Publishing; 2019.

Halpin Y, Terry LM, Curzio J. A longitudinal, mixed methods investigation of newly qualified nurses' workplace stressors and stress experiences during transition. J Adv Nurs. 2017;73(11):2577–86.

Harris C, Griffin MTQ. Nursing on empty: compassion fatigue signs, symptoms, and system interventions. J Christ Nurs. 2015;32(2):80–7.

Hart MD. A Delphi study to determine baseline informatics competencies for nurse managers. CIN: Computers, Informatics, Nursing. 2010;28(6):364–70.

Health Do. Framework for safe nurse staffing and skill mix in general and specialist medical and surgical care settings in Ireland 2018: London Department of Health; 2018.

Hegney DG, Craigie M, Hemsworth D, Osseiran-Moisson R, Aoun S, Francis K, et al. Compassion satisfaction, compassion fatigue, anxiety, depression and stress in registered nurses in Australia: study 1 results. J Nurs Manag. 2014;22(4):506–18.

Hegney DG, Rees CS, Osseiran-Moisson R, Breen L, Eley R, Windsor C, et al. Perceptions of nursing workloads and contributing factors, and their impact on implicit care rationing: a Queensland, Australia study. J Nurs Manag. 2019;27(2):371–80.

Heslop L. Status of costing hospital nursing work within Australian casemix activity-based funding policy. Int J Nurs Pract. 2012;18(1):2–6.

Hewko SJ, Brown P, Fraser KD, Wong CA, Cummings GG. Factors influencing nurse managers' intent to stay or leave: a quantitative analysis. J Nurs Manag. 2015;23(8):1058–66.

Hodge MB, Romano PS, Harvey D, Samuels SJ, Olson VA, Sauvé MJ, et al. Licensed caregiver characteristics and staffing in California acute care hospital units. J Nurs Adm. 2004;34(3):125–33.

Holyoake D-D, Searle K. Cyberchondria: emerging themes for children's nurses in the Internet age. Nurs Child Young People. 2015;27(5):34.

Hooper C, Craig J, Janvrin DR, Wetsel MA, Reimels E. Compassion satisfaction, burnout, and compassion fatigue among emergency nurses compared with nurses in other selected inpatient specialties. J Emerg Nurs. 2010;36(5):420–7.

Hovenga E. Patient Assessment and Information System (PAIS). 1996.

Hughes RG, Bobay KL, Jolly NA, Suby C. Comparison of nurse staffing based on changes in unit-level workload associated with patient churn. J Nurs Manag. 2015;23(3):390–400.

Hurst K. Selecting and applying methods for estimating the size and mix of nursing teams: a systematic review of the literature commissioned by the Department of Health: Nuffield Institute for Health; 2003.

Hussey P, Adams E, Shaffer FA. Nursing informatics and leadership, an essential competency for a global priority: eHealth. Nurse Lead. 2015;13(5):52–7.

Independent Hosptial Pricing Authority. National hosptial cost data collection: Australian public hospitals cost report 2013–2014 Round 18. Australia: Independent Hosptial Pricing Authority; n.d.

Jenkins B, Warren NA. Concept analysis: compassion fatigue and effects upon critical care nurses. Crit Care Nurs Q. 2012;35(4):388–95.

Jennings BM. Turbulance. Hughes R, ed. Rockville, MD: Agency for Helathcare Research and Quality; 2007.

Junttila JK, Koivu A, Fagerström L, Haatainen K, Nykänen P. Hospital mortality and optimality of nursing workload: a study on the predictive validity of the RAFAELA Nursing Intensity and Staffing system. Int J Nurs Stud. 2016;60:46–53.

Kalisch BJ, Landstrom GL, Hinshaw AS. Missed nursing care: a concept analysis. J Adv Nurs. 2009;65(7):1509–17.

Kane RL, Shamliyan TA, Mueller C, Duval S, Wilt TJ. The association of registered nurse staffing levels and patient outcomes: systematic review and meta-analysis. Med Care. 2007a:1195–204.

Kane RL, Shamliyan T, Mueller C, Duval S, Wilt TJ. Nurse staffing and quality of patient care. Evid Rep Technol Assess (Full Rep). 2007b;151(1):115.

Kennedy C, Tracey F. An integrated approach to sustainability and delivery of improved health outcomes for Children's Health Queensland community based services and programs. Int J Integr Care (IJIC). 2018;18

Kirgan M, Golembeski S. Retaining an aging workforce by giving voice to older and experienced nurses. Nurse Lead. 2010;8(1):34–6.

Kutney-Lee A, Wu ES, Sloane DM, Aiken LH. Changes in hospital nurse work environments and nurse job outcomes: an analysis of panel data. Int J Nurs Stud. 2013;50(2):195–201.

Labrague LJ, McEnroe-Petitte DM, Leocadio MC, Van Bogaert P, Cummings GG. Stress and ways of coping among nurse managers: an integrative review. J Clin Nurs. 2018;27(7–8):1346–59.

Lachev T, Price E. Applied Microsoft Power BI: bring your data to life! Prologika Press; 2018.

Lawler J. Behind the screens: Nursing, somology, and the problem of the body. Melbourne: Churchill Livingstone; 1991.

Leary A, Cook R, Jones S, Smith J, Gough M, Maxwell E, et al. Mining routinely collected acute data to reveal non-linear relationships between nurse staffing levels and outcomes. BMJ Open. 2016;6(12):e011177.

Lu H, Zhao Y, While A. Job satisfaction among hospital nurses: a literature review. Int J Nurs Stud. 2019;94:24–31.

Lytvyak E, Dieleman L, Halloran B, Huang V, Kroeker K, Peerani F, et al. A130 tableau dashboard as a quality improvement and strategic driving tool in the IBD outpatient setting: early experience from IBD Centre of excellence at the University of Alberta hospital. J Can Assoc Gastroenterol. 2018;1(suppl_1):225–6.

Macken L, Hyrkas K. Retention, fatigue, burnout and job satisfaction: new aspects and challenges. J Nurs Manag. 2014;22(5):541.

MacKusick CI, Minick P. Why are nurses leaving? Findings from an initial qualitative study on nursing attrition. Medsurg Nurs. 2010;19:6.

Manzano García G, Ayala Calvo JC. Emotional exhaustion of nursing staff: influence of emotional annoyance and resilience. Int Nurs Rev. 2012;59(1):101–7.

Maŕc M, Bartosiewicz A, Burzyńska J, Chmiel Z, Januszewicz P. A nursing shortage – a prospect of global and local policies. Int Nurs Rev. 2019;66(1):9–16.

McHugh MD, Berez J, Small DS. Hospitals with higher nurse staffing had lower odds of readmissions penalties than hospitals with lower staffing. Health Aff. 2013;32(10):1740–7.

McMullan M. Patients using the Internet to obtain health information: how this affects the patient – health professional relationship. Patient Educ Couns. 2006;63(1–2):24–8.

McPake B, Mahal A. Addressing the needs of an aging population in the health system: the Australian case. Health Syst Reform. 2017;3(3):236–47.

Moore LW, Sublett C, Leahy C. Nurse managers' insights regarding their role highlight the need for practice changes. Appl Nurs Res. 2016;30:98–103.

Morley C, Unwin M, Peterson GM, Stankovich J, Kinsman L. Emergency department crowding: a systematic review of causes, consequences and solutions. PLoS One. 2018;13(8):e0203316.

MSSS H, AAA C. The nursing shortage impact on job outcome (the case in Sri Lanka). J Competitiveness. 2015;7(3)

Najimi A, Goudarzi AM, Sharifirad G. Causes of job stress in nurses: a cross-sectional study. Iran J Nurs Midwifery Res. 2012;17(4):301.

National Health Service. National Health Service careers: Healthcare assistant 2015.

National Quality Board. Supporting NHS providers to deliver the right staff, with the right skills, in the right place at the right time: safe, sustainable and productive staffing: National Quality Board (NQB); 2016.

Needleman J. Nursing skill mix and patient outcomes: BMJ Publishing Group Ltd; 2017.

Needleman J, Buerhaus P, Mattke S, Stewart M, Zelevinsky K. Nurse staffing and patient outcomes in hospitals: Harvard School of Public Health Boston; 2001.

Needleman J, Buerhaus P, Mattke S, Stewart M, Zelevinsky K. Nurse-staffing levels and the quality of care in hospitals. N Engl J Med. 2002;346(22):1715–22.

Needleman J, Buerhaus P, Pankratz VS, Leibson CL, Stevens SR, Harris M. Nurse staffing and inpatient hospital mortality. N Engl J Med. 2011;364(11):1037–45.

Nolte AG, Downing C, Temane A, Hastings-Tolsma M. Compassion fatigue in nurses: a metasynthesis. J Clin Nurs. 2017;26(23–24):4364–78.

HIMSS Nursing Informatics Awareness Task Force. An emerging giant: nursing informatics. Nurs Manag. 2007;38(3):38–42.

O'Brien-Pallas L, Irvine D, Peereboom E, Murray M. Measuring nursing workload: understanding the variability. Nurs Econ. 1997;15(4):171–83.

Okwaraji F, En A. Burnout and psychological distress among nurses in a Nigerian tertiary health institution. Afr Health Sci. 2014;14(1):237–45.

van Oostveen CJ, Ubbink DT, Mens MA, Pompe EA, Vermeulen H. Pre-implementation studies of a workforce planning tool for nurse staffing and human resource management in university hospitals. J Nurs Manag. 2016;24(2):184–91.

Phillips JP. Workplace violence against health care workers in the United States. N Engl J Med. 2016;374(17):1661–9.

Power A, Kirwan G. Cyberpsychology and new media: a thematic reader: Psychology Press; 2013.

Punnakitikashem P, Rosenberber JM, Buckley-Behan DF. A stochastic programming approach for integrated nurse staffing and assignment. Lie Transactions. 2013;45(10):1059–76.

Queensland University of Technology. Business planning framework: nursing resources: Brisbane Queensland Health; 2001.

Qureshi SM, Purdy N, Neumann WP, editors. Simulating the impact of patient acuity and nurse-patient ratio on nurse workload and care quality. Congress of the international ergonomics association: Springer; 2018.

Rankin J, McGuire C, Matthews L, Russell M, Ray D, Research LBC, et al. Facilitators and barriers to the increased supervisory role of senior charge nurses: a qualitative study. J Nurs Manag. 2016;24(3):366–75.

Remus S, Kennedy MA. Innovation in transformative nursing leadership: nursing informatics competencies and roles. Can J Nurs Leadersh. 2012;25(4):14–26.

Roche M, Duffield C, Aisbett C, Diers D, Stasa H. Nursing work directions in Australia: does evidence drive the policy? Collegian. 2012;19(4):231–8.

Roche MA, Duffield C, Friedman S, Dimitrelis S, Rowbotham S. Regulated and unregulated nurses in the acute hospital setting: tasks performed, delayed or not completed. J Clin Nurs. 2016;25(1–2):153–62.

Rosow E, Adam J, Coulombe K, Race K, Anderson R. Virtual instrumentation and real-time executive dashboards: solutions for health care systems. Nurs Adm Q. 2003;27(1):58–76.

Rosser LH, Kleiner BH. Using management information systems to enhance health care quality assurance. J Manag Med. 1995;9:27–36.

Rothmann S, Van Der Colff J, Rothmann J. Occupational stress of nurses in South Africa. Curationis. 2006;29(2):22–33.

Royal College of Nursing. The UK nursing labour market review 2018. London: Royal College of Nursing; 2017.

Schubert M, Glass TR, Clarke SP, Aiken LH, Schaffert-Witvliet B, Sloane DM, et al. Rationing of nursing care and its relationship to patient outcomes: the Swiss extension of the International Hospital Outcomes Study. Int J Qual Health Care. 2008;20(4):227–37.

Scott RD. The direct medical costs of healthcare-associated infections in US hospitals and the benefits of prevention; 2009.

Scott A, Timmons S. Tensions within management roles in healthcare organisations. Nurs Manag. 2017;24(1):31–7.

Sensmeier J. Make the most of health IT. Nurs Manag. 2016;47(12):32–5.

Sermeus W, Aiken LH, Van den Heede K, Rafferty AM, Griffiths P, Moreno-Casbas MT, et al. Nurse forecasting in Europe (RN4CAST): rationale, design and methodology. BMC Nurs. 2011;10(1):6.

Sheppard K. Compassion fatigue: are you at risk? Am Nurse Today. 2016;11(1):53–5.

Smiley RA, Lauer P, Bienemy C, Berg JG, Shireman E, Reneau KA, et al. The 2017 national nursing workforce survey. J Nurs Regul. 2018;9(3 Supplement)

Snavely TM. A brief economic analysis of the looming nursing shortage in the United States. Nurs Econ. 2016;34(2):98–101.

Squillace MR, Rosenoff E, Remsburg RE, Bercovitz A, Branden L. An introduction to the national nursing assistant survey. 2007.

Stanley D. Leadership and management. Chichester, UK: John Wiley & Sons; 2016.

Stewart W, Terry L. Reducing burnout in nurses and care workers in secure settings. Nurs Stand. 2014;28(34):37–45.

Strudwick G, Nagle L, Kassam I, Pahwa M, Sequeira L. Informatics competencies for nurse leaders: a scoping review. J Nurs Adm. 2019a;49(6):323–30.

Strudwick G, Booth RG, Bjarnadottir RI, Rossetti SC, Friesen M, Sequeira L, et al. The role of nurse managers in the adoption of health information technology: findings from a qualitative study. J Nurs Adm. 2019b;49(11):549–55.

Taylor B, Yankey N, Robinson C, Annis A, Haddock KS, Alt-White A, et al. Evaluating the Veterans Health Administration's Staffing Methodology model: a reliable approach. Nurs Econ. 2015;33(1):36.

Tierney SJ, Seymour-Route P, Crawford S. Weighted staffing plans for better prediction of staffing needs. J Nurs Adm. 2013;43(9):461–7.

Twigg D, Duffield C. A review of workload measures: a context for a new staffing methodology in Western Australia. Int J Nurs Stud. 2009;46(1):132–40.

Twigg D, Duffield C, Bremner A, Rapley P, Finn J. The impact of the nursing hours per patient day (NHPPD) staffing method on patient outcomes: a retrospective analysis of patient and staffing data. Int J Nurs Stud. 2011;48(5):540–8.

Twigg DE, Myers H, Duffield C, Pugh JD, Gelder L, Roche M. The impact of adding assistants in nursing to acute care hospital ward nurse staffing on adverse patient outcomes: an analysis of administrative health data. Int J Nurs Stud. 2016;63:189–200.

U.S Bureau of Labour Statistics. Occuaptional outlook handbook United States: U.S Bureau of Labour Statistics; 2013.

Unruh LY, Fottler MD. Patient turnover and nursing staff adequacy. Health Serv Res. 2006;41(2):599–612.

Vermeir P, Vandijck D, Degroote S, Peleman R, Verhaeghe R, Mortier E, et al. Communication in healthcare: a narrative review of the literature and practical recommendations. Int J Clin Pract. 2015;69(11):1257–67.

Vespa J, Armstrong DM, Medina L. Demographic turning points for the United States: population projections for 2020 to 2060: US Department of Commerce, Economics and Statistics Administration, US …; 2018.

Ward L, Fenton K, Maher L. The high impact actions for nursing and midwifery 8: ready to go – no delays…last in our series. Nurs Times. 2010;106(34):16–7.

Weggelaar-Jansen AMJ, Broekharst DS, De Bruijne M. Developing a hospital-wide quality and safety dashboard: a qualitative research study. BMJ Qual Saf. 2018;27(12):1000–7.

Welsh Government. Nurse Staffing Levels Act 2016. Cardiff: Welsh Government; 2016.

Westra BL, Delaney CW. Informatics competencies for nursing and healthcare leaders. AMIA annual symposium proceedings: American Medical Informatics Association; 2008.

Williams J, Smith AP. Stress, job satisfaction and mental health of NHS nurses. Contemporary Ergonomics and Human Factors 2013. 95: ROUTLEDGE in association with GSE Research; 2013. p. 95–102.

Wise S, Duffield C. Has the search for better leadership come at the expense of management? Int J Nurs Stud. 2019;97:A1–2.

World Health Organization. Global strategy on human resources for health: workforce 2030. Geneva, Switzerland: WHO; 2016.

World Health Organization. Global health workforce statistics: Geneva World Health Organisation; 2018.

Yazici HJ. The role of communication in organizational change: an empirical investigation. Inf Manag. 2002;39:539–52.

Chapter 10
Data Privacy and Security

Ross Fraser

Abstract This chapter begins by explaining why health information privacy is important, both to nurses and to patients. The concept of privacy is complex and it is common to think of privacy as interchangeable with security. This is untrue and this chapter will introduce readers to the definitions of privacy, personal health information, health information custodians, and security-related terms such as authentication, authorization, and audit trails. The concept of personal health information (PHI) is explored in relation to its collection, use, disclosure, and retention. The rationale for privacy, implicit and deemed consent, and withholding and revoking consent are also presented. Other approaches to protecting privacy are described, including developing a privacy policy, designating a privacy officer, de-identification of personal information, and pseudonomization. Information security is surveyed, including international standards and current areas of concern. The chapter closes by exploring how nurses can contribute to the protection of privacy.

Keywords Privacy · Security · Consent · Health information custodian · Data steward · De-identification · Pseudonymization · GDPR · User enrolment · User authentication · Audit · Ransomware

Key Concepts
- Privacy
- Security
- Informational Consent
- Health information custodian
- Data steward

Electronic Supplementary Material The online version of this chapter (https://doi.org/10.1007/978-3-030-58740-6_10) contains supplementary material, which is available to authorized users.

R. Fraser (✉)
Sextant Inc., Toronto, ON, Canada
e-mail: ross.fraser@sextantsoftware.com

© Springer Nature Switzerland AG 2021
P. Hussey, M. A. Kennedy (eds.), *Introduction to Nursing Informatics*, Health Informatics, https://doi.org/10.1007/978-3-030-58740-6_10

- De-identification
- Pseudonymization
- User enrolment
- User authentication
- Audit

Learning Objectives for the Chapter

1. Describe attitudes on concepts such as privacy and person in contemporary society.
2. Explain key factors impacting patient privacy and the confidentiality of personal health records.
3. Examine the concept of informational consent from the perspective of express, implied and deemed consent.
4. Discuss the impact of data breaches and explain the impact of hacking of patient electronic records using examples from practice.
5. Describe the fair information practices that have evolved to protect personal privacy.
6. Explain the basic principles of computer security and how they apply to the protection of personal health information.

10.1 Introduction

Informational privacy is best thought of as a human right. Currently, in most jurisdictions, laws and customs do not yet afford personal health information the same level of protection as is accorded to rights such as security of the person, freedom from arbitrary search and seizure, or the right to vote. An increasing body of law and jurisprudence in western democracies, however, recognizes the importance of ensuring that individuals have basic rights in relation to their own personal information.

As has been argued in previous chapters, the provision of modern healthcare is a multidisciplinary endeavour. Perforce, then such a coordinated process requires the exchange of patient information among the members of the patient's healthcare team (see Chap. 5 for a discussion of document exchange). Nurses ask patients to share information about health, work, home, social life, sex life, and emotional state. Patients comply because of their implicit assumption that this information will remain confidential; i.e., that it will be shared with a limited audience and only for certain purposes related to the patient's healthcare.

This chapter includes a brief overview of how thinking about privacy has evolved since the 1970s and how societies have come to view privacy and the protection of personal information, including personal health information. It defines some common terms used in contemporary discussions of patient privacy and describes the basic privacy principles that underpin contemporary thinking about informational privacy. Since health records are typically stored electronically instead of on paper, we also survey the techniques used to secure personal health information in digital format and discuss some issues that arise from the computer technology now in use. We discuss the challenges to healthcare providers in maintaining the privacy and security of personal health information. Finally, we discuss the role of nurses in maintaining the privacy and security of personal health information.

Throughout this chapter, the discussion will focus almost exclusively on the protection of personal information, especially personal health information. This type of protection complements, but is distinct from, maintaining the privacy of the person. The latter issue is important to healthcare providers, since the cultural norms that inform a patient about what constitutes invasion of personal privacy may be very different from those informing the healthcare providers treating the patient. While most cultures place special emphasis on privacy of the person in respect to the genitals, there is wider variation in the emphasis given to privacy of buttocks or breasts, and great variation in the cultural significance attached to viewing a woman's face. Healthcare providers are usually sensitive to such issues—traditional hospital gowns notwithstanding. In any event, the relevant issues are typically dealt with effectively by ensuring that physical examinations are conducted in private and by respecting a patient's wishes about the gender of the examining healthcare provider or about the additional presence of a person of specified gender to act as witness or chaperone. Protecting the confidentiality of personal health information is a much more complex undertaking than protecting privacy of the person. As we shall see below, the definition of what constitutes personal health information can itself be the subject of debate. The technical challenges involved in maintaining the confidentiality and availability of the information may be daunting, and the information collected may need to be securely protected for decades. The focus of the rest of the chapter will therefore be on informational privacy: i.e., the protection of personal information. Yet the reader must remain aware that however much patients may care about the confidentiality of their records, they care just as much—if not more—about the privacy and sanctity of their own persons.

10.2   Why Patient Privacy Matters

For an effective relationship to exist between healthcare providers and their patients, patients must believe that the information they provide will remain confidential. Patients may otherwise withhold information critical to their treatment and care. Ask yourself the following questions:

1. Given that men with paedophile tendencies make up 4 percent or more of the adult male population (Hall 1995; Cloud 2002), do you believe that men with paedophilic urges should seek counselling and treatment before those urges overwhelm them? Or are the risks entailed by such secret desires becoming public knowledge so great that such men should never discuss them with a healthcare provider and hence never obtain treatment?

2. Given that alcohol and drug abuse affects as much as 15 percent of the adult workforce (Frone 2006) and that functioning alcoholics and individuals struggling with drug addiction may hold senior positions in corporations, government, and the military, which society would you feel safer living in: one in which such individuals continue to work and live without recourse to effective treatments because disclosure of their condition might irreparably harm their careers? Or one in which such individuals seek out treatment, secure in the knowledge that their drug or alcohol problems will not become public knowledge?
3. Should adolescents be able to openly discuss HIV/AIDS prevention strategies with their healthcare providers, even if it means discussing intimate details of their sexuality, or should they instead avoid such discussions on the assumption that such details might become publicly known and hope instead that they'll be able to get all of the information they need from the Internet?
4. In the midst of a pandemic, should you be able to disclose symptoms and seek testing while trusting in the ability of healthcare professionals to trace contacts and determine the source of your infection without revealing your identity to others? Or should you instead fear catastrophic consequences such as losing your job, alarming neighbours, or being shunned by local merchants—in short, should you remain silent and hope that your symptoms remain mild?

Privacy may not matter to every patient, but as the questions above indicate, it matters a great deal to patients whose treatment and care impact the health of an entire society. How healthcare providers handle patient privacy can therefore play an important role in shaping the kind of society in which we live. As healthcare providers with extended access to patients, nurses have a vital role to play in building trust, encouraging patients to be entirely forthcoming about healthcare issues that concern them, and reassuring those patients that their healthcare information will remain confidential.

While the need to assure patients that their privacy would be protected existed long before their health records were computerized, the introduction of electronic health records has considerably increased public concern about the confidentiality of personal health information and likewise increased the concern of nurses and other healthcare professionals. There are several reasons for this. Firstly, there is truth in the old adage that 'to err is human but to really screw things up requires a computer.' Computerization has allowed losses of confidentiality to occur on an industrial scale. Whereas loss of paper records rarely involved more than a few thousand records, privacy breaches involving electronic records routinely involve tens of thousands of records in a single breach. While paper-based records have been lost to fires and floods, electronic health record systems have also been rendered unavailable and access to electronic records temporarily lost or permanently destroyed. The list of incidents over the last two decades is long and dishonourable and the reasons for the breaches are diverse:

- **Failure to adequate protect paper records**—an American health insurance company settled a lawsuit for US$17 million over a 2017 data breach in which the privacy of 12,000 patients was compromised after letters mailed to the patients revealed through the clear window of the envelopes that the patients had been taking drugs for HIV (Gordon 2018). Ironically, the letters had been mailed in response to the settlement of a previous privacy breach.

- **Failure to adequately dispose of paper records**—the United Kingdom Information Commissioner's Office (ICO) ordered Belfast Health and Social Care Trust to pay a £225,000 fine after determining that the organization had breached the UK Data Protection Act by closing a hospital in 2006 and leaving behind patient medical records, X-rays, scans, lab results, and unopened pay-slips; all abandoned in the empty hospital building (Connolly 2012). On several occasions, trespassers subsequently gained access to the site and took photographs of the records and posted them online.
- **Failure to adequately protect electronic records**—Cyber attacks by hackers on an American university hospital in 2017 breached the personal health records of 417,000 patients (Davis 2018). Dozens of similar attacks, some of breathtaking scope, now happen each year. In 2015, Anthem, Inc. disclosed that hackers had broken into its servers and stolen records containing personal information for 78.8 million people (Anthem 2015). The compromised information included names, birthdates, social security numbers, and medical IDs. Anthem was required to pay a US$16 million settlement for what had become the largest health data breach in American history.
- **Failure to adequately dispose of electronic records**—The UK ICO fined Brighton and Sussex University Hospitals £325,000 after highly sensitive personal data belonging to tens of thousands of patients and staff was stolen and sold on eBay (Guardian Government Computing 2012). The data, including some relating to HIV and genito-urinary patients as well as information referring to criminal convictions and suspected offences, had been stored on hard drives sold on the Internet auction site in October and November 2010.
- **Failure to comply with established policies**—personal health data of tens of thousands, possibly hundreds of thousands of Canadians were accessed without proper authorization, including information on the mental, physical and sexual health of individuals, as well as lifestyle and use of health services. In the most serious cases, the British Columbia provincial government notified 38,486 individuals of the breaches (Canadian Broadcasting Corporation 2013). In three separate instances in 2010 and 2012, health information was saved on USB sticks and shared with university researchers or with contractors. Proper permissions had not been obtained and suitable procedural protocols had not been devised.
- **Staff misconduct**—in 1996, a state public health worker in Florida sent the names of 4000 HIV positive patients to two Florida newspapers (Stein 1997; Jurgens 2001)
- **Loss of systems availability**—in 2012, dozens of hospitals across the US lost access to electronic medical records for five hours during a computer outage that was caused by human error (Terhune 2012). Within minutes of the outage, doctors and nurses reverted to writing orders and notes by hand, but in many cases no longer had access to patient information previously saved in electronic records, potentially compromising patient care.

- **Loss of data**—in 2009, a computer hacker successfully compromised a health database used by pharmacies and doctors to track narcotics and painkiller prescriptions and stole records of more than eight million patients (Krebs 2009). The hacker then demanded a $10 million ransom from the state of Virginia, which the state government refused to pay. There have been many more examples in the years since. Russian hackers held an Australian medical centre to ransom in 2012 after encrypting thousands of patient health records and then demanding $4,000 to decrypt them (Hicks 2012). A California-based health service provider permanently closed in 2019 after it failed to recover patient records that were encrypted in a ransomware attack, stating that it would be impossible to rebuild its medical records and resume its practice (Srinivas 2019). An Ohio urology clinic also suffered a ransomware attack in 2019 after hackers breached its IT system and left all its patient data encrypted. A US $75,000 ransom was paid to unlock the data.

If the recent past is any indication, patient privacy and the confidentiality of personal health records will remain in the news and hence in the public's awareness for many years to come.

There is a final argument that is sometimes made to minimize the importance of privacy: that inter-generational shifts in attitudes have taken place and that young people are not concerned about their privacy (or, at least, they are less concerned than their parents' generation were). The evidence for such statements is equivocal. Inter-generational shifts in attitudes to privacy can be highly context-dependent, and the willingness of young people to share certain forms of personal information in online forums such as Facebook or Twitter cannot be taken as an indication that they care less about the privacy of their healthcare information. Certainly, societal attitudes shift over time in regard to what one might normally consider confidential. In 1968, Canadian gay men and lesbians were still subject to criminal prosecution for having consensual sex with their partners. In 2005, thirty-seven years later, such couples could legally marry anywhere in Canada. This shift in societal attitudes in that country has had an obvious impact on the importance placed on the confidentiality of sexual orientation as recorded in personal health records. Yet such liberalized attitudes are highly variable. The percentage of the American public opposed to abortion in 2019 is essentially identical to what it was in 1995 (Pew Research Center 2019) and the importance placed on the confidentiality of medical abortions may therefore not be very different in the U.S. now than it was a quarter of a century ago.

10.3 Definitions

Some terms are inevitably encountered in any robust discussion of privacy and information security and they are included in the discussion that follows. While nearly all of these terms are also used outside of healthcare, some have special meaning for healthcare providers. Where this is the case, additional discussion is provided on the use of these terms in healthcare settings.

Participants in a nursing informatics conference in Toronto in 2013 were asked to provide a definition of **privacy**. After much lively discussion, they defined it as the right of individuals and organizations to decide for themselves when, how, and to what extent information about them is transmitted to others. It is as good a definition as can be found in many privacy-related discussions, and more relevant to nursing than most.

Consent is an agreement, approval, or permission given voluntarily by a competent person that permits some act(s) for some stated purpose(s) (Adapted from Black's Law Dictionary 2009). For example, a patient may consent to having their personal health information collected by a clinic or consent to its disclosure to a third party (e.g., an insurance provider). Note that in this chapter, consent will always be used to refer to **informational consent** (i.e., consent to share or disclose information) as opposed to consent to treatment and care. Although consent for treatment and consent to collect, use or disclose health information are sometimes bundled together on the same patient consent form, they are distinct concepts. A patient may consent to an abortion but not consent to her personal health information being disclosed or used outside the clinic: indeed, she may insist that it not be. Conversely, a patient may consent to participation in a medical research project on sexual practices and sexually transmitted diseases without consenting to (or having any expectation of receiving) treatment.

Informational consent can take one of several forms. **Express consent** is an explicit (usually written) instruction from the patient—a voluntary agreement regarding what is being done or proposed that is unequivocal and does not require any inference or assumptions on the part of the healthcare organization or healthcare provider seeking consent. **Implied consent** is a voluntary agreement that can be reasonably determined through the actions or inactions of the patient. For example, if a patient voluntarily provides a urine sample to a diagnostic laboratory for the purpose of performing a lab test requested by the patient's healthcare provider, it can reasonably be inferred that the patient has consented to information related to the test being disclosed by the lab to the healthcare provider (otherwise, why bother to provide the urine sample and perform the tests?) In most jurisdictions, implied consent is sufficient for the collection, use and (limited) disclosure of personal health information.

Some jurisdictions have statutory provisions for **deemed consent**: under certain stated conditions, the law permits organizations to act as if the patient has consented, regardless of whether or not the patient has actually done so; the patient has no right to withdraw or withhold consent. This may include disclosures of personal health information for the purpose of mandatory reporting of certain infectious diseases, or to allow healthcare providers to comply with certain professional ethical practices.

A patient may **withhold consent** by expressly stating that s/he does not consent to a particular activity. Withholding consent occurs when a patient indicates that s/

he does not consent to the sharing of personal health information previously collected.

A patient may also **withdraw consent** previously given (also referred to as a patient **revoking consent**). Withdrawing or revoking consent occurs when a patient who has expressly provided consent or where consent has previously been implied revokes that consent at some later date.

A patient's **circle of care** (Information and Privacy Commissioner of Ontario 2015) refers to the persons participating in, and the activities related to, the provision of health care to the patient. This includes healthcare providers involved with necessary but incidental activities such as laboratory work or professional consultation. The term is sometimes used in privacy discussions and even privacy policies of healthcare organizations; e.g., when promising not to share a patient's personal information outside their circle of care without the patient's express consent.

A **health information custodian** (sometimes called a **data steward**) is an individual or organization that collects, uses, or discloses personal health information for the purposes of patient treatment and care, medical billing, health system planning and management, or health research. Depending on a jurisdiction's law or policy, any of the following entities may be considered a health information custodian:

- healthcare providers, i.e., professionals licensed or registered to provide health services
- Ministries or Departments of Health for a country, state, province, municipality or other governmental jurisdiction
- regional health authorities (where such entities exist)
- hospitals, nursing homes or other identified health care facilities
- pharmacies (and pharmacists, who are included above under healthcare providers)
- boards of health, agencies, committees and other organisations identified in jurisdictional regulations (e.g., a mental health board, cancer care board, etc.) and
- ambulance operators and paramedics.

Not every jurisdiction has privacy laws protecting personal health information. Where law and policy do not clearly outline custodial responsibilities in the collection, use and disclosure of personal health information, healthcare providers may need to look to their professional associations, licencing bodies, or colleges for guidance about their professional responsibilities.

A **privacy officer** is an individual who oversees activities related to the development, implementation, maintenance of, and adherence to an organization's policies and procedures covering the privacy, confidentiality and sometimes security of personal information. In many jurisdictions, it is now standard practice for large healthcare organizations such as hospitals to have a designated privacy officer. Privacy officers oversee access to personal health information by patients and their families. They also ensure patients are notified of their privacy rights. They educate staff about privacy responsibilities and provide privacy oversight and review of the organisation's information handling practices. They also respond to questions and complaints from patients and the public concerning the organization's information privacy practices. Privacy officers may also be required to periodically review and revise organizational privacy policies and practices in order to ensure currency with industry best practices and legislative developments.

Anonymity allows the subjects in a database to remain nameless and unidentified. Patient anonymity is frequently found in research databases and in data that consists of statistical summaries.

If data is anonymised, the data subject(s) cannot be identified by the recipients of the data. The process of anonymising data involves removing any information that identifies the patient or any information that could be utilized, either alone or with other information, to identify the patient. This process of **de-identification** is typically a non-trivial undertaking: it consists of taking steps necessary to ensure that the anonymised data cannot be utilized, either alone or with other information, to identify a patient. A variety of statistical techniques may need to be employed to ensure successful de-identification: i.e., to ensure that the risk of re-identification has been reduced to an acceptably low level.

Anonymity can also apply to users of information systems. Truly anonymous access to an online service is only obtained when each individual instance of system access cannot be linked over time to later access to the same or other online services (i.e., users are not asked to register or log in to such systems, nor is repeated access over time by a user tracked by means of web browser cookies or other such technical means).

Pseudonymity allows the subjects in a database to be tracked over time while remaining nameless. Pseudonyms (e.g., patient X, patient Y, etc.) are attached to records in place of names, addresses and other public identifiers. Users of online services can also be given pseudonyms, or choose their own, during user registration, allowing them to maintain a consistent pseudonymous presence from one online encounter to another. Many web sites allow users to remain pseudonymous. Note that much discussion of anonymity is actually a discussion of pseudonymity and many users claiming to want online anonymity actually want online pseudonymity (e.g., in blogs, on Twitter, etc.).

The terms anonymous and anonymity are often used when the terms pseudonymous and pseudonymity should be used instead. Truly anonymous patient data is typically useless in a long-term longitudinal study, as new data collected on a given patient cannot be matched up with data collected on the same patient the previous year or the year before (all the patients are anonymous). Rather, such databases are typically pseudonymous: data collected last year on patient 13786 is linked to new data collected from patient 13786. Such schemes require some trusted party or methodology to reliably and consistently derive the pseudonym (13786) from personal identifiers such as patient name, address, birthdate, etc. This process of **pseudonymization** is said to be **irreversible** if, after identifiable data have been processed to produce pseudonymous data, it is computationally infeasible to trace back to the original identifier from the pseudonym.

Every information system used in healthcare requires that users be identified, registered as new users, and authorized to access various types of data (e.g., patient demographics, billing data, or lab test results) or to perform various types of services (registering a new patient, writing a prescription, or ordering a lab test). **User identification** (sometimes referred to as **user identity verification**) is done once during **user registration** prior to allowing an individual to access an information system. Identification answers the question "who are you?" and is an essential part of the user registration process.

User enrolment is done once for each online service or computer program within an organization that a registered user is authorized to access. User enrolment answers questions such as: "what information repositories do you need to access?" and "do you need to edit records as well as view them?" Once enrolled, a user has the **authorization** to access the relevant data or services.

User authentication is done each time a user logs into a computer system or program. User authorization attempts to securely answer the question "is the person logging into the system really you?"

Auditing is done by keeping **audit log** files (sometimes referred to as an **audit trail**) that record *which* users have done *what* and *when*. An audit log answers, for each user, the questions "what information have you accessed?", "what changes to information have you made?", "what actions have you performed? (printing records, transferring records, merging records, etc.)" and "when were these actions performed?"

10.4   What Constitutes Personal Health Information?

Personal health information is information about an identifiable individual that relates to the physical or mental health of the individual, or to provision of health services to the individual. It may include:

- information about registration of the individual for the provision of health services, including name, address, phone numbers and other contact details, plus other demographic information such as birthdate,
- information about payments or eligibility for health care insurance,
- a number or other identifier assigned to an individual to uniquely identify the individual for health care purposes,
- information about the individual that is collected in the course of the providing the individual with health services,
- information derived from the testing or examination of a body part or bodily substance (e.g., a lab test result or diagnostic image), or
- identification of healthcare providers involved in the provision of healthcare to the individual.

Personal health information does not include information that is anonymised, either by itself or when combined with other available information (see above for a discussion of anonymity).

10.5   What Determines the Sensitivity of Personal Health Information?

In the past, there has been a tendency to treat certain types of clinical information as more or less sensitive than other types. For example, tests revealing HIV status were considered more sensitive than other lab test results. Encounter records were thought more sensitive than demographic data and mental health records were felt to be more sensitive than other encounter records. Such attempts to build a hierarchy of sensitivity levels within personal health information are fraught with challenges. Firstly, the patient ultimately decides which data is most sensitive. To a woman escaping an abusive partner, the confidentiality of information about the treatment of her broken arm may be of little concern, but the confidentiality her new address at a women's shelter may be of vital importance. Someone treated for a drinking problem may consider a list of allergies to be of no consequence but would consider a disulfiram prescription in the medication history to be highly confidential. The mere presence of a patient's name in the registry of a cancer clinic would indicate to others that the patient had cancer—an inference that the patient may not want anyone outside the circle of care to make.

The belief that personal health information admits of degrees ('not confidential,' 'somewhat confidential,' 'highly confidential') and that these can be determined beforehand by information system designers is largely a myth. Personal health information—all of it—should be treated as confidential, not shared outside the patient's circle of care without the patient's express consent except where permitted or required by law. It must be protected by reasonable technical and administrative safeguards throughout its entire useful lifetime, and then securely disposed of when no longer needed.

10.6   A Brief History of Informational Privacy

Fair Information Practice was a term initially proposed in a report prepared in 1973 on behalf of the US Secretary of Health (Hare 1973a). The report was written in response to the growing use of data processing systems containing information about individuals. Its lasting contribution to privacy was the development of a code of fair information practices for record-keeping organizations collecting personal data. By contemporary standards, these practices are straightforward: that there be no databases containing personal information whose very existence is secret; that individuals have the right to find out what type of information is held about them and what it is used for; that personal information collected for one purpose must not be subsequently used for another purpose without obtaining the individual's consent; that there be some procedure allowing an individual to correct or amend a record of personal information about that individual; and that organizations creating, using, maintaining or disseminating records of identifiable personal data must assure the reliability of the data for their intended use and must take reasonable steps to prevent misuse of the data (Hare 1973b). These recommendations subsequently provided the foundation for the US Federal Privacy Act of 1974.

In 1980, the Council of Europe adopted a *Convention for the Protection of Individuals with Regard to Automatic Processing of Personal Data* (Council of Europe 1981a). It extended somewhat the Fair Information Practice core principles and included (modest) special provisions for "personal data concerning health or sexual life" (Council of Europe 1981b). In the same year, the Organisation for Economic Cooperation and Development (OECD) proposed *Guidelines on the Protection of Privacy and Transborder Flows of Personal Data* (Organization for Economic Co-Operation and Development 1999). These OECD Guidelines, the Council of Europe Convention, and the 1995 European Union Data Protection Directive (European Union 1995) all built upon the Fair Information Practices as core principles, revising and extending the original concepts. The OECD guidelines influenced subsequent privacy law and policy in many countries, including Canada (Holmes 2006), Australia (Clarke 2000), the UK (Smith 1994), and others.

Contemporary approaches to patient privacy continue to evolve.

10.7   Privacy Principles

While the OECD *Guidelines on the Protection of Privacy and Transborder Flows of Personal Data* have influenced both law and policy on the protection of personal information, the eight principles in the *Guidelines* have been further elaborated upon in several countries to incorporate nuances that were not explicit in the original. Below we will first examine the ten privacy principles in the *Model Code for the Protection of Personal Information* (Canadian Standards Association 1996), published by the Canadian Standards Association in 1996 and later incorporated into Canadian laws that protect personal health information. With minor variations, these principles can also be seen in the laws in Europe, Australia, New Zealand, and other countries. Some aspects of these principals can also be seen in the US Health Insurance Portability and Accountability Act of 1996 (US Government Printing Office 1996). Later, we will examine the core principles of the European General Data Protection Regulation (GDPR), a European Union directive that, 20 years after the Canadian principles were written, expanded upon these privacy principles and added several new principles relevant to healthcare and the protection of personal health information. The GDPR has also had a marked impact globally and has influenced national and regional legislation in non-European jurisdictions such as California, Hong Kong, and Israel.

As core principles, the ten Canadian principles established in 1996 facilitated an easily recognisable and exemplary approach to data protection. These ten principles are stated below in a form that emphasizes their relation to personal health information. Similarly worded principles have formed the basis of subsequent legislation and regulation in other countries, and so our discussion will not be limited to Canada:

1. **Accountability for information**: Organizations that collect, use or disclose PHI are responsible for the personal health information in their custody or care.

    A named individual within the organization should be responsible for facilitating organizational compliance with applicable data protection legislation and organizational privacy policies.

2. **Identifying purposes for collection, use and disclosure of information**: To allow patients to make appropriate decisions about their PHI, it is important that they be made aware of the purposes for which this information is being collected, used, and disclosed.

There are many legitimate purposes for collecting personal health information; indeed, an international standard classification of such purposes has been developed (ISO/TS 14265: Health Informatics – Classification of purposes for processing personal health information 2011). These purposes include:

- providing clinical care to an individual
- providing emergency care to an individual
- supporting care activities for the individual within the healthcare organisation
- enabling medical billing and/or permissions from a funding party for providing health care services to the patient)
- health service management and quality assurance
- education for health care professionals
- public health surveillance and disease control (i.e., monitoring populations for significant health events and then intervening to provide health care or preventive care to relevant individuals)
- public safety emergency (i.e., protecting the public in a situation in which there is significant risk that is possibly not health-related)
- population health management (i.e., monitoring populations for health events, trends or outcomes in order to inform strategy and policy)
- research
- market studies to support the discovery of product-specific knowledge
- law enforcement (enforcing jurisdictional legislation or assisting forensic investigation) and
- patient use (in support of the patient's own interests).

Personal health information collected for the purposes of treatment and care cannot generally be used for unrelated purposes (e.g., for clinical research) unless the patient consented to these additional purposes at the time of collection. Specific jurisdictions may have exceptions in law or regulation that permit such secondary uses without obtaining express consent from each patient.

3. **Consent**: An organisation should be able to demonstrate that it is in compliance with applicable laws and that the patient can reasonably be expected to know that

information about them was going to be collected and used for defined purposes. In order for an instance of consent to be valid, it must:

- be given by the individual to whom the information relates if she or he is capable of consenting at the time of consenting or by a substitute decision-maker;
- relate to the information in question;
- not be obtained through deception or coercion;
- be knowledgeable (i.e. it must be reasonable in the circumstances to believe that the patient knows the purposes for which the information is being collected, used, or disclosed, that the patient has had the opportunity to withhold consent—if that is what the patient wants—and that the patient has been informed of the reasonable consequences of such action).

The last point deserves elaboration. A balance needs to be found between either demanding blanket access to all available personal health information, or allowing patient consent restrictions to stand in the way of effective treatment. Patients need to understand that restrictions they place on the disclosure of their personal health information may impact the quality of their care. Healthcare providers, for their part, need to understand that refusing to treat a patient unless the patient allows the unrestricted collection, use and disclosure of his/her personal health information not only shows disrespect for patient privacy but also holds patients to ransom ("give use all your data or we won't treat you.") The cost of striking the necessary balance need not be burdensome: a brief but well-written notice to patients (e.g., posted in waiting rooms) can go far towards streamlining the administration of patient consent while at the same time enhancing patient trust.

4. **Limiting collection** (also referred to in European Union regulations as **data minimization**): Organisations should limit collection of personal health information to that which is necessary for the identified purposes; i.e. personal health information should not be collected indiscriminately.

Historically, many fields of data (e.g., religion and race) were collected in patient records, even in cases where they had little or no bearing on treatment and care. While there may be jurisdictional laws that mandate the collection of certain information (e.g., race) for statistical and public health surveillance purposes, designers and implementers of electronic health record systems need to carefully review the relevance of the data collected and limit collection to what is needed.

5. **Limiting use, disclosure and retention**: Once organisations identify the purposes for which they collect personal information and then seek consent, as appropriate, from patients to collect information for these purposes, these organization should only use, disclose and retain information for the same purposes. In the European Union's regulations, retention is referred to as the **storage limitation principle**.

Personal health information should not be collected for one purpose (e.g., treatment and care), and then used for another (e.g., research) without first obtaining the consent of the patient for the new use. When a later use is found for data, this new use is sometimes called a **secondary use**. Secondary uses usually require express patient consent, but there may be certain exemptions in local laws or regulations.

6. **Accuracy** (referred to in European Union regulations as the **right to rectification**): The need for accuracy as a fair information practice is particularly relevant in the delivery of healthcare. Patients are typically aware of the need to provide accurate information in order to ensure that healthcare is delivered in a safe, efficient and effective way. Personal health information needs to be sufficiently accurate, complete and up-to-date to minimize the possibility that inappropriate information is being used to make a decision about a patient. Of particular concern to healthcare organizations is ensuring that patients are properly identified and that the subject of the data is actually the patient in question.

7. **Safeguards**: By implementing information security safeguards, organisations protect personal health information against loss and theft, as well as unauthorised access, disclosure, copying, use, and modification. These safeguards are discussed further in the section below. In the European Union regulations, safeguards are referred to as the **integrity and confidentiality principle**, and elsewhere as the **security principle**.

8. **Openness**: It should be possible for concerned patients to know the purposes for which information about them is collected, used, and disclosed. Also, they should have access to an overview of the technical and administrative safeguards that are in place to ensure the confidentiality of that information. At a minimum, the organizations' privacy policy should be available to patients.

9. **Individual access**: Patients should have the right to access their own personal health information so that they can assure its accuracy, and amend inaccurate or incomplete information. This may require mediated access: i.e., patients may need to go over their record with a healthcare provider to understand the meaning of the information contained therein. Patients may also need counselling, as appropriate, to ensure that potentially disturbing information is reviewed appropriately and sensitively. Nurses are sometimes called upon to perform this counselling function.

10. **Challenging compliance** (referred to in European Union regulations as the **right to object**): The right of a patient to lodge a privacy complaint against an organization was first articulated when the *Fair Information Practices* were promulgated more than forty years ago (Federal Trade Commission (US) n.d.).

The General Data Protection Regulation, a substantial revision of the European Data Directive that was passed by the European Union in 2016, has added several new or enhanced privacy principles to this established list of principles:

11. **Right of erasure**: Under Article 17 of the GDPR, individuals have the general right to have their personal data erased. This is also known as the "right to be forgotten." This right is not absolute and only applies in certain circumstances, for example, where the personal data is no longer necessary for the purpose for which it was originally collected, or where the individual has withdrawn their

consent. Importantly, the erasure applies to both online systems and to backup data. But broad exceptions strictly limit this right in the case of personal health information. The right of erasure does not apply if processing of the data is necessary for public health purposes (e.g., protecting against serious threats to health such as pandemics, or ensuring high standards of quality and safety of drugs or medical devices); or if the processing is necessary for the purposes of preventative or occupational medicine under the responsibility of a healthcare professional (e.g., where the processing is necessary for medical diagnosis, for the provision of health or social care, or for the management of health or social care systems or services).

12. **Breach notification**: Article 33 of the GDPR specifies that individuals have, under somewhat circumscribed conditions, the right to know if a serious privacy breach has occurred that involves their personal information. The right is tentative but follows on such rights being established in law in Australia (Office of the Australian Information Commissioner n.d.), Canada (Privacy Commissioner of Canada 2018), the US (National Conference of State Legislatures 2020), and many other jurisdictions.

13. **Lawful basis**: The GDPR specifies that the processing of personal information must be based on at least one of (a) consent (the individual has given clear consent to process their personal data for a specific purpose), (b) contract (the processing is necessary for a contract with the individual, or because they have asked for specific steps to be taken before entering into a contract), (c) legal obligation (the processing is necessary to comply with the law), (d) vital interests (the processing is necessary to protect someone's life), (e) public task (the processing is necessary to perform a task in the public interest or for official functions that have a clear basis in law), or (f) legitimate interests (the processing is necessary for the legitimate interests of the data processor or the legitimate interests of a third party, unless there is a good reason to protect the individual's personal data which overrides those legitimate interests). Provision (f) does not apply to a public authority processing data to perform an official task.

14. **Data Portability**: In a similar vein to the U.S. Health Insurance Portability and Accountability Act of 1996 (HIPAA), the GDPR also introduces a right to data portability. This allows individuals to obtain and reuse their personal data for their own purposes across different services. It therefore allows patients to move, copy or transfer personal data from one IT system to another in a safe and secure way, without affecting the data's usability.

The GDPR also sets a high standard for consent, continuing an international trend that has progressed over the last 20 years. It requires explicit (as opposed to implied) consent for the collection and processing of personal health information. Patient consent must be explicitly obtained for each purpose for which data has been collected and is being used (typical purposes being treatment and care, or medical research). Consent must be a specific, freely given, plainly worded, and unambiguous affirmation by the patient; an online form with consent options that default to opt-in is in violation of the GDPR. The GDPR also addresses an important issue for the treatment of adolescents: when are they old enough to issue informational consent directives? The answer it gives is 16 years old, with some additional specific provisions for patients as young as 13 years old (European Parliament 2016).

10.8   Privacy Policy

It has become common for organizations to formulate a privacy policy and make it available to the public. Healthcare organizations are active participants in this trend. Even where nurses are not involved in the development of the policy, they, like all staff, should be familiar with it.

There is no universally agreed-upon format or outline for an organizational privacy policy in healthcare. Good policies typically contain most or all of the following components:

- a broad description of the types of personal information held—but not an exhaustive list of data fields (e.g., contact information, diagnostic test data, or lists of currently active prescriptions)
- a description of the purposes for which the information is collected, used, and disclosed (e.g., treatment and care, fundraising, clinical research)
- a statement about how the information is used (e.g., during patient consultation and diagnosis)
- a commitment to maintain the confidentiality of the information (e.g., an assurance that the organization is committed to respecting personal privacy, safeguarding confidential information and ensuring the security of personal health information within its custody)
- a non-technical description of the security steps taken to protect confidential information when it is stored or transmitted
- a description of the circumstances under which personal information will be disclosed to third parties (e.g., to an IT service provider securely hosting the data on a central server or providing external processing),
- a description of the circumstances under which data is depersonalized (i.e., anonymised or pseudonymised) or aggregated (e.g., for the purpose of gathering and reporting healthcare statistics) and
- contact information and procedures to follow for individuals who have questions about the privacy of their data or who have a complaint.

10.9   Information Security Principles

Maintaining the confidentiality of information is one of three primary goals of information security. The other two goals are maintaining the integrity of data (i.e., preventing information from being corrupted, either unintentionally or maliciously) and maintaining the availability of information systems and data either in the face of environmental disasters such as equipment failures, fires, floods, or power outages; or in the face of hostile actions such as denial of service attacks on systems by hackers or disgruntled employees. Information security specialists typically pursue all three goals in tandem. While privacy concerns often focus attention on data confidentiality, the continuous availability of systems and data is equally essential for healthcare operations. As noted above in Sec. 10.2, many health organizations have been struck by ransomware, a form of computer virus that encrypts the data in a system to make it inaccessible to the system's users. System administrators are then met with a ransom demand to unlock the data. Ransomware works because data backup often doesn't—hospitals and other large healthcare organizations have thus sometimes failed to ensure the ongoing availability of their healthcare systems and data.

Effective information security is a chain with many links: many separate safeguards are required to ensure that the confidentiality of data is maintained. The resulting security is only as good as the weakest link(s) in the chain. There are so many links in the information security chain that a series of international standards was developed to catalogue them and describe their effective use. The best known of these standards are ISO 27001 (*Information technology—Security techniques—Information security management systems—Requirements*) (ISO 27001 2013) and ISO 27002 (*Information technology—Security techniques—Code of practice for information security controls*) (ISO 27002 2013), published by the International Organization for Standardization. While these standards are not specific to any particular industrial sector, a healthcare-specific guideline for information security, ISO 27799, was developed in 2006 and revised in 2016 (ISO 27799 2016). All of these standards break down the task of providing information security into 14 specific areas. Each is described below.

1. **Information Security Policy**: Every organization collecting, using, or storing personal health information should have a security policy, appropriate to the jurisdiction in which the organization operates. Security is far too complex— and security incidents can unfold far too quickly—for staff to make up procedures as they go along. A robust security policy deals with all of the areas below that are relevant to the organization's operations.
2. **Organizing Information Security**: Like the first privacy principle above (accountability for information), good information security requires that there be a named individual responsible for security (sometimes called a chief information security officer) within any organization that hosts an electronic health record system or other large repository of personal health information. Reporting responsibilities for security incidents also need to be clear and unambiguous.
3. **Asset Management**: Organizations need to be aware of all their information assets, including data repositories and also the systems, software and hardware on which they run. When faced with the Y2K bug in the late 1990s, many healthcare organizations realized that they did not have an adequate inventory of system and data repositories—even when such systems and data were critical to patient treatment and care.

4. **Human Resources Security**: Organizations need to ensure that staff members: are aware of information security threats and concerns; prevent damage from security incidents and malfunctions caused by human error; and reduce the risks to information security from theft, fraud or misuse of facilities.

5. **Access Control**: This includes the identification of users during user registration, the assignment of access privileges that determine which information resources and services these users can access, their subsequent authentication during log in, and their authorisation prior to being granted access to specific services and data. Access control is intended to prevent unauthorised access to information systems as well as to ensure information security when users are accessing data via mobile computing and networking facilities.

6. **Cryptography**: Encryption is an enormously important aspect of maintaining data confidentiality but the topic is also highly technical and has, in the past, been fraught with errors made by those who thought they understood cryptography but were subsequently proved wrong. Expert advice is needed to ensure that cryptography is properly applied to protect data in transit and in storage.

7. **Physical and Environmental Security**: Physical security prevents unauthorised access, damage and theft of equipment or information storage media. Environmental security protects against damage or compromise of assets and interruption to business activities from fires, floods, and other environmental disasters.

8. **Operations Security**: Operations security ensures the correct and secure operation of information processing facilities; protects the integrity of software and information; maintains the integrity and availability of information processing; minimizes the risk of systems failures; safeguards information in databases and supporting infrastructures; prevents damage to information assets; and prevents loss, modification or misuse of information or documents exchanged between organisations. Data security aims to protect the confidentiality, integrity and availability of all data stored in data repositories.

9. **Communications Security**: Communications security aims to protect (principally via encryption) the confidentiality and integrity of data and messages transmitted from, or to, or within an organization.

10. **Information Systems Acquisition, Development and Maintenance**: Information systems need to be developed with security in mind: security must be an integral component of information systems: baked-in like the flour in a cake, not layered on later, like icing. If security is an afterthought, the information system will not be robustly secure.

11. **Supplier Relationships**: Many healthcare organizations have turned to third-party service providers and cloud computing to deliver their information systems. As the computer rooms of the 1970s were replaced by Internet connections to vast commercial data centres built in the 2010s, the importance of the supplier relationships with third party data centre and network providers (Amazon, Microsoft, CloudFlare, and others) have become ever more important. Healthcare organizations can turn to suppliers to provide systems, applications and databases, but these organizations retain the obligation to ensure that ade-

quate controls are in place to maintain the confidentiality, data integrity, and availability of personal health information. That responsibility cannot be outsourced.

12. **Information Security Incident Management**: Security incident management builds an organizational infrastructure for reporting security incidents and suspected weaknesses. In doing so, it minimizes the damage from security incidents and malfunctions. Security incidents within healthcare organizations need to be managed effectively, and improvements need to be implemented to prevent future occurrences. Nurses, like all healthcare providers, have an important role to play in reporting (suspected) security breaches.

13. **Information Security Aspects of Business Continuity**: The demands placed on healthcare organizations can be onerous: environmental problems such as hurricanes that are notorious for sharply increasing the demand for emergency medical services are at the same time tests of the ability of information systems to remain operational in adverse circumstances. Components of disaster recovery such as data backup can entail unique information security challenges: copies of backed-up data, for example, are just as confidential as the original data.

14. **Compliance**: Organizations must comply with the laws that their respective jurisdictions have enacted to protect personal health information. An important component of information security is ensuring that the steps taken to secure the collection, use, disclosure, and retention of personal health information meet the minimum requirements set out by law and regulation.

10.10   Limits to Privacy

Maintaining the implied trust that exists between patients and their healthcare providers requires that the reasonable expectations of both groups be met. It is reasonable for a gynaecologist to ask a patient whether an abortion had previously been carried out. It is almost entirely unreasonable that this question be posed by a dentist. What, then, constitutes a reasonable request for personal health information? For patients, such privacy-related assessments are often founded on the patient's perception of a need-to-know. Will surrendering personal information help my healthcare provider make a more accurate diagnosis? Is the information needed to allow better decisions to be made about my treatment? Will it help my care team assess the outcome? To the extent that patients believe the answer is "yes", they are more likely to comply with attempts to collect such information.

Patient perceptions of the healthcare provider's need-to-know may therefore need to be addressed in the structuring of intake procedures and the related forms that gather needed personal information. Nurses involved in intake play an important role in reassuring patients that requests for personal information are reasonable; i.e., that the information requested is needed by healthcare providers to perform the tasks of assessment, diagnosis, or treatment—tasks that will directly benefit the patient. Conversely, "just fill in the form" is never a good answer to the question "why are you asking me these personal questions"?

Not all patient privacy concerns can be addressed realistically. A common concern of patients is whether a friend, neighbour, or relative who works as a healthcare provider will be able to access the patient's personal health data (Gostin 2001). When the healthcare provider in question is also a staff member of the facility collecting the information, it may be difficult to place restrictions on their access to such data. An important role is played in this situation by the operation of an audit log that records all accesses to all records by all users of an electronic medical record system. Regular review of audit logs goes far towards eliminating the problem of inappropriate access to records, and it thus helps in the enforcement of professional standards.

Finally, patients may have unrealistic expectations about the granularity or grouping of data fields in the their records. They may naively assume that information about a specific condition such as HIV/AIDS can be easily masked ("don't disclose the AIDS flag") whereas the information they are concerned about may be evident from many data sources (e.g., treatment for HIV/AIDS may be evident from summary care records, diagnostic test results, prescription medications, and counselling records, among others). Moreover, most medical record systems cannot block access to data on a field-by-field basis. Patients need to be informed about both the extent and the format of the information they are concerned about so that their privacy concerns can be realistically assessed.

10.11   Privacy of Healthcare Providers

While the focus of this chapter has been on patient privacy, healthcare providers also have legitimate privacy concerns. Perhaps primary among those concerns is whether data collected for one purpose (e.g., patient wait-time management) can later be used for a different purpose (e.g., ranking healthcare providers as identifiable professionals on their timely delivery of healthcare services). In some jurisdictions, data collected on healthcare professionals by healthcare organizations is explicitly excluded from consideration as personal information. In others, the distinct is not clear-cut.

Nurses, like other healthcare professionals, are also patients. Most healthcare professional associations demand a clear delineation between data collected on healthcare providers as professionals rendering healthcare services, and data collected on healthcare providers as patients undergoing treatment. Organizations must be careful to ensure that the rights of nurses and other healthcare professionals as patients are not compromised by their involvement as professionals and staff in the very organizations responsible for their treatment.

10.12 The Role of Nurses in Maintaining the Privacy and Security of Personal Health Information

This chapter has discussed several areas of privacy administration in which nurses can fulfil an important role:

- In the formation and review of institutional privacy policies: healthcare institutional policies need to accommodate the workflow of all healthcare providers, not just those of physicians. Nurses need to ensure that privacy policies are both robust and practicable. They should be empowered to provide appropriate feedback when this is not the case.
- During patient admission and at other times during the course of treatment and care when information is elicited from patients: patients need trustworthy advice about what types of personal information will be collected from them, and for what purpose and uses. How long will this information be retained? How will its confidentiality be protected? To whom will it be disclosed and why? These questions deserve informed answers and nurses should be prepared to provide them.
- In the creation of patient education materials that clearly explain how personal health information is collected, used, retained and disclosed, and how that information is protected while being held.
- In inculcating patient trust: nurses can provide a supportive atmosphere in which patients can disclose deeply personal information that is sometimes painful to divulge. This is arguably the most important activity that nurses carry out in relation to an individual patient's privacy. It is a task for which nurses are perhaps most uniquely suited.

By diligently carrying out these activities when assigned, nurses maintain a venerable tradition. The oldest ethical guide for the nursing profession was provided by Canadian-born Lystra Gretter in 1893 and known as the Florence Nightingale pledge: "… I will do all in my power to maintain and elevate the standard of my profession, and will hold in confidence all personal matters committed to my keeping and all family affairs coming to my knowledge in the practice of my profession …" (Cabrera et al. 2000). One hundred and twenty-five years later, nurses still uphold this pledge, even as electronic systems and complex networks extend the reach of their care.

10.13 Review Questions

1. What is the difference between anonymity and pseudonymity?
2. If you were conducting a longitudinal study, which is the best approach to adopt: collection of anonymous patient data or collection of pseudonymous patient data?
3. What you would consider to be the key characteristics of personal information?
4. Is a health card number or patient chart number considered personal health information or are they just numbers that, absent a name or other information, do not need to be kept confidential?

5. Put the following record detail in the order of sensitivity and classify whether the data detail is sensitive or not? a) HIV Status of an individual b) health encounter detail of a GP assessment of a patient with a possible chest infection. c) demographic data d) mental health assessment history data detail.
6. What are the main goals of information security?

10.13.1   Answers

1. **Anonymity** allows the subjects in a database to remain nameless and unidentified. Patient anonymity is frequently found in research databases and in data that consists of statistical summaries. **Pseudonymity** on the other hand, allows the subjects in a database to be tracked over time while at the same time remaining nameless. Pseudonyms (e.g., patient X, patient Y, etc.) are attached to records in place of names, addresses and other public identifiers. Users of online services can also be given pseudonyms, or choose their own, during user registration, allowing them to maintain a consistent pseudonymous presence from one online encounter to another.
2. **It is better to use pseudonymity**. The terms anonymous and anonymity are often used when the terms pseudonymous and pseudonymity should be used instead. Truly anonymous patient data is typically useless in a long-term longitudinal study, as new data collected on a given patient cannot be matched up with data collected on the same patient the previous year or the year before (all the patients are anonymous). Rather, such databases are typically pseudonymous: data collected last year on patient 13,786 is linked to new data collected from patient 13,786. Such schemes require some trusted party or methodology to reliably and consistently derive the pseudonym (13786) from personal identifiers such as patient name, address, birthdate, etc. This process of pseudonymization is said to be irreversible if, after identifiable data have been processed to produce pseudonymous data, it is computationally infeasible to trace back to the original identifier from the pseudonym.
3. Personal health information is information about an identifiable individual that relates to the physical or mental health of the individual, or to provision of health services to the individual. It may include:

   a. information about registration of the individual for the provision of health services, including name, address, phone numbers and other contact details, plus other demographic information such as birthdate,
   b. information about payments or eligibility for health care insurance,
   c. a number or other identifier assigned to an individual to uniquely identify the individual for health care purposes,
   d. information about the individual that is collected in the course of the providing the individual with health services,
   e. information derived from the testing or examination of a body part or bodily substance (e.g., a lab test result or diagnostic image), or

f. identification of healthcare providers involved in the provision of healthcare to the individual.

Personal health information does not include information that is anonymised, either by itself or when combined with other available information.

4. Health card numbers and patient chart numbers that are identified as such are still considered personal health information because they can be used to link records together from multiple data sources (e.g., a database of records with only health card numbers and diagnoses linked to a database of records containing only patient health card numbers and contact information). These data linkages can often associate identifying information (name, address, etc.) with clinical information (test results, diagnoses, etc.). Many jurisdictions explicitly protect health card numbers in their health data privacy laws.

5. The belief that personal health information admits of degrees of sensitivity ('not confidential,' 'somewhat confidential,' 'highly confidential') and that these can be determined beforehand by information system designers is largely a myth. Personal health information—all of it—should be treated as sensitive and confidential and not shared outside the patient's circle of care without the patient's express consent except where permitted or required by law. It must be protected by reasonable technical and administrative safeguards throughout its entire useful lifetime, and then securely disposed of when no longer needed.

6. The main goals of information security are to (1) maintain the confidentiality of data, (2) maintain data integrity during the transmission, processing and storage of that data, and (3) maintain the availability of information systems and data either in the face of environmental disasters such as equipment failures, power outages, etc.; or in the face of hostile actions such as denial of service attacks carried out against systems by hackers or disgruntled employees.

Glossary

Access control The identification of users during user registration, the assignment of access privileges that determine which information resources and services these users can access, their subsequent authentication during log in, and their authorisation prior to being granted access to specific services and data

Anonymity Term used which allows the subjects in a database to remain nameless and unidentified

Audit Auditing is done by keeping audit log files (sometimes referred to as an audit trail) that record which users have done what (accessed information or performed actions on information on specific patient records) and when (date of access; number of times record was accessed).

Circle of care A term used which refers to the persons participating in, and the activities related to, the provision of health care to the patient

Consent An agreement, approval, or permission given voluntarily by a competent person that permits some act(s) for some stated purpose(s). Adapted from Black's Law Dictionary (9th edition), 2009

GDPR European General Data Protection Regulation (GDPR), a European Union directive that, 20 years after the Canadian principles were written, expanded upon these privacy principles and added several new principles relevant to healthcare and the protection of personal health information

Health information custodian A health information custodian (sometimes called a data steward) is an individual or organization that collects, uses, or discloses personal health information for the purposes of patient treatment and care, medical billing, health system planning and management, or health research

PHI Personal health information

Privacy The right of individuals and organizations to decide for themselves when, how, and to what extent information about them is transmitted to others NI Conference 2013 Toronto

Pseudonymity A term used which allows the subjects in a database to be tracked over time while at the same time remaining nameless

Pseudonyms Term used such as patient x or patient y which are attached to records instead of names, addresses and other public identifiers.

Ransomware A form of computer virus that encrypts the data in a system to make it inaccessible to the system's users. System administrators are then met with a ransom demand to unlock the data.

Security Physical protection of data using such means as firewalls, encryption, user credentials, and other physical means

User authentication User authorization attempts to securely verify the identify of the person logging into the system

User enrolment User enrolment registers each person for specific functionality in an online service or computer program within an organization that a registered user is authorized to access. Once enrolled, a user has the authorization to access the relevant data or services. Not all users will have access to all modules or components of a service or program as access is typically based on the "need to know" principle.

References[1]

Adapted from Black's Law Dictionary (9th edition); 2009. ISBN-13: 9780314199492.

Mathews A. Anthem. Hacked database included 78.8 million people. Wall Street Journal, 24 Feb 2015. https://www.wsj.com/articles/anthem-hacked-database-included-78-8-million-people-1424807364.

Cabrera E, Papaevangelou H, Mcparland J. Patient's autonomy, privacy and informed consent. IOS Press; 2000. ISBN 1586030396, 9781586030391.

Canadian Broadcasting Corporation. B.C. privacy breach shows millions affected. CBC News, 14 Jan 2013. https://www.cbc.ca/news/canada/british-columbia/b-c-privacy-breach-shows-millions-affected-1.1342374.

Canadian Standards Association. Model code for the protection of personal information (CAN/CSA-Q830-96). 1996. https://laws-lois.justice.gc.ca/eng/acts/p-8.6/page-11.html.

[1] Note: All web references were last accessed on May 4, 2020.

Clarke R. Beyond the OECD guidelines: privacy protection for the 21st century. Cyber Security and Information Systems Information Analysis Center (CSIAC). Rolling Meadows, IL: Jan; 2000.

Cloud J. Pedophilia. Time Magazine, 29 April 2002. http://content.time.com/time/magazine/article/0,9171,232584,00.html.

Connolly ML. Belfast Trust fined £225,000 over patient records breach. BBC, 19 Jun 2012. https://www.bbc.com/news/uk-northern-ireland-18497161.

Council of Europe. Convention for the protection of individuals with regard to automatic processing of personal data. Strasbourg; 28 Jan 1981a. https://www.coe.int/en/web/conventions/full-list/-/conventions/treaty/108.

Council of Europe. Convention for the Protection of Individuals with Regard to Automatic Processing of Personal Data. Strasbourg; 28 Jan 1981b, article 6. https://www.coe.int/en/web/conventions/full-list/-/conventions/treaty/108.

Davis J. 417,000 Augusta University Health patient records breached nearly one year ago. Healthcare IT News, 17 Aug 2018. https://www.healthcareitnews.com/news/417000-augusta-university-health-patient-records-breached-nearly-one-year-ago.

European Parliament. General data protection regulation. 27 Apr 2016, Article 8. https://eur-lex.europa.eu/legal-content/EN/TXT/?qid=1532348683434&uri=CELEX:02016R0679-20160504.

European Union. Data Protection Directive (95/46/EC), 1995. https://ec.europa.eu/eip/ageing/standards/ict-and-communication/data/directive-9546ec_en.

Federal Trade Commission (US). Fair Information Practice Principles (FIPs), s. 5. Enforcement/Redress. Washington, DC; n.d. https://web.archive.org/web/20090205180646/http://ftc.gov/reports/privacy3/fairinfo.shtm.

Frone MR. Prevalence and distribution of alcohol use and impairment in the workplace: a U.S. national survey. J Stud Alcohol. 2006;67:147–56. https://www.jsad.com/doi/abs/10.15288/jsa.2006.67.147

Gordon E. Aetna agrees to pay $17 million in HIV privacy breach. NPR, 17 Jan 2018. https://www.npr.org/sections/health-shots/2018/01/17/572312972/aetna-agrees-to-pay-17-million-in-hiv-privacy-breach.

Gostin LO. National health information privacy regulations under the health insurance portability and accountability act. JAMA. 2001;285(23):3015–21. https://doi.org/10.1001/jama.285.23.3015. http://jama.jamanetwork.com/article.aspx?articleid=193930

Guardian Government Computing. ICO fines Sussex trust £325,000 for data breach. The Guardian, 1 June 2012. https://www.theguardian.com/government-computing-network/2012/jun/01/ico-data-breach-brighton-nhs.

Hall, et al. Sexual arousal and arousability to pedophilic stimuli in a community sample of normal men. Behav Ther. 1995;26:681–94. http://www.sciencedirect.com/science/article/pii/S0005789405800395

Hare WH. Records, computers and the rights of citizens: Rand Corporation; 1973a. http://www.rand.org/pubs/papers/2008/P5077.pdf

Hare WH. Records, computers and the rights of citizens: Rand Corporation; 1973b. p. 3. http://www.rand.org/pubs/papers/2008/P5077.pdf

Hicks S. Russian hackers hold Gold Coast doctors to ransom. ABC News, 11 Dec 2012. http://www.abc.net.au/news/2012-12-10/hackers-target-gold-coast-medical-centre/4418676.

Holmes N. The right to privacy and parliament. Library of Parliament (Canada); Feb 2006.

Information and Privacy Commissioner of Ontario. Circle of care: sharing personal health information for health-care purposes; Aug 2015. https://www.ipc.on.ca/wp-content/uploads/Resources/circle-of-care.pdf.

ISO 27001: Information technology – Security techniques – Information security management systems – Requirements. International Organization for Standardization; 2013. https://www.iso.org/standard/54534.html.

ISO 27002. Information technology – security techniques – code of practice for information security controls. International Organization for Standardization. 2013; https://www.iso.org/standard/54533.html

ISO 27799: Health informatics – Information security management in health using ISO/IEC 27002. International Organization for Standardization, 2016. https://www.iso.org/standard/62777.html.

ISO/TS 14265: Health Informatics – Classification of purposes for processing personal health information. International Organization for Standardization; 2011. https://www.iso.org/standard/54547.html.

Jurgens R. HIV testing and confidentiality: final report. Canadian HIV/AIDS Legal Network & Canadian AIDS Society. 2001; http://www.aidslaw.ca/site/hiv-testing-and-confidentiality-final-report/?lang=en

Krebs B. Hackers break into Virginia health professions database, Demand Ransom. Washington Post, 4 May 2009. http://voices.washingtonpost.com/securityfix/2009/05/hackers_break_into_virginia_he.html.

National Conference of State Legislatures. Security Breach Notification Laws. 8 Mar 2020. https://www.ncsl.org/research/telecommunications-and-information-technology/security-breach-notification-laws.aspx

Office of the Australian Information Commissioner. Notifiable data breaches; n.d. https://www.oaic.gov.au/privacy/notifiable-data-breaches/.

Organization for Economic Co-Operation and Development. Guidelines on the protection of privacy and transborder flows of personal data. Last modified Jan 1999. http://www.oecd.org/internet/ieconomy/oecdguidelinesontheprotectionofprivacyandtransborderflowsofpersonaldata.htm.

Pew Research Center. Public opinion on abortion: views on abortion, 1995–2019. Pew Research Center; 29 Aug 2019. https://www.pewforum.org/fact-sheet/public-opinion-on-abortion/.

Privacy Commissioner of Canada. What you need to know about mandatory reporting of breaches of security safeguards. Oct 2018. https://www.priv.gc.ca/en/privacy-topics/business-privacy/safeguards-and-breaches/privacy-breaches/respond-to-a-privacy-breach-at-your-business/gd_pb_201810/.

Smith GK. Privacy in the information age: De Montfort University; Apr 1994.

Srinivas R. 7 times ransomware became a major healthcare hazard. CISO Magazine, 14 Nov 2019. https://www.cisomag.com/7-times-ransomware-became-a-major-healthcare-hazard/.

Stein L. The electronic medical record: promises and threats; web security: a matter of trust. Web J. 1997;2(3) https://dl.acm.org/doi/abs/10.5555/275079.275101

Terhune C. Patient data outage exposes risks of electronic medical records. Los Angeles Times, 3 Aug 2012. http://articles.latimes.com/2012/aug/03/business/la-fi-hospital-data-outage-20120803.

US Government Printing Office. Health insurance portability and accountability act, 1996. https://www.govinfo.gov/content/pkg/PLAW-104publ191/html/PLAW-104publ191.htm.

Chapter 11
The Role of the Informatics Nurse

Lynn M. Nagle

Abstract Over the past 2 decades, the scope of practice for nurses in informatics roles has been evolving and shifting in response to the needs of health care organizations. While informatician practice has been seldom consistently defined or circumscribed in terms of role responsibilities and scope, the work has significantly contributed to the evolution and dissemination of information and communication technology (ICT) across the globe. Further the advent of formalized education in nursing and health informatics has led to the establishment of associated credentials and situated informatics as a specialty within nursing and other health professions. In this chapter, the author will review the types of informatics roles that have been assumed by nurses working in the field of informatics, key role functions, and a perspective on the essential leadership roles and potential areas of specialization for the next generation of nurse informaticians.

Keywords Nurse informatician · Informatics role · Informatics specialist · Analyst Information and communication technology · Health informatics

Learning Objectives for the Chapter
1. Describe the types of roles and responsibilities assumed by nurses working in the field of informatics.
2. Identify the importance of the nursing perspective in the field of health informatics and nursing informatics as a specialty.

Electronic Supplementary Material The online version of this chapter (https://doi.org/10.1007/978-3-030-58740-6_11) contains supplementary material, which is available to authorized users.

L. M. Nagle (✉)
Director of Digital Health and Virtual Learning, Faculty of Nursing, University of New Brunswick, Fredericton, New Brunswick, Canada

Lawrence S. Bloomberg Faculty of Nursing, University of Toronto, Toronto, Canada

Arthur Labatt Family School of Nursing, Western University, London, Canada
e-mail: lnagle@nagleassoc.ca

3. Discuss efforts focused on the development of informatics competency development (e.g., certification).
4. Consider current informatics practice domains and potential role functions for the future.

11.1 Introduction

The various roles, practice and competencies of nurses in informatics have been evolving for several decades. Similarly, academic opportunities and credentials in the field have become increasingly available and sought after by nurses. From the 1960s through the 1980s, information and communication technology (ICT) initiatives in health care organizations were almost exclusively led by traditional information technology (IT) and or telecommunications departments. When deemed necessary, clinicians, often nurses, were seconded for a period of time to bring a clinical perspective to ICT discussions. Anecdotally, these positions were largely time limited and focused mostly on system implementation and user training. These incidental assignments often came with the designation of *IT nurse* as the titles nurse informatician, informatics specialist or informaticist were uncommon until the emergence of formal programs of study and opportunities to obtain formal certification. More often than not, nurses were engaged after ICT choices and designs were finalized, with little consideration for the potential impacts on the daily work of the largest group of health care providers, nurses.

Today a majority of healthcare organizations recognize that successful implementation and adoption of ICT necessitates the inclusion of all clinician perspectives and not just that of physicians. Furthermore, studies are demonstrating that organizations with the foresight to involve nurses and other clinicians at the outset of ICT initiatives, including the acquisition and design phases, are more likely to achieve success in adoption and use (Ash et al. 2003; Ash and Bates 2005; Leatt et al. 2006; Studer 2005; Warm and Thomas 2011). While a wide variety of "informatics" positions are often filled by nurses, consistency and clarity of what constitutes the *work* of these positions is lacking. Over the years, many unique position descriptions have been created with an array of titles, roles and responsibilities. Nursing positions in informatics run the gamut from the unit-based "*nurse super user*" to the organizational executive level, "*Chief Information Officer*" (CIO) or nurse executive position of "*Chief Nursing Informatics Officer*" (CNIO). Accompanying the variability of work is a range of requisite experience, education and associated competencies even among those with similar titles. However, the finding of variability in the work of informatics' nurses is not unique to nursing and has been recognized as an area needing greater specificity and uniformity in healthcare practice (Hersh 2006; McLane and Turley 2011; Smith et al. 2011). In this chapter, the author provides an overview of informatics as a nursing specialty, and the various roles, responsibilities, and activities assumed by nurse informaticians. Although not formally sanctioned by any regulatory body, the title *nurse informatician* will be used as the default reference to nurses working in informatics in order to provide illustrations within the context of this chapter. Additionally, speculation on directions for future informatics roles for nurses is offered for the reader's consideration.

11.2   Informatics as a Specialty in Nursing

> ...a specialty that integrates nursing science, computer science, and information science to manage and communicate data, information, and knowledge in nursing practice. Nursing informatics facilitates the integration of data, information, and knowledge to support patients, nurses, and other providers in their decision-making in all roles and settings. This support is accomplished through the use of information structures, information processes, and information technology (Staggers and Thompson 2002).

Small groups of nurses interested in informatics and its potential application to practice, education, administration and research began organizing internationally in the 1960s. Organized international and national gatherings of nurses occurred over many years in several nations long before nursing informatics became formally recognized as a specialty (Scholes et al. 2002). In the early years, a contingent of nurses organized as a special interest group of the International Medical Informatics Association (IMIA) and became established as the Nursing Informatics Special Interest Group (IMIA NI-SIG). The IMIA NI-SIG currently serves as a unifying body supporting networking and collaboration among nurse informaticians around the globe, while also advancing the practice and research of informatics. Table 11.1 reflects the current goals and objectives of the NI-SIG which are each supported by specific activities and challenges to the community.

In 1992, the American Nurses Association (ANA) recognized the specialty of nursing informatics, publishing *The Scope of Practice for Nursing Informatics* (American Nurses Association 1994) and *The Standards of Practice for Nursing Informatics* (American Nurses Association 1995). These were subsequently revised into a single publication in 2008 to reflect the scope and standards of practice and professional performance for the informatics nurse specialist; a 2nd edition was published in 2016 (American Nurses Association (ANA) 2016). See Table 11.2 for the overarching dimensions of the ANA nurse informatics specialist standards for practice and professional performance.

In the late 1980s, Canadian nurses working in informatics were initially organized as the Nursing Informatics—Special Interest Group (SIG) of the Canadian Organization for the Advancement of Computers in Health (COACH). Disbanded in 2001, this group was reconstituted in 2002 as an independent corporate entity, the Canadian Nursing Informatics Association (CNIA). A year later, the CNIA was granted Affiliate Group status with the Canadian Nurses Association (CNA), formally recognizing the specialty within the Canadian nursing community. Shortly thereafter, the CNIA became the COACH nominee to the represent Canadian nurses on the IMIA NI-SIG. During the last decade, although CNIA members have been

Table 11.1 IMIA Special Interest Group—nursing informatics goals & objectives

Goals and Objectives

The focus of IMIA-NI is to foster collaboration among nurses and others who are interested in Nursing Informatics to facilitate development in the field. We aim to share knowledge, experience and ideas with nurses and healthcare providers worldwide about the practice of Nursing Informatics and the benefits of enhanced information management.

Specific Objectives

- Explore the scope of Nursing Informatics and its implication for health policy and information handling activities associated with evidence based nursing practice, nursing management, nursing research, nursing education, standards and patient (or client) decision making and the various relationships with other health care informatics entities.
- Identify priorities or gaps and make recommendations for future developments in Nursing Informatics
- Support the development of Nursing Informatics in member countries and promote Nursing Informatics worldwide.
- Promote linkages and collaborative activities with national and international nursing and healthcare informatics groups and nursing and health care organisations globally.
- Provide, promote and support informatics meetings, conferences, and electronic communication forums to enable opportunities for the sharing of ideas, developments and knowledge.
- To participate in IMIA working group and special interest groups to present a nursing perspective.
- Develop recommendations, guidelines, tools and courses related to Nursing Informatics. Encourage the publication and dissemination of research and development materials in the field of Nursing Informatics
- To support and work with patients, families, communities and societies to adopt and manage informatics approaches to healthcare.
- Ensure the group is more visible by providing up to date information on the web site enabling external groups e.g. WHO, ICN to access as required.

Last updated: 07 Dec 2012; Accessed 1 Mar 2020 at: https://imia-medinfo.org/wp/imia-ni-goals-objectives/

IMIA-NI International Medical Informatics Association—Nursing Informatics

invited to participate in several international initiatives, they have been most active in the development of national health data standards, core informatics competencies for basic nursing curricula, resources for nurse educators and formal education and certification programs in Canada.

Although beyond the scope of this chapter, nurses working in informatics have continued to organize worldwide and are convening regularly to network and address shared issues and challenges in national and international meetings and conferences. IMIA member and non-member countries are invited to participate in a number of scientific meetings (e.g., Medinfo, International Nursing Informatics Congress, European Federation for Medical Informatics), which take place every 2–3 years in a variety of locations. In the early days, these forums were commonly the venue by which a majority of nurses obtained the foundations of their training and education in informatics. For nurses from countries in which informatics learning options are few or non-existent, this is likely still their primary means of garnering informatics knowledge.

Table 11.2 Informatics nurse specialist standards of practice and professional performance

Standards of Practice
1. Assessment
2. Problem and issues identification
3. Outcomes identification
4. Planning
5. Implementation
5a. Co-ordination of activities
5b. Health teaching and health promotion and education
5c. Consultation
6. Evaluation
Standards of Professional Performance
7. Education
8. Professional practice evaluation
9. Quality of practice
10. Collegiality
11. Collaboration
12. Ethics
13. Research
14. Resource utilization
15. Advocacy
16. Leadership

Adapted from: American Nurses Association (ANA) (American Medical Informatics Association 2020)

11.3 Specialty Preparation, Certification and Competencies

In conjunction with the recognition of nursing informatics as a specialty, several college and university based programs were launched in the early 90s, offering individuals an opportunity to obtain a wide variety of certificates, diplomas and undergraduate and graduate degrees focused in informatics. Today there are numerous programs with varied areas of focus, duration and terminal credentials but each is intended to provide nurses and others with the specialized knowledge and skills needed to become effective informaticians. Over the last 10 years, many online program offerings have also been developed further extending the reach of continuing education opportunities. The American Medical Informatics Association (AMIA) maintains a comprehensive inventory of US and internationally based informatics program and course offerings on their website (American Medical Informatics Association 2020). Similarly, the Canadian health informatics association, Digital Health Canada, maintains a listing of educational opportunities targeting individuals with technical and/or clinical backgrounds (Digital Health Canada 2020). In addition to these education offerings, there are now a number of professional journals that have a specific focus on issues of practice and research in nursing informatics including: (a) *CIN: Computers, Informatics, Nursing* and (b) the

Online Journal of Nursing Informatics. Although the publication of nurse informaticians' work is not limited to these journals, they do offer nurses opportunities to publish their experiences and learnings from practice, education and research with a nursing audience in mind.

In addition to taking formal programs of study, those with health informatics expertise may realise a nationally recognized professional designation upon successful completion of national certification examinations. Among these is the Health Information Management Systems Society (HIMSS) designation of Certified Professional in Healthcare Information and Management Systems (CPHIMS) (Health Information Management Systems Society 2020). A Canadian variation of this credential, CPHIMS-CA, is also offered for interested individuals with clinical or technology backgrounds. Upon successful completion of the certification exam, individuals receive a credential signifying that they have the health informatics "skills, knowledge and abilities to perform safely and effectively in a broad range of practice settings" (Digital Health Canada 2020). While the ANA has afforded nurses the option of securing a Board certification in nursing informatics for several years now (American Nurses Credentialing Center (ANCC) n.d.) this type of nursing specific professional certification is not widely available to nurses in other countries. In addition to nursing and informatics education credentials, many nurses have also completed a course of study and exam to achieve a Project Management Professional® (PMP) certification in response to the demand for project leadership skills within healthcare settings. With the establishment of nursing informatics organizations and the creation of opportunities to complete formal informatics education offerings, informatics has achieved recognition as a specialty within nursing (Warm and Thomas 2011; McLane and Turley 2011; Health Information Management Systems Society 2017). Nonetheless many nurses remain unaware of the potential career opportunities in the field and often encounter these by chance rather than design. Until core informatics competencies become integrated into the curricula of all entry level nursing programs, informatics may not even be recognized by many nurses as a specialty option. Increasing awareness and knowledge of informatics within the broader nursing community continues to be a key area of focus for many nursing informatics specialty groups.

Beyond a specialization in informatics, there are key competencies essential for individuals in all areas of nursing practice and others specific to those in leadership positions. The delineation of core entry-to-practice informatics competencies for all registered nurses has been undertaken by several countries (Association of Schools of Nursing 2012; Honey et al. 2017; Nagle et al. 2014). In particular, a recent publication by members of the IMIA-NISIG (Goosen and Murphy 2017), provides a comprehensive overview of informatics competency requirements for now and into the future. Further to these efforts, informatics competency self-assessment tools for student nurses, registered nurses, registered practical nurses, ((Kleib and Nagle 2018a; and nurse leaders, (Collins et al. 2017; Yen et al. 2017; Strudwick et al. 2019a; Strudwick et al. 2019b) are currently in development and/or being tested for their psychometric properties. Despite these efforts, systematic integration of core informatics competencies into undergraduate nursing curricula remains inconsistent and simply lacking in many schools of nursing. A recent national study of Canadian schools of nursing revealed that a majority of undergraduate programs have limited informatics content but on a positive note, there is a willingness among faculty to address these gaps (Nagle et al. 2018). There is no doubt that core informatics competency is fundamental for the delivery of safe, quality practice by all nurses and other healthcare providers in the twenty first century.

11.4   Domains of Nurse Informatician Work

According to an earlier paper by McLane and Turley (McLane and Turley 2011), *"informaticians are prepared to influence, contribute to, and mold the realization of an organization's vision for knowledge management"* (p. 30). This remains an apt description today as many individuals, including nurses, have attained credentials that denote their knowledge, expertise and experience in the field of health informatics. Over the years, many nurses have moved into senior executive positions including the role of Chief Information Officer; some of the challenges for a nurse in this role have been described previously (Nagle 2000). Roles for nurses have actually evolved to the extent that executive positions with the designation of CNIO have been established in some health care organizations. Recognition of the essential role of informatics savvy nurse leaders has led to continued advocacy for more CNIO positions and the development of informatics competency among nurse leaders (Kennedy and Moen 2017; Kannry et al. 2016; Nagle 2016). It is most common to find nurses specializing in the field of informatics referred to as informaticists, informaticians, informatics nurse specialists and/or clinical informatics specialists, sometimes but not always, denoting that they have advanced training or a credential in informatics. However, despite the emergence of informatics specific educational offerings and positions, many nurses do not have formalized training and often find themselves in informatics roles for which they are ill-prepared. And as was found in a recent HIMSS survey, a majority of nurse informaticians continue to derive much of their knowledge and experience through on-the-job training (Health Information Management Systems Society 2017).

Nurse informaticians can be found working within health care organizations, leading and participating in ICT initiatives. Others have secured roles working in government and legislative bodies, advancing standards, policy and strategic initiatives. In academic settings, nurses are advancing informatics education and research and informing innovations in teaching and learning. And still others have been recruited by ICT software and hardware developers and suppliers to bring their expertise to bear on the evolution of technology solutions to support clinical care delivery. The evolution of nurse informatician roles has occurred as a direct result of the need to converge nursing expertise with the knowledge of informatics to better inform systems design, implementation, education, and evaluation. Their knowledge and skills have been acknowledged as integral to the effective implementation of ICT as well as effective information and knowledge management (Warm and Thomas 2011; McLane and Turley 2011; Smith et al. 2011).

Informatics roles in practice settings have been widely varied in scope and function but have largely focused on components of the system lifecycle (e.g., design, implementation, training, and evaluation). Hersh (Hersh 2006) underscored the ill-defined relationship between the practice of informaticians and job titles. McLane and Turley (McLane and Turley 2011) highlighted the intricacy and complexity of the knowledge and skills required by organizations endeavouring to deliver on an ICT agenda that will lead to safer, more effective care and also support clinical practice.

According to Sewell (Sewell 2019) "There are two roles in informatics: the informatics specialist and the clinician who must use health information technology. This means in essence that every nurse has a role in informatics" [p4]. However, for the purpose of this chapter, the roles and responsibilities of nurse informaticians will be highlighted using broad categories of informatics practice domains. Table 11.3 provides a synthesis of seven domains of informatician work:

1. Leadership
2. ICT Life Cycle Management
3. Health System Use
4. Entrepreneurship
5. Vendor Support
6. Education
7. Research

11.5 Leadership

Notwithstanding the fact that all informatics roles require an element of leadership capacity, for the purpose of this discussion, the domain is applied to those roles that are typically senior positions within healthcare organizations, ICT companies or government. These individuals typically provide strategic or operational oversight of organizational, regional and national ICT solutions. They may provide expert consultation on issues of ICT strategy, including support for the processes of acquisition, deployment, implementation, evaluation and education. Some nurses in these senior roles may focus on issues of advocacy or political action to drive broad ICT or health and professional policy directions. To date, the number of nurses recognized for their informatics expertise at government and policy tables has been limited but there is clearly an opportunity and need for the voice of nurses to be heard. The concept of *change leadership* is an essential role function for the senior nurse informatician such that the ICT vision, strategy and solutions, management teams and supporting actors and activities are provided with explicit and committed executive support. Titles such as Chief Information Officer, CNIO, Vice-President or Director of Nursing Informatics, Nurse Informatics Consultant or Advocate are most commonly used to designate these positions.

Table 11.3 Domains and areas of focus for nurse informaticians

Domain	Areas of focus
Leadership	Strategy
	Strategic planning
	Change leadership
	Consultation
	Advocacy
	Political action
	Health policy
	Customer relations
ICT life cycle management	Systems analyses
	Workflow
	Process improvement
	Usability
	Ergonomics
	Socio-cultural
	Functional specification
	Acquisition
	Application design
	Data representation
	Terminology
	Standards development
	Interoperability/integration
	Implementation
	Change management
	Education
	Competency assessment
	Training & education
	Evaluation
	Formative
	Summative
	Systems support
Health system use	Data analytics
	Aggregate reporting
	Utilization management
	Decision support
	Generation of new knowledge
	Use of data, information, and knowledge
	Outcomes Management
	Quality Improvement
	Ethical use
	Protection of privacy
Entrepreneurship	Software/hardware solution development
	Consulting

(continued)

Table 11.3 (continued)

Domain	Areas of focus
Vendor support	Product development
	Sales
	Customer support
Education	Curriculum/course development & delivery
	Competency assessment
	ICT innovation in education
Research	Conduct of research focused on applications of informatics in practice, education, and/or administration

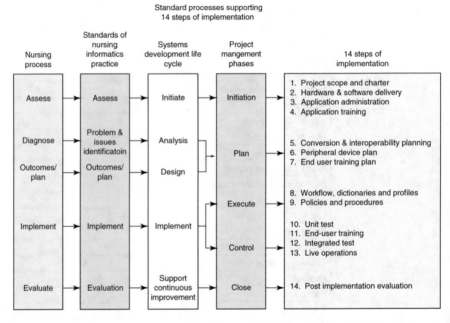

Fig. 11.1 Standard processes supporting 14 steps of implementation (With permission © McGraw Hill)

11.6 ICT Life Cycle Management

Smith and Tyler (Smith and Tyler 2011); p78] described the system development life cycle (SDLC) as comprised of five phases: initiation, analysis, design, implementation, and continuous improvement or support (Fig. 11.1). Further they illustrated the alignment of the SDLC with the standards of nursing informatics practice (see Table 11.2), the project management process and the nursing process.

The roles encompassed within this domain constitute by far, a majority of positions currently filled by nurse informaticians. Given the breadth and depth of activities needed to manage the ICT life cycle, these roles typically vary widely in title, scope of responsibility and employers' requisite qualifications. The work of nurses in this area may include:

- providing oversight (e.g., project management) or hands-on involvement in the tasks of information gathering and analyses to inform ICT functional specifications for solution acquisitions and designs;
- process mapping and analyses of current and desired future states;
- supporting or engaging in application design and build activities;
- assuring the use of data and interoperability standards;
- usability testing;
- ergonomic evaluation;
- developing methods and tools for initial and ongoing user support, training and education;
- leading and supporting evaluation activities, formative and summative;
- system optimization focused on increasing productivity and efficiency with ICT use;
- reviewing, revising, and developing relevant practice related ICT policies.

These work efforts are largely focused on getting the solution functionality and supporting processes and infrastructure optimally designed to achieve successful clinician adoption and integration into practice. Each of the core work elements requires oversight, expertise, and iterative engagement of the targeted user community. To this end, project management, clinical expertise, and skilled change management are necessary ingredients to success. Not all nurse informaticians will have the experience, skill, and knowledge to contribute to all aspects of the ICT lifecycle, but in the course of time and with experiential practise, it is likely that most will garner exposure and an understanding of each dimension. The work of systems analyses is typically undertaken by a combination of technical and clinical experts. Nurse analysts will generally focus on the clinical systems pre- and post-ICT, starting with activities to inform the solution acquisition through to understanding the chosen solution's impact on clinical and associated business processes. The work usually encompasses the capture and documentation of clinical operations in the context of specific settings and is inclusive of all clinicians and non-clinicians for whom a new technology will potentially change or impact the flow of their day to day activities.

Expertise in the areas of data standards, terminologies, and systems interoperability (See Chaps. 2, 5 and 6) is of utmost importance but as yet not well understood by many clinicians. The adoption and use of clinical data standards among nurses are particularly challenging as the use of standardized language is a foreign concept to most. Perhaps the most universally understood and applied standard is the rubric of the nursing process, but the standardized terminologies that underpin the documentation of the steps are less so (e.g., nursing diagnosis, interventions, outcomes). The integration nursing data standards and codification of these in electronic health records is an area needing the engagement of many more nurse informaticians, given that a future which includes comparable, analyzable and reportable nursing relevant metrics depends upon it.

The area of human factors encompasses a myriad of socio-technical issues not the least of which is the usability of ICT solutions. As a division of cognitive psychology, in the context of informatics human factors is largely concerned with human-machine or human-computer (i.e., devices and applications) interactions. The emphasis on human factors has emerged in recent years as a consideration that is germane to the ultimate success of ICT deployment. Nurses working in this area will concern themselves not only with the cognitive impact of ICT solutions on nurses' and others' work but also with the physical or ergonomic design issues (e.g., workstation height, lighting).

Role designations such as Project Manager, Data/Terminology/Standards Specialist, Application Specialist, Nurse Informatics Specialist, Clinical Informatics Specialist, Business/Clinical Process Analyst, Usability Specialist, Nurse Ergonomist, ICT Policy and Procedure Manager are examples of some of the commonly used titles associated with these responsibilities.

11.7 Health System Use

The area of health system use is emerging to likely be the most important focus of health informaticians' work in the years ahead. Health system use reflects the shift from the investment and development in information systems to the analysis and use of data to inform business and clinical decisions. Health data analytics may inform or drive reactive, proactive or retrospective actions or decisions. The increasing sophistication of health information systems is affording decision-makers, managers, and clinicians the capacity to make better informed decisions to achieve both short and long term outcomes. In addition to the phrase health system use, the terms *business intelligence* and *clinical intelligence* are being increasingly applied to describe the processes and outputs of this work. The outputs may be driven by specific business, clinical or research questions, focused on specific financial or clinical performance metrics and outcomes, and often encompass the provision of benchmarking and performance measurement reports. In its most basic application, health information use can occur at the patient/client, unit/program, organizational, regional or national level. In this regard, one might deem the staff nurse or nurse manager as the first level of user, focused on the use of clinical data, information and knowledge to inform clinical or management practice decisions respectively.

Although it is still early days for ICT supported clinical decision-making, nurses have been using tools such as nursing workload management systems for more than three decades. Originally designed to support staffing decisions based upon patient acuity scores, these tools became pervasive in healthcare during the 1980s and 90s. (For additional information about these systems, refer to Chap. 9) While not commonly used to adjust daily staffing levels, the data from these systems have been used to track patient acuity, a proxy for the costs of nursing care, and often to guide organizational decisions about issues such as staff mix. Nurses supporting the implementation and use of these systems were typically designated as the *vendor name* (e.g., Medicus™, GRASP™), *workload* or *systems* nurse. Commonplace among the nursing workforce, these were likely the first informatics nurses found in clinical settings, but the position titles did not denote the importance of their activities as data managers and custodians, assuring data quality, reliability and completeness of workload data. These roles continue to exist in many health care organizations today, but as clinical system vendors are beginning to design tools to generate nursing workload and patient acuity as bi-products of clinical documentation, they may well become unnecessary in the future and subsumed by the work of the nurse informatician.

At local levels, many health care provider organizations have acquired business analytic software tools that support the mining and analysis of data to inform business and clinical decisions. Considering broader levels of system use, data and information from health information systems can support program quality and safety improvements, planning and resource allocation, clinical utilization review, and management of public health issues and substantially support health services research. At present, these are the most common applications to which the term health system use is being applied. Health system use analyses are being conducted at regional, national and international levels to inform funding directions, health policy, and overall health system improvements. In some countries, national data repositories have been created to house data for these purposes (e.g., Canadian Institute of Health Information [CIHI], National Database of Nursing Quality Indicators® [NDNQI®], Institute for Clinical Evaluative Sciences [ICES]). For examples of national reports being generated by CIHI go to Chap. 8. While not necessarily solely staffed by nurse informaticians, many health care organizations have dedicated departments delivering analytic outputs in the form of performance dashboards or scorecards. The supporting roles are commonly referred to by titles such as Decision Support Analyst, Business Analyst, Clinical Decision Support Analyst and Quality and Safety Improvement Officer.

11.8 Vendor Support

In recent years, vendors, particularly those developing software solutions to support clinical care, have begun to recognize the invaluable perspectives and knowledge of nurses to inform the design of tools that are deemed to be useful in support of practice. Nurses working for software and hardware companies often find themselves attending sales meetings and informatics conferences, conducting product demonstrations for prospective clients, and supporting healthcare customers post-sales. Others have assumed roles focused on product design, development and functional evaluation activities. Positions such as Nursing Product Consultant, Sales Representative, Application Specialist and, in some large software organizations, senior level positions (e.g., Chief Nursing Officer or VP Nursing) are not uncommon.

11.9 Education

Nurse educators have been introducing the concepts of informatics to students in undergraduate and graduate programs for many years. Despite the number of faculty early adopters in this area, a majority of nursing schools still have limited or no informatics content in the undergraduate nursing curricula.

> *Whether recognized or not, in today's world, informatics is simply a part of every faculty member's tool kit. Therefore, it should not be offered or developed as a separate course. Rather it should be integrated with approaches to the theoretical and practical teachings in every course.* [(Nagle 2007), p24]

Typically offered as a single course, elective or required, the need to integrate informatics content as a thread throughout entry level nursing programs remains significant. Because of its niche nature to date, there are a limited number of nursing faculty who have a comfort level with the delivery of informatics content. Despite many informatics concepts being central to basic nursing practice (e.g., evidence-informed decision-making), it would seem that many educators see informatics as a wholly separate area of expertise. Albeit the practice of a nurse informatician is quite different from that of a bedside nurse, they are conceptually and practically interconnected. But until informatics becomes explicit and integral to the work of practitioners and educators, it is likely that the number of nurse informatician educators in schools of nursing will remain few in number. See Chaps. 14 and 15 for a detailed discussion on informatics and education.

In practice however, the role of the nursing informatician in educating and training clinicians in the use of ICT solutions is much more common. The assumption of these responsibilities by clinical nurse educators is not necessarily included with the delivery of other types of clinical teaching. Rather ICT education and training is commonly separate and within the purview of those in the role of "system educators" who may or may not have clinical backgrounds. These educators typically report to the IT or informatics department. In addition to these roles, it is common for unit-based or program-based nurses to be designated as "super users" to provide staff with ongoing support following the implementation of a new solution. These are often nurses who have expressed an interest or affinity for technology but not always; at times individuals are conscripted into these roles—not usually a successful strategy.

11.10 Research

Over the years, nurse researchers have committed entire careers studying the concepts and practice of informatics in nursing (See Chaps. 12, 13 for more on research in nursing informatics). Relative to other areas of nursing research, the extent of informatics nursing research being conducted world-wide is growing. But there is a need for considerably more research in the field and additional evidence to advance our informatics knowledge base. Within each of the domains of *Leadership, ICT Life Cycle Management, and Health System Use* as highlighted in Table 11.3, there are as yet many unanswered questions regarding ICT effectiveness, efficiency, outcomes and overall benefits to nursing and the health care system as a whole. The future development of researchers in the field will be largely dependent upon there being an increased recognition of informatics within the academic arena. Budding researchers will need the guidance and mentoring of nurse educators with informatics and research expertise.

11.11 Entrepreneurship

Over the years, many enterprising nurses have undertaken the creation of an independent business operation. The scope of these businesses has encompassed the provision of expertise to support any of the previously described domains of informatics work. Most commonly nursing informatics consultants have supported the work of ICT vendors and health care organizations lacking the requisite knowledge and experience to successfully execute an ICT acquisition, deployment and/or evaluation. The nurse informatics consultant is typically a seasoned practitioner who has an established track record in the field and viewed by actual and prospective clients as a valuable and trusted advisor. As previously discussed, nurses working solo or in partnership with other companies, have also led or contributed to the design, development, and distribution of proprietary software products to support the clinical, administrative, research and educational work of other nurses.

In this section, the key domains that may provide the focus of a nurse informatician's work have been broadly described and summarized. Table 11.4 provides the reader with a further synthesis of various role functions, position titles and some of the activities associated with each. Although the delineation and separation of some role functions may not be consistent within or among health care organizations, this discussion is intended provide a simplified framework of the types of work that the nurse informatician may undertake. Neither the position titles nor designated activities are meant to be authoritative or prescriptive, but representative of a specialty that is in evolution.

11.12 Nurse Informatician Roles for the Future

Across the globe, the healthcare industry continues to wrestle with clinician acceptance and full integration of ICT solutions into the processes of care delivery. Although seemingly protracted, the duration of this journey is not surprising and the evolution of systems will continue for many years to come. However, at this juncture it is important to rethink the role of nurse informaticians for the next decade. Some organizations have created formal informatics leadership positions or

Table 11.4 Role focus, position titles and activities

Role focus	Position titles	Activities
Change leadership	Chief information officer	Strategic planning
	Chief nursing informatics	Innovation
	Officer	Sponsorship
	Director nursing	Team building
	Informatics	System acquisition and funding
	Consultant	Health policy & political action
	Advocate	
Change management	Project manager	Operational management
	Informatics nurse specialist	Problem-solving
	Informatician	Budget management
	Informaticist	Team building
		User relationship management
		Vendor management
Systems analyses	Clinical analyst	Process analysis
	Business analyst	Standards
	Application specialist	System acquisition
	Usability specialist	Application design & build
	Nurse ergonomist	Human factors testing
	Data standards specialist	Ergonomics
	Interoperability specialist	Evaluation
Implementation	Informatics nurse	User support
	Application support specialist	Application support
		Device support
Education	Systems educator/trainer	Education
	Nurse educator	Training
		Support
		Orientation
Evaluation	Informatics researcher	Pilot testing
	System user	Interative design/usability testing
	Informatics specialist	Formative/summative System optimization
Systems support	Informatics nurse	Ongoing support in use of ICT
	Nurse educator	Program/department/unit based
	Nurse super user	
	Application support	
System use	**Nurse as:**	Nurse as knowledge worker
	Data gatherer	Outcomes management
	Information user	Evidence-based practice
	Knowledge user	
	Knowledge generator	

dedicated informatics departments, and most continue to designate a small number of willing individuals to represent the clinical perspective within ICT initiatives. Additionally, a majority of nurses continue to derive their knowledge and expertise via the school of hard knocks as the *informatics* or *IT nurse* within an organization. Until the core concepts and competencies of informatics become embedded within the undergraduate curricula of the health professions and recognized as essential for current practice in every setting, this landscape is unlikely to change. The specialty has been recognized within the profession for more than 3 decades, but the essential nature of nursing informatics roles has yet to be widely recognized and embraced by academia and healthcare organizations.

Heightened concerns for safety and quality have been directly linked to the need for timely access to information and evidence to support optimal clinical decision-making. In the context of increasingly ICT enabled clinical environments equipping nurses with advanced informational support, there is a place for informatics in the work of all nurses (Nagle 2016; Nagle et al. 2007). However, in contemplating future roles for nurse informaticians, it is important to consider that the evolving context of ICT use in healthcare delivery organizations (see Chaps. 2, 14, and 15) will likely include:

(a) organizations and providers reaching greater levels of maturity in their use of systems, necessitating an enhanced understanding of meaningful use among clinicians;
(b) increased integration of ICTs across care sectors (e.g., acute care, primary care, long-term care, home care)
(c) citizens taking an increasingly active role in managing their health and health information;
(d) expanded virtualization of health service delivery (e.g., telehomecare, mHealth, telehealth, cloud computing);
(e) increased emphasis on cost containment to assure that services are accessible and affordable;
(f) inclusion of genomic information as core data within electronic health records will introduce new ethical issues;
(g) increased use of artificial intelligence (AI) and robotics in the delivery of health services.

These emerging contexts will necessitate the evolution of nurse informatician roles to contend with the resultant issues that will surely arise. Envision the nurse informatician who specializes in the virtualization of care, robotics nurse, nurse genomic ethicist, personal health record nurse specialist, AI nurse specialist, health data integration and continuum of care and cost management expert, to mention but a few. For further discussion of future informatician roles and responsibilities, see Nagle and colleagues (Nagle et al. 2017). The authors anticipate new roles for nurse informaticians in the face of a universal, aging demographic characterized by sustained chronic, complex conditions, consumerism, ubiquitous technology and virtual-connected care. In particular, they highlight the need for new dimensions of informatics expertise in the areas of data science or "big data", robotics, artificial intelligence, genomics and perhaps even within new settings such as outer space. Each of these areas invite the development of new informatics knowledge and know-how, much of which is as yet unknown.

Imagining the world beyond today's reality, consider a future that allows for the extension of healthcare services to address the needs of developing nations and underserved communities and the potential to address current health inequities. In the context of healthcare delivery throughout the world, and perhaps beyond, consider the possibilities for the future, and appreciate that nurse informaticians are well situated to provide critical roles and responsibilities for many years to come. Chapters 13, 14, and 15 presents a vision of the future and how nursing informatics will support professional practice, advocacy, and the delivery of optimal client care.

11.13   Review Questions

1. Identify some of the roles and responsibilities assumed by nurses working in the field of informatics.
2. In your opinion, why is a nursing perspective is valuable to the work of health informatics.
3. What opportunities currently exist to obtain formal and informal education in the field of nursing/health informatics?
4. Describe some of the current informatics practice domains and potential role functions for the future.

11.13.1   Answers

1. Nurses interested in the field of informatics today will likely find opportunities in the following areas:

   - Practice
   - Academia
   - Government
   - Consulting

2. Nurses understand the processes of care delivery across all healthcare settings. Without a nursing perspective, health technology solutions may not provide the appropriate functionality or data and information to effectively and appropriately inform clinical decision-making.
3. Nurses may acquire informatics expertise formally and informally. Nurses commonly acquire knowledge and experience on the job but may also derive learnings from networking with colleagues at conferences and workshops. Many college and university programs offer certificates, diplomas, and undergraduate and graduate degrees focused in informatics. In some countries (e.g., Canada and

US), nurses may acquire a formal certification in health informatics (e.g., CPHIMS). Competencies have been developed in several countries for entry-to-practice and nurse leaders.

4. Today informatics practice domains may include the following: Leadership, ICT life cycle management, health system use, entrepreneurship, vendor support, education and research. In the future, nurse informaticians will likely be needed in the areas of: data science, artificial intelligence, robotics, genomics and perhaps space aeronautics, to name a few.

Glossary

AMIA American Medical Informatics Association

Business intelligence The use of data and information to inform decision impacting any aspect of a business

Clinical intelligence The use of data and information to inform decisions that are specifically clinical in nature

CNIA Canadian Nursing Informatics Association

CNIO Chief Nursing Informatics Officer

CPHIMS Certified Professional in Healthcare Information and Management Systems

Health informatics The intersection between health care, information management and information technology

HIMSS Health Information Management Systems Society

HSU Health System Use, where information is aggregated and analyzed to inform decisions

IMIA NI-SIG International Medical Informatics Association Nursing Informatics Special Interest Group

IMIA International Medical Informatics Association

PMP Project Mangement Professional, a professional credential granted by Project Management International (PMI)

SDLC Systems Development Life Cycle

References

American Medical Informatics Association. Academic informatics programs. 2020. Accessed at: https://www.amia.org/education/programs-and-courses. Accessed 26 Feb 2020.

American Nurses Association. Scope of practice for nursing informatics. Washington, DC: ANA; 1994.

American Nurses Association. Standards of practice for nursing informatics. Washington, DC: ANA; 1995.

American Nurses Association (ANA). Nursing informatics:Scope and standards of practice. 2nd ed. Silver Spring: Nursesbooks.Org; 2016.

American Nurses Credentialing Center (ANCC). (n.d.). Nursing informatics. At: https://www.nursingworld.org/our-certifications/informatics-nurse/. Accessed 26 Feb 2020.

Ash JS, Bates DW. Factors and forces affecting EHR system adoption: report of a 2004 ACMI. discussion. J Am Med Inform Assoc. 2005;12:8–12.

Ash JS, Stavri PZ, Dykstra R. Implementing computerized physician order entry: the importance of special people. Int J Med Inform. 2003;69:235–50.

Canadian Association of Schools of Nursing. Nursing Informatics Entry-to-Practice Competencies for Registered Nurses, Ottawa, ON: Author; 2012. At: http://www.casn.ca/2014/12/casn-entry-practice-nursing-informatics-competencies/; Accessed 20 Feb 2020.

Collins S, Yen PY, Phillips A, Kennedy MK. Nursing Informatics Competency Assessment for the Nurse Leader: The Delphi Study. J Nur Admin. 2017;47(4):212–8.

Digital Health Canada. Health informatics education. 2020. https://digitalhealthcanada.com/core-hi-education/. Accessed 26 Feb 2020.

Goosen W, Murphy J, editors. Forecasting Informatics Competencies for Nurses in the Future of Connected Health. Amsterdam: IOS Press; 2017.

Health Information Management Systems Society (HIMSS). HIMSS 2017 nursing informatics workforce survey. 2017. At: https://www.himss.org/resources/2017-himss-nursing-informatics-workforce-survey. Accessed 26 Feb 2020.

Health Information Management Systems Society (HIMSS). Health IT certifications. 2020. At: http://www.himss.org/health-it-certification?navItemNumber=13588. Accessed 26 Feb 2020.

Hersh W. Who are the informaticians? What we know and should know. J Am Med Inform Assoc. 2006;13(2):166–70.

Honey MLL, Skiba DJ, Procter P, Foster J, Kouri P, Nagle LM. Nursing informatics competencies for entry to practice: the perspective of six countries. Stud Health Technol Inform. 2017;232:51–61.

Kannry J, Sengstack P, Thyvalikakath TP, et al. The Chief Clinical Informatics Officer (CCIO): AMIA task force report on CCIO knowledge, education, and skillset requirements. Appl Clin Inform. 2016;7(1):143–76.

Kennedy MA, Moen A. Nursing leadership and informatics competencies: Shaping transformation of professional practice. In: Goosen W, Murphy J, editors. Forecasting Informatics Competencies for Nurses in the Future of Connected Health. Amsterdam: IOS Press; 2017. p. 197–206.

Kleib M, Nagle LM. Development of the Canadian Nurse Informatics Competency Assessment Scale (C-NICAS) and evaluation of Alberta's Registered Nurses' self-perceived informatics competencies. Com Inf Nur. 2018a;36(7):35–358.

Kleib M, Nagle LM. Factors Associated with Canadian nurses' informatics competency. Com Inf Nurs. 2018b;36(8):406–15.

Leatt P, Shea C, Studer M, Wang V. IT solutions for patient safety: best practices for successful implementation in healthcare. Healthc Q. 2006;9(1):94–104.

McLane S, Turley J. Informaticians: how they may benefit your healthcare organization. J Nurs Adm. 2011;41(1):29–35.

Nagle LM. Nurses *Carpe Diem*. In: One step beyond: the evolution of technology and nursing. Proceedings of 7th International Congress Nursing Informatics Conference on CD, Auckland, 2000.

Nagle LM. Everything I know about informatics, I didn't learn in nursing school. Can J Nurs Leadersh. 2007;20(3):22–5.

Nagle LM. The importance of being informatics savvy. Can J Nurs Leadersh. 2016;28(4):1–4.

Nagle LM, Crosby K, Frisch N, Borycki E, Donelle L, Hannah K, Harris A, Jetté S, Shaben, T. Developing entry-to-practice competencies for registered nurses. Proceedings 12th International Congress on Nursing Informatics, 2014, Taipei, Taiwan.

Nagle LM, Sermeus W, Junger A. Evolving role of the nursing informatics specialist. In: Goosen W, Murphy J, editors. Forecasting informatics competencies for nurses in the future of connected health. Amsterdam: IOS Press; 2017. p. 212–21.

Nagle, LM, Furlong, K, Kleib M. (Eds). Study of digital health in Canadian schools of nursing: curricula content and nurse educator capacity. 2018. Ottawa, ON: Canada Health

Infoway. At: https://www.infoway-inforoute.ca/en/component/edocman/resources/reports/benefits-evaluation/3716-study-of-digital-health-in-canadian-schools-of-nursing. Accessed 26 Feb 2020.

Scholes M, Tallberg MA, Pluyter-Wenting E. International nursing informatics: a history of the first forty years: 1960–2000. London: British Computer Society; 2002.

Sewell J. Informatics and nursing: opportunities and challenges. 6th ed. Philadelphia: Wolters Kluwer—Lippincott Williams & Wilkin; 2019.

Smith K, Tyler DD. Systems life cycle: planning and analysis. In: Saba VK, McCormick KA, editors. Essentials of nursing informatics. 5th ed. New York: McGraw-Hill; 2011. p. 77–92.

Smith SE, Drake LE, Harris J-G, Watson K, Pohlner PG. Clinical informatics: a workforce priority for 21st century healthcare. Aust Health Rev. 2011;35:130–5.

Staggers N, Thompson CB. The evolution of definitions for nursing informatics: a critical analysis and revised definition. J Am Med Inform Assoc. 2002;9(3):255–61.

Strudwick G, Nagle LM, Kassam I, Pahwa M, Sequeira L. Informatics competencies for nurse leaders: a scoping review. J Nurs Admin. 2019a;49(6):323–30.

Strudwick G, Nagle LM, Morgan A, Kennedy MA, Currie LM, White P. Adapting and validating nurse leader informatics competencies in the Canadian context: Results of a Delphi study. Int J Med Inform. 2019b;129:211–8.

Studer M. The effect of organizational factors on the effectiveness of EMR system implementation: what have we learned? Healthc Q. 2005;8(4):92–8.

Warm D, Thomas B. A review of the effectiveness of the clinical informaticist role. Nurs Stand. 2011;25(44):35–8.

Yen PY, Phillips A, Kennedy MK, Collins S. Nursing informatics competency assessment for the nurse leader: Instrument refinement, validation, and psychometric analysis. J Nurs Admin. 2017;47(5):271–7.

Chapter 12
Researching Nursing Informatics in a Digital Age

Tracie Risling, Gillian Strudwick, and Richard Booth

Abstract To ensure that nurses are able to practice in evidence informed environments, nursing research has become an essential part of the profession. This chapter provides a foundational overview of the research process commonly used in nursing study, while highlighting how informatics can contribute to the research process but also be a researched topic in itself. The chapter begins with a detailed description of the common steps taken when conducting nursing research for both nursing informatics and other topics. Then, a number of ways nursing informatics can be used to support the research process itself are given using practical examples. The chapter concludes with a discussion of current and future opportunities for nursing informatics research.

Keywords Nursing informatics research · Nursing research · Quantitative methods · Qualitative methods · Mixed methods research

Learning Objectives for the Chapter
1. Explain nursing research and research methods.
2. Discuss qualitative, quantitative and mixed methods research.

Electronic Supplementary Material The online version of this chapter (https://doi.org/10.1007/978-3-030-58740-6_12) contains supplementary material, which is available to authorized users.

T. Risling (✉)
College of Nursing, University of Saskatchewan, Saskatoon, SK, Canada
e-mail: tracie.risling@usask.ca

G. Strudwick
Centre for Addiction and Mental Health, Toronto, Ontario, Canada

Institute of Health Policy, Management and Evaluation, University of Toronto, Toronto, ON, Canada
e-mail: gillian.strudwick@camh.ca

R. Booth
Arthur Labatt Family School of Nursing, Western University, London, ON, Canada
e-mail: rbooth6@uwo.ca

© Springer Nature Switzerland AG 2021
P. Hussey, M. A. Kennedy (eds.), *Introduction to Nursing Informatics*, Health Informatics, https://doi.org/10.1007/978-3-030-58740-6_12

3. Describe at least two areas influencing the futue of nursing informatics research.
4. Introduce emerging technologies impacting nursing research such as artificial intelligence (AI) and machine learning (ML).
5. Review the importance of compassionate care in nursing informatics intervention and research.

12.1 Introduction

With the increased digitalization of all aspects of the nursing role and healthcare over the last few decades, the influence on nursing research has begun to be felt in all domains of knowledge generation and inquiry. Historically, while nursing informatics has existed for numerous years as a specific topic within the body of nursing literature, the growing importance and presence of digital technologies in all aspects of life and work has resulted in a paradigm shift toward *how* these forms of innovation and informatics can be used as a supportive mechanism (Polit and Beck 2012), to extend, and at times, underpin many forms of nursing research activities. Insomuch as, the increased presence and visibility of informatics in the workplace and society has subtly offered nurses new and important opportunities to leverage the functionalities of these technologies to assist in many types of research activities, including information aggregation, data collection, and knowledge dissemination. While using supportive elements of informatics to conduct research has become commonplace in nursing research, it is important to appreciate that the topic of nursing informatics also exists as its own nursing specialty, and the foci of significant research activities by numerous scholars and practitioners worldwide (Sidani and Braden 2011; Peters et al. 2015).

For instance, the recent increased adoption of electronic medical records (EMR) and other digitalized record keeping systems have opened entirely new fields of inquiry to nursing scholars. With the increased ability to query, trend, and aggregate datasets arising from disparate locations, nursing researchers now have the opportunity to generate micro- and macro- interpretations related to population health, wellness, and other areas of inquiry relevant to the nursing role and health (Levac et al. 2010). To date, there is a growing body of nursing researchers who use healthcare administrative data arising from EMR and other digitized record systems to generate insights and other clinical recommendations to support practice (Levac et al. 2010; Arksey and O'Malley 2005). Further, the increased use of digital community technologies has also afforded researchers new and novel mechanisms from which to interact with vulnerable individuals and populations. For instance, the use of mobile technology to support individuals experiencing mental illness and homelessness is a novel approach that leverages the use of communication technology in a proactive fashion to support the wellbeing of individuals (Canadian Agency for Drugs and Technologies in Health 2018).

As outlined above, while nursing informatics can act as a supportive mechanism to conduct and apply nursing research, the topic can also be subject of its own inquiry (Trust MKP 2002). The discipline of nursing informatics has a long history of generating evidence related to the use of digital technology to support the nursing role and client care. While research focused on nursing informatics is broad and diverse, a few common traits do exist that span most inquiry in this area. For instance, as described by Matney et al. (Munhall 2012), the philosophical foundations of all nursing informatics research encapsulate concepts related to *data, information, knowledge*, and *wisdom*. Further, Matney et al. outlines that nursing informatics inquiry is appreciative of different philosophical and ontological lenses from which to explore the core concepts of data, information, knowledge, and wisdom. This philosophical and ontological plurality and receptivity can be viewed throughout published nursing informatics literature – including researchers that seek to rigorously evaluate technology systems used by nurses through post-positivist or objectivist methods (e.g., (Creswell and Clark 2007; Barnard and Sandelowski 2001)); while, other researchers prefer to utilize interpretive and constructivist approaches to better understand the experiences, workflow, and other fluid interpretations of human-technology interactions (e.g., (Kaminski 2011; Strudwick 2015)). Regardless of the philosophical or ontological approaches, research exploring specific aspects of nursing informatics will likely continue on into the future as distinct sub-set of other nursing research and continue to provide valuable insights to inform aspects of practice and healthcare delivery. Therefore, due to the multidimensional nature from which nursing informatics can both influence aspects of nursing research, and/or be the foci of nursing research, efforts will be taken in this chapter to provide a fulsome range of descriptions that accentuates these potentials and implications for the future.

12.2 Section 1: Steps in the Research Process

Nursing research is conducted on a variety of different topics that are important to the profession. This includes research on topics of relevance to those in clinical practice, administration/management, education, research, regulatory and other settings. This research is essential to the generation of evidence that nurses can use to make informed decisions in their respective roles. While the methods used by nursing researchers vary significantly based on the topic being studied, the general process that nursing researchers use to approach research is often quite similar. This section of the chapter will provide an overview of the common steps used by nursing researchers when engaging in research. This section applies to both research that is about nursing informatics, or uses nursing informatics approaches, as well as non-nursing informatics topics. The following section will provide examples of how the research steps outlined in this section apply specifically within a nursing informatics context.

12.2.1 Overview of the Nursing Research Process

The research process typically begins with the identification of a key issue, topic or problem relevant to nurses (Polit and Beck 2012). It then involves a series of investigative techniques to understand what is already known about the topic, and what aspects of the topic remain unknown. From this point, nursing researchers identify a need to conduct research to answer or address an important gap in what is known about a particular topic, problem or aspect of a topic. Often a series of research questions are then developed to address the particular gap identified from the literature review. A number of methods are then selected, designed and carried out to answer the research questions. The data obtained from this process is then analyzed, interpreted and discussed in the context of the original problem or topic, as well as the literature. These findings are then shared to those who would benefit from knowing the research results, traditionally through journal articles and conference presentations. The steps in a typical nursing research process are shown in Table 12.1, and are detailed in the remaining part of this section of the chapter.

12.2.2 Step 1: Identify a Key Issue, Topic or Problem Relevant to Nurses

The first step in the nursing research process is to identify a key issue, topic or problem that is relevant to nurses and that is important to address. This issue could be relevant to nurses working in clinical practice, administration/managerial, education, informatics, research and other settings. Key issues, topics or problems that need to be addressed could range from identifying appropriate nursing interventions to prevent pressure ulcers (Sidani and Braden 2011), to uncovering the appropriate

Table 12.1 Steps of the nursing research process

Step	Research Process Activity
1	Identify a key issue, topic or problem relevant to nurses
2	Conduct a review of the literature
3	Develop research questions that address the gaps identified in the literature
4	Select an appropriate theoretical framework
5	Determine the methods required to carry out the research
6	Collect the research data based on the methods determined in step 5
7	Perform data analysis
8	Interpret and discuss the results
9[a]	Conduct knowledge translation activities

[a]it may be appropriate to conduct knowledge translation activities during different steps in the research process

compliment of nurse staffing that would yield the best patient outcomes in a particular care setting, to identifying how best to educate nursing students to learn to use a new form of technology to deliver care. As the environments in which nurse's practice evolve, nursing research will continue to ask and answer important questions for the profession.

A common place to identify a key issue, topic or problem relevant to nurses is in their place of work, whether it be clinical, administration/managerial, educational or otherwise. It may be that nurses in these various settings are required to make important decisions, but lack (or are not aware of) the appropriate evidence to do so in an informed way. This lack of evidence may serve as a motivation for nurses to identify a key issue, topic or problem that they wish to pursue through formal research.

12.2.3   Step 2: Conduct a Literature Review

Once a key issue, topic or problem has been identified, a review of the literature can be done. The goal of the literature review is to uncover all that is known about the key issue, topic or problem that may help to identify how to solve it. It may be that research has already been completed that addresses the key issue, topic or problem, and that no further steps in the research process need to take place. So as long as the research that addresses the area of interest was done in a scientifically rigorous and appropriate way, it may be that the findings can be directly applied to the original problem or issue. Where gaps in the research exist that would prevent the application of appropriate findings, the nurse would proceed to step 3, which is to develop research questions.

There are different types of literature reviews that can be done to find out more about a key issue, topic or problem. These include traditional, narrative, integrated, rapid, scoping and systematic reviews (Peters et al. 2015; Levac et al. 2010; Arksey and O'Malley 2005). Each has their own specific methods and steps for conducting the literature review. However, while there are several established methods for conducting literature reviews, most follow a similar approach. This approach involves searching electronic databases and identifying articles within that may address the key issue, topic or problem, and then appraising the research to determine if the findings may be applicable to address the issue or problem. Common electronic databases that are searched among nursing researchers include (but are not limited to):

- CINAHL: The Cumulative Index of Nursing and Allied Health Literature
- PubMed
- PsycInfo
- Medline
- Scopus
- Google Scholar

- EMBASE
- Cochrane Library
- ERIC: Education Resources Information Center
- Joanna Briggs Institute

As well as the electronic databases listed above, depending on the focus of the research, it may be appropriate to utilize a database that is specific to another scientific domain. For example, to identify articles that discuss the design of a health related technology, it may be valuable to search an engineering database like Engineering Village. Many nursing schools are affiliated with academic libraries and librarians with knowledge of the many databases available to search. Consulting with a librarian can support the identification of the most appropriate databases to search for a given topic.

Each of the previously listed electronic databases that may be relevant to nursing is searched in a different way. Some (e.g. Medline) require the use of keywords and Medical Subject Headings (MeSH), combined together through a series of symbols called 'Boolean operators'. Others (e.g. google scholar) allow for text to be searched more similarly to how searches are done in a regular web based search engine like google. It's important to know how to search these electronic databases appropriately in order to yield the best results, including how to use Boolean operators if necessary. Often these databases have online tutorials, or instructions available that can be used to support successful use. As well, some educational institutions, healthcare organizations and libraries offer supports (e.g. librarians) and courses or tutorials to assist in the successful use of these electronic databases.

In addition to literature reviews of academic databases, there are also 'grey' literature reviews that are conducted to identify sources of important information that may not be found in traditional academic library environments. Grey literature sources can include websites, briefing notes, newsletters, government reports, conference presentation and beyond (Canadian Agency for Drugs and Technologies in Health 2018). These sources may contain information that was not formally written in a research article that could address the key issue, topic or problem. A common method for searching the grey literature is through web search engines such as google, or through searching organizational intranet sites. Depending on the key issue, topic or problem being investigated, including a grey literature search may be appropriate. One way to identify if a grey literature search may be worth conducting is to ask yourself, 'could the answer to my key issue, topic or problem be found in a report, website or conference presentation?' If the answer to this question is 'yes', it is likely worth conducting a grey literature search.

Once academic or grey literature is identified that may address or provide important information related to the key issue, topic or problem, it is important to conduct an appraisal of its quality. If a study is identified that addresses the issue in a problematic way or the scientific approach is not done well, the findings may not be relevant or useful to you. Several tools to support nurses in appraising academic articles exist. For example, the Critical Appraisal Skills Programme (Trust MKP 2002), developed in the United Kingdom, is one such resource that offers nurses free worksheets with key questions to ask when appraising research studies. The worksheets can be found at the following web address: https://casp-uk.net/casp-tools-checklists/

12.2.4   Step 3: Develop Research Questions That Address the Gaps Identified in the Literature

The next step in the research process is to develop a clear set of research questions that address the gaps that have been identified from the literature review conducted in the previous step. The research questions are what will be answered once the research has been conducted, and analyzed. One of the most important steps in the research process is to ensure that the research questions are clear, and addressable through nursing research. The research questions will then be used to identify the appropriate methods that would answer these questions. Thus, if the research questions have not been articulated well, are too vague, or are easy to misinterpret, it could lead to fatal flaws in the overall research. Once research questions are initially written, it's often useful to seek the feedback of others, particularly those with nursing research expertise. Another perspective in reviewing these questions is often helpful to support the 'honing in' on the best wording and use of language in the development of these research questions.

12.2.5   Step 4: Select an Appropriate Theoretical Framework

Once the research questions have been developed, a theoretical framework can be identified that appropriately addresses these questions. While not all health related research utilizes theoretical frameworks, it is common in nursing research to ground the research in a theoretical framework that helps to provide a basis for the research approach. There is not one ideal framework that is appropriate for all studies carried out by nurses. There are many different frameworks and models and the selection of any one of these is typically topic dependent. Depending on the topic, frameworks may be chosen from the nursing discipline, or others such as psychology, public health, sociology, gender studies and beyond.

In qualitative research, it is also common for studies to be reflective of the worldview that a researcher brings to their research. A worldview is often described as the way someone understands the world and the phenomenon they are studying (Munhall 2012). In some qualitative research studies, the researchers will explicitly discuss their worldviews within the context of their work.

12.2.6   Step 5: Determine the Methods Required to Carry Out the Research

In step 5, the methods that are required to carry out the research are determined. The selected methods are largely chosen based on the research question being asked (Polit and Beck 2012). Open-ended research questions that are exploratory in nature tend to be answered best through qualitative research approaches and methods, whereas research questions that are answerable by a more definitive and closed-ended response typically use quantitative approaches and methods. Mixed methods are used when the research questions require both quantitative and qualitative approaches to answer them (Creswell and Clark 2007).

Once the approach (qualitative, quantitative or mixed methods) is selected, the sample, setting and data sources can be identified (if appropriate) to address the research questions. In research involving human subjects, the sample is the population which is studied for the purpose of the research. Commonly in nursing research, the sample consists of a group of patients with a similar condition (e.g. women with diabetes), or nurses themselves. The place or context in which the research takes place is called the setting. In nursing research, the setting is commonly a clinic, hospital, or community setting. Data sources vary widely in nursing research. In many forms of research, it is common for the data source to be a human participant themselves with data obtained through interviews and focus groups or by instruments or tools delivered through a questionnaire or survey, for example. The subject or participant could be a patient, family member, nurse etc. In other kinds of research, the data source could come from a non-human source like nursing documentation in an electronic health record, step counts on a pedometer, a heart rate monitor, staffing databases and beyond. It is important that the sample, setting and data source(s) are appropriately matched to the research questions so that these questions can be adequately answered. There are many different data sources that may answer a research question. Carefully considering how well the information is contained in the data source, as well as the feasibility of accessing the data source are key questions that should be thought about when selecting these sources.

In many settings it is a required step to write a research proposal summarizing steps 1 through 4, and detailing the specific methods that would be used in step 5. If money is required to execute the research, this research proposal may be read by potential funders like a granting agency, a donor or senior leadership at an organization where the research may take place. In addition, it is standard practice in many organizations around the world to have the research proposal reviewed and approved by a Research Ethics Board prior to conducting the research. This is to ensure the research is carried out in an ethical way.

12.2.7 Step 6: Collect the Research Data Based on the Methods Determined in Step 5

In Step 6, the methods identified and approved by the Research Ethics Board are carried out. If the research involves human subjects, recruitment of potential subjects occurs during this step. These participants are typically required to provide informed consent before they participate in the research, which communicates that they understand what they are being asked to do, along with any risks or benefits.

For research involving secondary data sources, during this step, researchers would obtain the various data sources and prepare the data for analysis.

Depending on the methods utilized, the outputs of the research at this step will vary. For example, focus groups and interviews will typically yield long transcripts of what was said by participants, whereas administrative secondary data may be captured on a spreadsheet. Artefacts from research may also include audio files, videos, photos, logbooks, reflection journals and artwork developed by participants. These outputs are dependent on the research methods used.

12.2.8   Step 7: Perform Data Analysis

The next step of the research process is data analysis. Techniques for data analysis vary depending on the type of research that was conducted. Various software tools have been created to support these analysis types. For example, for quantitative data analysis there are a variety of different statistical software programs, and for qualitative studies there is software that can support the organization of themes and coded categories. Ensuring that the right analytical methods are used is important in accurately and sufficiently answering the research questions.

12.2.9   Step 8: Interpret and Discuss the Results

Once the data has been analyzed, the next step is to interpret and situate the findings back into the literature, as well as the context in which the key issue, topic or problem was identified. When the results of the research are available, it is often important to ask if there are any key decisions, practices or policies that should modified as a result? In addition, researchers may also ask what other questions have been identified as a result of the research that was conducted? It is not uncommon for additional research questions to be uncovered as a result of the research process in itself.

12.2.10   Step 9: Conduct Knowledge Translation Activities

In some studies, the knowledge gleaned from the research activities is shared with those who would benefit from it after the study has been completed. In other studies, there is a more integrated approach, where knowledge translation occurs throughout the research process. Traditional knowledge translation activities that take place once a study is completed include an academic publication in a scientific journal, and a conference presentation. Other activities may include web-based seminars (e.g. webinars), factsheets, briefing notes, presentation at stakeholder meetings, social media campaigns, the development of videogames to share the information, websites, toolkits, and beyond.

In nursing clinical practice, it is often a challenge to ensure that the latest evidence is incorporated into routine practice. One way to support knowledge translation in these settings is to regularly review and update practice related policies and subsequent education/training for nurses based on the latest evidence. This would require an organizational commitment to ensure the appropriate resourcing and staff with expertise to review and update these policies regularly.

12.3   Section 2: How Nursing Informatics Can Be Used Throughout the Research Process

Nursing informatics can be viewed as both a topic of study, as well as an approach to support the conduction of good quality nursing research. This section of the chapter outlines how nursing informatics approaches can be utilized to support the various steps in the nursing research process, with a special emphasis on step 5, which is to determine the methods required to carry out the research.

12.3.1   Step 1: Identify a Key Issue, Topic or Problem Relevant to Nurses

Informatics is changing nursing education, practice, and research. As technology continues to flow into nursing environments potential research topics increase correspondingly. The expanding use of electronic health records (EHRs) in nursing care is a good example of this. As EHR data became more commonly used around the world, nurses began to identify research priorities associated with this technology. These included, the urgent need to standardize data across records and systems, the impact of the use of this technology on existing work practices and patient relationships, and emerging ideas about what could potentially be done with the large amount of patient and nursing data being created in these records. From these few examples dozens of related research questions could, and in fact have been generated in nursing informatics as detailed further in Chaps. 3 and 11.

In general, the rapid pace of digital development tends to provide consistent opportunities or need for informatics research. Because of this, new researchers may be overwhelmed in choosing a topic or problem to study, as opposed to trying to find an area of research. A good starting point for all researchers is to examine the literature, in particular looking for any systematic or rapid reviews that have been done on their topic or within their practice area of interest.

Researchers in all disciplines are also increasingly interacting with each other on social media and in other online communities, further examples of which are highlighted in Chap. 14 on Knowledge and Social Networks. Not surprisingly, these digital connections tend to be heavily used by informatics researchers. New researchers should establish their own networked communities using platforms such as Twitter, ResearchGate, Mendeley or Google Scholar as a starting point in their research. Find and follow nursing informatic and research organizations on Twitter and keep up to date on current hashtags to easily find information, for examples #Nurses4HIT and #NursingInformatics.

12.3.2 Step 2: Conduct a Literature Review

The purpose and value of online databases in conducting a comprehensive literature review has already been detailed, and librarians can be very valuable team members or resources in this work. In addition to the use of Medical Subject Headings (MeSH) or other subject key words, informatics researchers can also take advantage of the work done to establish standardized nursing data. Along with the long-standing presence of NANDA International, the global source of standardized nursing diagnoses, researchers can also pull literature search terms from SNOMED International or ICNP, the International Classification for Nursing Practice. The increasing development of data standards is not just benefitting the technical advancement of electronic health communication, it is also uniting informatics researchers around the world by aligning their terminology and associated research questions.

There are further ways to promote connectivity using other digital supports during a literature review. Even standard citation management software programs are now likely to offer ways for teams to share data and information. Mendeley has prioritized global collaboration and networking in its citation product, and EndNote also supports team interaction and sharing. Many of the databases used to complete reviews will send data to these other tools, making the work of the researcher much more efficient.

Lastly, another issue that nursing informatics researchers can face during the literature review phase is managing the volume of information gathered. Even when researching very new technologies there are typically large bodies of literature that have to be included in a review at least initially. Try searching the terms internet or mobile application in any of the databases you have learned about and you will quickly see the challenge informatics researchers must learn to manage. While the combining of key search terms can help to reduce the numbers in a literature search, informatics researchers doing systematic review work may want to harness the power of digital review management tools such Rayyan QCRI, or Covidence to aid them in their work.

More recently, informatics researchers have also begun to explore the opportunities that machine learning, a form of artificial intelligence, or natural language processing may present to automate parts of the literature review process. Although additional study is needed to compare the efficiency and accuracy of computers versus human researchers in sorting and classifying items in a large literature review, there is emerging evidence to support this automation in managing extensive data.

12.3.3   Step 3: Develop Research Questions That Address the Gaps Identified in the Literature

The development of a research question can begin as early as the first step in the research process. Very often researchers begin with a question in mind related to their topic or problem of interest. It is also common however, for that research question to evolve or be refined during the literature review process as specific detail about where additional studies are needed is revealed. In nursing informatics research, this is also the time to consider whether or not the emerging question is philosophical, theoretical, or more practical in nature. For example, nursing has long debated the introduction of technology in terms of how it impacts the art and science of nursing, the very essence of how we approach care. Barnard and Sandelowski (2001) noted that nursing had taken "professional ownership of the space between technology and patient, and the responsibility for maintaining humane care in technological environments" thereby becoming mediators or a bridge between these two forces (Barnard and Sandelowski 2001). This philosophical debate is still a part of nursing informatics research today. But, in addition, there are research questions that focus on the development of new technologies for nursing practice, and/or the evaluation of such tools as they are introduced into care environments. These kinds of practical questions or studies are typically called applied research.

Once you have established the foundation for your research question you can review the published work of other researchers and see how they have constructed similar questions. This is where connections established through social media or research platforms such as Mendeley will be valuable. If you are wanting to connect with community members, patients, or potential users of the technology of interest there are online brainstorming tools or meeting sites such as GroupMap or Zoom that may be useful. If you are holding meetings in person or online to refine research questions or ideas you can use additional digital tools such as Poll Everywhere or Mentimeter to allow participants to vote or help evolve the final research question(s).

12.3.4   Step 4: Select an Appropriate Theoretical Framework

Nursing informatics research tends to be complex and like other study can benefit from the use of general theoretical framework to guide the work. Nursing theory has produced dozens of potential frameworks that may be useful in informatics research, but because this work often requires a more interdisciplinary approach, it is worthwhile to consider theoretical contributions from other disciplines. Nursing informatics researchers have long partnered and/or borrowed approaches from psychology, computer science, and engineering. As a starting point consider two well-known theoretical approaches to the uptake and use of technology, Rogers Diffusion of Innovation Theory (Kaminski 2011) and the Unified Theory of Technology Acceptance and Use (Strudwick 2015).

The diffusion of innovation theory presents five technology uptake categories innovators (enthusiasts), early adopters (visionaries), early majority (pragmatists), late majority (conservatives), and laggards (skeptics) in a bell-shaped curve that predicts how acceptance of new innovations will progress in a population (Kaminski 2011; Rogers 2003). Nursing informatics researchers can use this framework to anticipate user needs or potential barriers to introducing new technologies.

Similarly, the Unified Theory of Technology Acceptance and Use or UTAUT is another framework that can be used to explore the uptake and integration of digital interventions (Venkatesh et al. 2003). This has been done by nursing informatics researchers as evidenced in an integrative review on technology acceptance in nursing by Strudwick (Rogers 2003). The various acceptance models in this review, including the UTAUT continue to be valuable approaches for supporting informatics research. It is important to note however, that these frameworks also continue to evolve, sometimes as rapidly as technology does itself. For example, the UTAUT has been updated to the UTAUT2 to allow researchers to reflect upon how variables such as age, gender and experience influence consideration of technology uptake and how sustained use is influenced by factors such as motivation, price and habit (Venkatesh et al. 2012).

These theoretical frameworks are only a small representation of what exists in the literature. Even with so many options to choose from, nursing informatics researchers may not find a theoretical foundation that aligns well with the work they are planning to do. In this case, there is also an ongoing innovation of these frameworks themselves. Risling and Risling (2020) united the qualitative nursing methodology Interpretive Description with key elements from the computer science software development lifecycle to create a research framework specific to the development of new health technologies or interventions. This is just one example of how nurses are collaborating with colleagues from other relevant disciplines to develop entirely new or blended theoretical approaches for informatics research.

12.3.5   Step 5: Determine the Methods Required to Carry Out the Research

To create a strong methodological foundation for a research project you first decide if you are going to using a quantitative, qualitative, or mixed-methods approach. Then you can consider what particular methodology or methodologies will best address the research questions you have identified. Only once these decisions are made do you want to consider what methods you will use to actually complete the research.

In informatics research common methods including data mining, online surveying, and even crowdsourcing. Data mining is not a new concept for nursing. Goodwin et al. (2003) highlighted the value of using this approach to build nursing knowledge in the early 2000s, identifying key machine learning tools as well as potential challenges to data mining in nursing (Goodwin et al. 2003). This method has become increasingly popular as the amount of electronic health data has expanded in clinical information systems. But data mining is not only restricted to healthcare records and systems, researchers are using other sources, such as posts in online community forums, or social media sites to collect large data sets as well. Computer programs can be set up to 'scrape' this data from platforms, like Twitter, creating very large data sets in a short period of time, depending on the topic. Analytic tools are then used to highlight meaningful patterns or relationships in the data sets by researchers.

The use of online survey tools is also not new, however there are more ways to reach potential participants and conduct these surveys as digital connectivity increases around the world. Universities and healthcare institutions will often have a preferred survey tool for research use, but very simple online polling is also built into common social media platforms such as Twitter™, Instagram™, and Facebook™. While these tools would not typically be used for formal research, they could be valuable in drawing participants into your survey.

Reaching out to a wide range of participants in the community is a key element of crowdsourcing, as well as in the movement that has now become known as citizen science. Basic crowdsourcing can be done through tools, such as Amazon Mechanical Turk™ which is a more formal marketplace. Then there are a number of citizen science projects, websites or applications such as Zooniverse™ which has connected millions of citizens to research projects of interest to them. While crowdsourcing can be an exciting method it is not something researchers should choose to do without understanding the challenges associated with it, such as potential biases and data reliability issues that may arise.

Finally, it is important to remember that researchers will be directed in the methods they use by the methodologies that have been selected to complete the research. Returning to the earlier methodological example uniting nursing and computer science, if you are doing research developing or evaluating a new technological intervention, then using methods from the software development cycle to collect data are needed. This work commonly includes usability testing, or an evaluation of how well the technology is accepted by users, and if it delivers the expected outcomes. Birnie et al. (2018) provide an excellent example of this in their research evaluating the usability of interactive virtual reality (VR) to reduce pain for children and adolescents undergoing cancer treatments (Birnie et al. 2018). In this research, the team worked with patients and practitioners to determine the ease of use, understanding and acceptability of the VR technology as well as examining how well it could be implemented in clinical care, and if its use resulted in any adverse effects (Birnie et al. 2018). This type of usability testing, very common in computer science, is starting to be used much more frequently in informatics research. Other types of tech data, such as detailed usage statistics from webpages or mobile applications are also more typically collected now in nursing led research.

12.3.6 Step 6: Collect the Research Data Based on the Methods Determined in Step 5

One of the benefits of employing data collection methods from computer science for nursing informatics research is that much of this reporting can be built right into the technological interventions under study. There are ethical considerations that must be followed if this data is being collected automatically however with all participants fully informed of what specific information, over what period of time will be collected, so that they can evaluate any privacy or confidentiality risks.

Automation of reports and data synthesis is one of the promoted benefits of expanding the use of technology in healthcare and nursing informatics researchers can certainly take advantage of this as well. Data may be compiled locally, nationally, or even globally in some instances, although more work on standardizing nursing data is needed in order to really capitalize on the potential of big data in nursing.

As data is collected, regardless of method, nursing informatics researchers are likely to use further electronic or digital tools to review, clean, and organize their data. Voice recognition software is making automatic transcribing more accurate and accessible, and there are numerous other software and web-based applications researchers can use to organize their data and prepare it for analysis. Extra consideration should be given to securely storing all of this data with the use of password protection, encryption, and secure cloud storage. These security procedures will likely need to be detailed in any research ethics application, with particular processes often dictated by the institute that the researcher is employed by and/or where the research is being conducted.

12.3.7 Step 7: Perform Data Analysis

There are computer tools to aid your data analysis no matter the methodological approach. SPSS™ is a statistical analysis software platform very commonly used in quantitative research. There are also digital tools for qualitative analysis, such as NVIVO™ or ATLAS.ti™ that support researchers in seeking patterns or themes in their data. When working with large or 'big data' sets, artificial intelligence (AI) or more often a subset of AI called machine learning, can also be used. Algorithms are used to support autonomous analysis or classification in machine learning and often output predictions, for example in McLean's (2018) work using machine learning to classify diabetics by risk and predict incident of foot ulcers. This type of predictive analysis is being seen more frequently in nursing informatics research identifying patient risks, staffing needs, and even future use of emergency or other health services.

Another tool to support analysis of nursing data is natural language processing or NLP. Using NLP is a means to process large amounts of narrative data and this is not a new approach in nursing informatics research. In 2009 nurse researchers were already using NLP techniques to extract data from nursing narratives (Hyun et al. 2009). Because a lot of nursing data is not standardized and is presented in long-hand or narrative form, advancing the use of NLP techniques is a valuable pursuit. Despite the early efforts in this area, much more refinement of this technique in nursing informatics focused research is needed.

There are other lower tech options for processing complex data sets that are still of value in digital health research. Visualization tools such as concept maps, social network analysis, or the newer application of journey mapping can also be considered. Concept mapping is a familiar tool to many nurses as it is often used by students in their clinical placements to organize patient data and priorities. Social network analysis is part of a methodological approach that reveals key players or networks and relationships in a visual data analysis. In informatics research this is often done to identify where the introduction of new technology will be supported or blocked in an organization.

Journey mapping is a newer approach in nursing informatics, more typically used in marketing or customer service research. Still it is a valuable addition to user-centred research by encouraging researchers to map out every interaction point that a patient or practitioner may have in encountering and using a new technology. These later types of analysis are particularly useful in planning for deployment of technological interventions and/or evaluating their impact especially in terms of quality improvement or other specific outcomes within a health system.

12.3.8   Step 8 Interpret and Discuss the Results

Nursing informatics research is rarely done in isolation and the results from the studies we do often needs to be interpreted and shared across diverse audiences. Whether you are partnered with patients, practitioners, institutions, technology or other industry partners, educators, policy makers and/or colleagues from any variety of disciplines there will be a point in your research process where you may want to seek expert opinion on your results. Some research processes, like Delphi studies or scoping reviews, have this kind of consultation built into the methodology. However, even if there is no methodological prompt, holding team meetings or sessions with collaborating partners is a worthwhile stop in this part of the research process. One of the key items that tends to be a subject of discussion at this point in any study is how to finalize the analysis and/or presentation of the data.

Much of our information is packaged and shared in digital formats today and this includes research results. However, there are a few interesting approaches that can be considered to improve the potential impact and translation of study findings. First, if large data sets have been used as part of the research concise data visualization models should be a part of the results. Data visualization has become almost an art form with specialized experts in this field but nursing also has a long history of engaging in visual data representations. Florence Nightingale represented data on mortality statistics from her field work in a visual chart which has come to be called the rose diagram, and nursing informatics researchers still recognize the value of this data visualization today (Monsen et al. 2015). Infographics, which are also increasingly used to share research results, can be built from multiple data visualizations.

Another tool borrowed from computer science and in particular software development that can extremely useful in finalizing and sharing data results in the use of personas. A persona is an archetypal representation of data and identified needs usually from particular user group that is identified in informatics research (LeRouge et al. 2013). Personas are short, fictional, biographies created from research results grouped into a collection of 'people' who then represent the themes in the study. Essentially, you use data to bring users 'to life' through personas, representing data sets through imagery and other characterizations (LeRouge et al. 2013). The use of personas can summarize key findings and also highlight priority needs and requirements for the implementation of informatics findings or developed interventions in an engaging way.

12.3.9   Step 9: Conduct Knowledge Translation Activities

When the findings of a study are finalized and packaged for release, it is important that research teams think about multiple ways that this information can be shared. Nursing informatics researchers are usually well connected through multiple digital platforms and further advantaged by well-developed digital literacy skills. Given this, nursing informatics research should be widely publicized and disseminated. While there is some very good translation work being done, this is an area that could be improved upon. Nursing journals tend to have lower impact factors than informatics or other disciplinary publications, but it is important to retain a connection to nursing audiences when conducting informatics research. Because this field of study is highly interdisciplinary it is also critical that nursing establish its informatics expertise across disciplines.

In order not to become overwhelmed by the needs related to knowledge translation in nursing informatics research it is important to create a detailed plan at the beginning of any project. While this plan will likely evolve as the research progresses having an early roadmap to the final destination will aid the research team in identifying knowledge translation opportunities during the journey. Any knowledge translation from a research project will include more traditional academic routes such as article publication and conference presentation, but nursing informatics researchers should also always consider novel ways to share their findings.

Harnessing digital skills to create whiteboard animations, social media campaigns, TikToks™, or contributions to newly emerging platforms should be a part of every research plan.

12.4 Section: 3: Current and Future Opportunities for Nursing Informatics Research

As noted, nursing informatics research is a fast-paced field and as technology rapidly evolves so does the opportunity to research the effects of it on nursing practice, people, and healthcare. One of the by-products of increasing connectivity in the world is the amount of data that is being produced. There is a rapid exponential increase in electronic data as technology becomes integrated into more parts of our lives and world. Data is being captured from every internet search, smart phone tap, wearable device, geo-locator, online purchase, and like, comment or tweet. In healthcare, EHRs, biomedical sensors, home and hospital monitoring tools, genomic study and other computer enhanced research further contributes to what many call a 'fire-hose' of data. Nursing informatics researchers are working with this data in many forms, from online sources like social media posting, to patient and practice data collected in care settings.

There will be an ongoing need for nursing informatics researchers to develop advanced analytic skills to continue to be leaders in producing meaningful analysis from these ever-expanding data sets. While partnering with colleagues who specialize in AI or machine learning is also an advantage, building foundational knowledge of these tools and basic processes in nursing is a necessity. Nursing is already a leader in advancing data standards work, contributing to the ICNP program and conducting work like the CHOBIC projects to standardize EHR data. This demonstrates a long-held understanding of what is needed for nursing data to be integrated and represented in computer driven systems.

Nursing informatics researchers must also be aware and responsive to what kind of data and study is most urgent. In addition to maintaining an in-depth familiarity with informatics literature, strong national and global networks of researchers are key in identifying needs and gaps as work progresses around the world. It is important that research addresses all specialty areas of nursing across education, practice, and administration. The Canadian Nursing Informatics Association continues to advance the idea that nursing informatics is nursing. Meaning, that in this digital age, all nurses no matter the area of practice are extensively engaged with technology and digital health.

Another area that is emerging strongly in nursing informatics research is patient-oriented or partnered research. Patients, like nurses, are on the receiving end of an increasing amount of healthcare technology and partnering with them to try and influence the design and development of these tools is essential to maximize use and positive health outcomes. Increased study incorporating journey mapping or user-centred design approaches are needed. However, user-centred or co-design should not just be pursued with patients, more nurses need to be engaged in this kind of research so that the impact of technology on their workflow, patient care and relationships can be studied further.

Ultimately, even when surrounded by technology, nursing and nursing informatics research is about people. Nursing informatics researchers are uniquely positioned to contribute data and findings that highlight aspects of both the art and science of the profession. Recent work on *Nursing and Compassionate Care in a Technological World* represents this kind of contribution (Strudwick et al. 2020). While reviewing current and future influences of AI in nursing the authors demonstrate the critical need for vigilant engagement by the profession in the advancement of this technology in order to ensure that this evolution does not disrupt the ethical, just, and compassionate care that is the essence of nursing (Strudwick et al. 2020).

12.5 Conclusion

The value nursing informatics brings to research has only begun to be felt in many areas of inquiry and knowledge generation. With the increasing digitalization of vast aspects of the nursing role and healthcare, the future appears bright in terms of using these forms of innovation to support the generation of knowledge and other inquiry activities important to nurses. In summary, this chapter has sought to explore the research process in light of viewing nursing informatics as both a supportive mechanism to extend and amplify current research activities conducted by nurses, while also reinforcing that nursing informatics can be the target of specific research inquiry. While both dimensions share similar methods, processes, and are commonly mutually synergetic, highlighting the importance of both is equally important. As a profession that has prided itself on advocacy, leadership, and human-centred care, all nursing research should remain cognizant of the potential power informatics can bring to knowledge generation and inquiry. Failing to appreciate contemporary reality would only serve to inhibit timely and relevant research generation to support human wellbeing and evolution of the nursing role to lead change within increasingly digitalized healthcare settings of the future.

12.6 Review Questions

1. Within nursing informatics research, how are philosophical and theoretical lenses applied or endorsed to support research conceptualization or activities?
2. How can nursing informatics be used in nursing research? Describe the process from which nursing informatics can act as a supportive mechanism in nursing research.

3. What is grey literature?

Discussion (take it online)

What are some contemporary opportunities for nursing research within the informatics discipline? How do you see these opportunities evolving over the coming decades with increased digitalization in all areas of society and healthcare?

Activities

1. Conduct a search of the literature on two of the electronic databases listed in Step 2 of Conduct a Literature Review of this chapter. Search under key words Nursing Informatics AND Research
2. Go to the critical appraisal skills programme https://casp-uk.net/casp-tools-checklists/

   Review the worksheets and select one. Use the worksheet checklist with a paper sourced from your literature review activity completed in activity one above.

12.6.1 Answers

1. As described by Matney et al. (Munhall 2012), the philosophical foundations of all nursing informatics research include concepts such as *data, information, knowledge*, and *wisdom*. Further, Matney et al. outlines that nursing informatics inquiry is appreciative of different philosophical and ontological lenses from which to explore the core concepts of data, information, knowledge, and wisdom. These different views, or lenses allow nursing informatics researchers to explore different aspects of technology in nursing such as evaluating technology systems, understanding digital experiences, and how technology impacts workflow, and other fluid interpretations of human-technology interactions.
2. The increased use of technology in the workplace and society has given nurses new opportunities to employ these technologies to assist in many types of research activities, including information aggregation, data collection, and knowledge dissemination. While using supportive elements of informatics to conduct research has become commonplace in nursing research, it is important to appreciate that the topic of nursing informatics also exists as its own nursing specialty.
3. 'Grey' literature reviews are conducted to identify sources of important information that may not be found in traditional academic library environments. Grey literature sources can include websites, briefing notes, newsletters, government reports, conference presentation and beyond. Information sourced from grey literature can contain information that was not formally written in a research article that could address the key issue, topic or problem you are investigating.

Glossary

CINAHL Cumulative Index of Nursing and Allied Health Literature

Data mining Semi-automatic exploration of large data sets, looking for meaning through patterns in the data

Grey literature Information sources outside of formal academic or peer reviewed journals (such as industry magazines, newspapers, social media, etc.)

Knowledge translation The synthesis, dissemination and exchange of knowledge by researchers to the targeted knowledge users

MEDLINE Database of biomedical literature

MeSH Medical Subject Headings is a vocabulary thesaurus used for indexing articles in PubMed

Mixed methods research The research approach combining both qualitative and quantitative research methods

NLP Natural language processing

Nursing research Systematic inquiry designed to generate evidence for the nursing profession, including nursing practice, education, administration, and informatics

PsychINFO Database of behavioural and mental health literature

Qualitative research Investigation of phenomena, typically in an in-depth and holistic fashion, through the collection of rich narrative materials using a flexible research design

Quantitative research Investigation of phenomena that lend themselves to precise measurement and quantification, often involving a rigorous and controlled design

UTAUT Unified Theory of Technology Acceptance and Use

References

Arksey H, O'Malley L. Scoping studies: towards a methodological framework. Int J Soc Res Methodol. 2005;8(1):19–32. Available from: http://www.tandfonline.com/doi/abs/10.1080/1364557032000119616

Barnard A, Sandelowski M. Technology and humane nursing care: (ir)reconcilable or invented difference? J Adv Nurs. 2001;34(3):367–75.

Birnie KA, et al. *Usability testing of an interactive virtual reality distraction intervention to reduce procedural pain in children and adolescents with cancer.* Journal of Pediatric Oncology Nursing. 2018;35(6):406–16.

Canadian Agency for Drugs and Technologies in Health. Grey matters: a practical tool for searching health-related grey literature [Internet]. 2018 [cited 2018 Nov 26]. Available from: https://www.cadth.ca/resources/finding-evidence/grey-matters

Creswell JW, Clark VLP. Designing and conducting mixed methods research. In 2007. p. 119–167.

Goodwin L, VanDyne M, Lin S, Talbert S. Data mining issues and opportunities for building nursing knowledge. J of Biomed Inf. 2003;36(4–5):379–88.

Hyun S, Johnson SB, Bakken S. Exploring the ability of natural language processing to extract data from nursing narratives. Comput Inform Nurs. 2009;27(4):215–25.

Kaminski, J. Theory in nursing informatics: diffusion of innovation theory. Canadian Journal of Nursing Informatics [Internet]. 2011;6(2). Available from: https://cjni.net/journal/?p=1444

LeRouge C, et al. User profiles and personas in the design and development of consumer health technologies. International Journal of Medical Informatics. 2013;82(11):E251–68.

Levac D, Colquhoun H, O'Brien KK. Scoping studies: advancing the methodology. Implement Sci. 2010;5(1):69. Available from: http://implementationscience.biomedcentral.com/articles/10.1186/1748-5908-5-69

McLean, A. Machine learning. Canadian Journal of Nursing Informatics. 2018. Available from: https://cjni.net/journal/?p=5857

Monsen KA, Peterson JJ, Mathiason MA, Ms K, Lee S, Chi CL, et al. Data visualization techniques to showcase nursing care quality. CIN - Computers Informatics Nursing. 2015;33(10):417–26.

Munhall P. Nursing research: a qualitative perspective. 5th ed. Sudbury, MA: Jones & Bartlett Learning; 2012.

Peters MDJ, Godfrey CM, Khalil H, McInerney P, Parker D, Soares CB. Guidance for conducting systematic scoping reviews. Int J Evid Based Healthc. 2015;13:141–6.

Polit D, Beck C. Nursing research : generating and assessing evidence for nursing practice. 9th ed. Philadelphia: Wolters Kluwer Health/Lippincott Williams & Wilkins; 2012.

Risling TL, Risling DE. Advancing nursing participation in user-centred design. Journal of Research in Nursing. 2020;25(3):226–38. https://doi.org/10.1177/1744987120913590.

Rogers EM. Diffusion of innovations. 5th ed. New York: Free Press; 2003.

Sidani S, Braden C. Design, evaluation and translation of nursing interventions. West Sussix: John Wiley & Sons, Ltd; 2011.

Strudwick G. Predicting nurses' use of healthcare technology using the technology acceptance model: an integrative review. CIN. 2015;33(5):189–98. Available from: https://nursing.ceconnection.com/ovidfiles/00024665-201505000-00004.pdf

Strudwick G, Wiljer D, Inglis F. Nursing and compassionate care in a technological world: a discussion paper. Toronto, ON: AMS Healthcare; 2020.

Trust MKP. Critical appraisal skills programme (CASP): making sense of evidence. Oxford: London (UK); 2002.

Venkatesh V, Morris M, David G, David F. User acceptance of information technology: toward a unified view. Manag Inf Syst Q. 2003;27:425–78.

Venkatesh V, Thong JYL, Xu X. Consumer acceptance and use of information technology: extending the unified theory of acceptance and use of technology. MIS Quarterly. 2012;36(1):157–78.

Chapter 13
Applied Informatics Research in Nursing for eHealth

Kaija Saranto and Ulla-Mari Kinnunen

Abstract In this chapter, the previous research priorities and defined topics are used to determine the present state of the art of applied nursing informatics. The aim is to describe how recent publications support previous nursing informatics research agendas. The Scopus database was searched to find studies focusing on Nursing Informatics and eHealth in the context of applied clinical informatics. The search yielded publications from the last decade (from 2010 until February 2020). The search results (N = 55) were analyzed and classified using the research topic areas (N = 20) defined by The Nursing Informatics International Research Network (NIIRN). The results revealed that the three highest number of publications of the search focused on "the development of decision support systems specific to nursing practice decisions," "the evaluation of the impact of HIT systems for nursing care on outcomes for patients", and the "evaluation of the impact of standardized nursing documentation content/meaning on the utility of information for feedback and quality improvement." One paper focused on "the development of electronic information systems providing real-time feedback to nurses about their practices/health care delivery to improve safety," which was previously assessed as the most important. Seven defined research areas had no publications. Future research should focus on the missing research priorities, such as the evaluation of quality, the use of telecommunications and social media, the design and management of databases, theory development, and the integration of genomic data. The present nursing informatics research agenda should be updated based on changes in practice and technological advancements. The results should be interpreted with caution, as the analysis purposefully focused on one journal specializing in applied clinical informatics. However, they indicate what we should focus on in applied nursing informatics and eHealth research in the future.

Electronic Supplementary Material The online version of this chapter (https://doi.org/10.1007/978-3-030-58740-6_13) contains supplementary material, which is available to authorized users.

K. Saranto (✉) · U.-M. Kinnunen
Department of Health and Social Management, University of Eastern Finland,
Kuopio, Finland
e-mail: kaija.saranto@uef.fi; ulla-mari.kinnunen@uef.fi

© Springer Nature Switzerland AG 2021   339
P. Hussey, M. A. Kennedy (eds.), *Introduction to Nursing Informatics*, Health
Informatics, https://doi.org/10.1007/978-3-030-58740-6_13

Keywords Nursing · Informatics · Research · Agenda · Research priority
Applied informatics · eHealth

Learning Objectives for the Chapter
1. Describe the key research topic areas for nursing informatics and eHealth.
2. Reflect the distribution of defined research topic areas during 1998–2013.
3. Assess how the latest research agenda corresponds to the published studies.
4. Define the limitations of the search results.
5. Discuss future research priorities.

13.1 Defining the Nursing Informatics Research Agenda for eHealth

The aim of this chapter is to describe how recent publications (2010–2020) support the nursing informatics agenda set for 2008–2018. Over the years, research agendas have been of interest among nursing informatics researchers (Brennan et al. 1998; Bakken et al. 2012; Dowding et al. 2013; Peltonen et al. 2016). At various times, distinct groups have identified important research topics following not only the overall adoption of Health Information Technology (HIT) but also the development of systems and devices, legislation, and guidelines to ensure confidentiality and the privacy of users and care providers (Block et al. 2011).

The evolving concepts in the field of nursing informatics have emphasized changes in research focus. Perhaps one of the broadest concepts is eHealth, which appeared in the informatics field in the late 1990s (Oh et al. 2005). In terms of nursing practice, the definition by Eysenbach (2001) is often used to describe the widespread use of the Internet and related technologies in health care. In his definition, "e" must not be interpreted only as electronic but also as education, encouragement, empowerment, evidence-based, ethics, and equity. Overall, eHealth means ways to improve efficiency, enhance quality, enable information flow, and extend the scope of health services. Eysenbach stresses that eHealth must not only be regarded as encompassing technical issues but as being more broadly connected to thinking, attitudes, and the commitment to improve health (Eysenbach 2001).

> eHealth characterizes not only a technical development, but also a state-of-mind, a way of thinking, an attitude, and a commitment for networked, global thinking, to improve health care locally, regionally, and worldwide by using information and communication technology. (Eysenbach 2001)

In the early 2000s, eHealth was closely connected to telehealth and mobile health solutions as technological tools emerged in health services. eHealth adoption began among professionals, but patients and their families were soon seen as important actors (Saranto et al. 2017; Koivunen and Saranto 2017). Related to the broad definition of eHealth, clinical decision support, mobile health, big data science, the evaluation and implementation of standardized terminologies, and education and competencies have been proposed as the five topic areas of nursing informatics research according to a broad international survey (Peltonen et al. 2016). Nursing informatics education and certification have been the leading factors in the implementation and use of technological tools and devices in nursing practice. It has also been obvious that nurses are working within an interdisciplinary context that requires partnership and collaboration not only in practice but also in the development and research of eHealth diffusion (Scott et al. 2017). However, nurses' participation in the development of HIT tools depends on their level of education and training. Nurses also need support from both colleagues and managers to practice on interdisciplinary teams (Brennan et al. 1998; Bakken et al. 2012; Dowding et al. 2013; Peltonen et al. 2016; Block et al. 2011; Oh et al. 2005; Eysenbach 2001; Saranto et al. 2017; Koivunen and Saranto 2017; Scott et al. 2017; Gassert and Salmon 1998; Kinnunen et al. 2019; Hübner et al. 2019).

One of the earliest nursing informatics research agendas was presented in 1992. Since then, research initiatives have been identified by several international and national expert panels (Bakken et al. 2012). The U.S. Public Health Service's National Institute of Nursing Research identified research priorities for nursing informatics in 1992, and the work continued with a Delphi survey in 1998 (Brennan et al. 1998). Many of these research initiatives have identified advances in health services and health informatics, helping patients shift from being passive recipients of care to active users of information technologies to support self-care. The implementation of electronic health records and the need for nursing language terms and taxonomies has been a research priority since the 1990s (Saranto et al. 2013).

Bakken et al. (2012) summarized the two previous initiatives (Brennan et al. 1998) to compile a nursing informatics research agenda for 2008–2018. Three new priority areas were defined in six research topics:

- User Needs

  - Identification of users' (nurses, patients, families) information needs

- Acquisition, Representation and Storage of Data, Information, and Knowledge

  - Develop, validate, and formalize nursing language terms, taxonomies, and classifications.
  - Design and management of nursing information databases for use in patient management, clinical records, and research

- Informatics Support for Nursing and Healthcare Practice

  - Technology development including decision support systems to support nursing practice (integrates human-computer interaction)

- Informatics Support for Patients/Families/Consumers

  - Patients' use of information technology
  - Consumer health informatics (New)

- Design and Evaluation Methodologies
  - Systems modeling and evaluation
- Use of telecommunications technology for nursing practice (New)
  - Professional practice issues (e.g., competencies, confidentiality) (New) (Bakken et al. 2012).

Parallel to Bakken's work, an international network implemented a study to find research priority areas for nursing informatics. The Nursing Informatics International Research Network (NIIRN) comprises a group of experts who are collaborating on developing internationally relevant research programs for nursing informatics. In 2012, NIIRN proposed international priorities for research in nursing informatics for patient care. The priorities were determined using an online survey of 468 respondents. Based on the survey results, 20 research topic areas were identified. The priorities were established based on the WHO world regions, Europe, the Western Pacific, South East Asia, the Americas, the Eastern Mediterranean, and Africa, thus representing the network participants. Although the ranking varied between the regions, the two highest-ranking topics were "the development of information systems that can provide real-time feedback" and "evaluation of the impact of HIT systems on patient outcomes." The two lowest-ranking topics were "theory development" and "the integration of genomic data into clinical information systems"(Dowding et al. 2013). Table 13.1 shows the 10 research priorities from 1998(Brennan et al. 1998) and the 20 research topic areas from 2012 (Dowding et al. 2013).

Both lists of research priorities (Table 13.1) are based on the consensus of individual researchers. Brennan (1998) argued that although already advanced in 1998, the missing topics in her list—imaging technology, formal education in health informatics, signal processing, and bioinformatics—may reflect their relevance to nursing practice. She also stressed the importance of interpreting the results as a national research agenda, prompting discussion on international research. Some 15 years later, the international Delphi panel prioritized 20 research topics, which included all the previously defined topics. However, due to the more descriptive wording of the topics, some previous topics could also be regarded a topic in the new list. Two examples are "patient use of information technologies, including consumer health informatics" and "technology development to support practice and patient care—decision support, human–computer interaction"(Dowding et al. 2013). In this chapter, all 20 research topic areas (Dowding et al. 2013) are used to determine the present state of the art of published applied nursing informatics and eHealth studies.

Table 13.1 NI Research priorities in 1998 and 2013

NI research priorities 1998 (N = 10) (Brennan al. 1998)	Rank	Research topic areas 2013 (N = 20) (Dowding al. 2013)	Rank
Standardized language/vocabularies—development, testing, mapping	1	The development of electronic information systems that can provide real-time feedback to nurses about their practices/health care delivery to improve safety	1
Technology development to support practice and patient care—decision support, human-computer interaction	2*	Evaluation of the impact of HIT systems for nursing care (e.g. EHR) on outcomes for patients (safer care, better patient outcomes)	2
Data base issues (architecture, construction, access, cost etc.)	2*	The development of decision support systems specific to nursing practice decisions	3
Systems evaluation issues—re-engineering nursing, effectiveness	3	Investigation of the impact of HIT systems for nursing care (e.g. EHR) on nurses' work practices and workflow	4
Using telecommunications technology for nursing practice telenursing, home care, etc.	4*	The design and management of nursing information databases for use in patient management, clinical records and research	5
Putting technology into practice—systems models, demonstrations, etc.	4*	Effective ways of training nurses in the use of HIT to support new care delivery models	6
Information needs of nurses and other clinicians	7	The identification of outcomes associated with the quality of nursing care that are important to patients, which can be used to evaluate the quality of care provided by nurses	7
Patient use of information technologies, including consumer health informatics	8*	Evaluation of the impact of e-prescribing systems on nursing care, medication safety and patient outcomes	8
Nursing intervention innovations for professional practice electronic delivery of nursing interventions, testing effectiveness	8*	The role of patient-held electronic records on participation in their care, and quality of care	9
Professional practice issues (competencies, confidentiality)	9	Evaluation of the impact of HIT systems for nursing care (e.g. EHR) on outcomes for staff (e.g. less documentation, faster documentation)	10
		Evaluation of the impact of standardized nursing documentation content/meaning on the utility of information for feedback and quality improvement	11
		Identification of users' (nurses, patients, families) health information needs to inform the design of HIT systems	12
		The role of mobile technology (e.g. use of smart phones, tablet devices) in supporting nurses deliver high quality and safe health care	13

(continued)

Table 13.1 (continued)

NI research priorities 1998 (N = 10) (Brennan al. 1998)	Rank	Research topic areas 2013 (N = 20) (Dowding al. 2013)	Rank
		Assessment of if and how decision aids for patients improves shared decision making between patients and nurses	14
		Investigation of how telecommunications technology and telehealth initiatives impact on nursing practice (e.g. in providing care to individuals in remote and rural areas)	15
		The development, validation and formalization of nursing language terms, taxonomies and classifications to support interoperability between HIT systems	16
		The development of more advanced methods for measuring the impact of HIT nurses' work and communication patterns	17
		Investigation of how social media (e.g. twitter, Facebook) may affect the ways patients interact with health care providers including nurses.	18
		Theory development to support the design of HIT that better meets the information and practice needs of nurses	19
		Integrating genomic data (information specific to the genetic makeup of patients) into the HIT systems used by nurses to inform nursing care content/meaning on the utility of information for feedback and quality improvement	20

*equal rank

13.1.1 The Review Process

A search of the Scopus database revealed various studies focusing on nursing, informatics, and eHealth in the context of applied clinical informatics, concepts that were also used as the keywords. Based on the published nursing research agenda in 1998 (Brennan et al. 1998), in 2012 (Bakken et al. 2012), and in 2013 (Dowding et al. 2013) the time frame was set as 2010–2020. The search result (N = 55) was extracted from the database, including bibliographic information for the papers and abstracts with keywords. The first screening of the titles revealed three papers that focused purely on medicine. Based on the abstracts, 10 papers that did not focus on nursing or patient care or that were more strategic in nature were identified. These were excluded. All the other studies were included in the review. Thus, 42 papers were accepted for the review (Fig. 13.1).

The papers were classified according to the research topic areas (N = 20) defined by NIIRN (Dowding et al. 2013). Papers were classified by the authors separately, and in four cases consensus was reached through discussion.

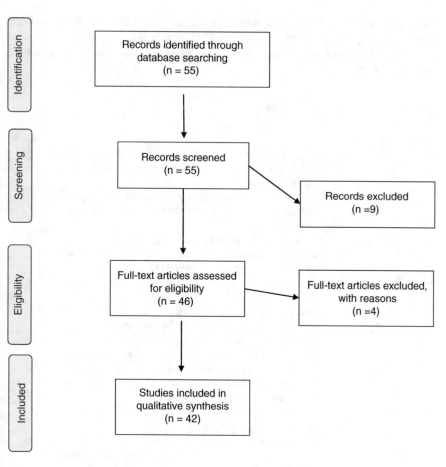

Fig. 13.1 Flowchart of literature search. (Moher et al. 2009)

13.1.2   Research Evidence Based on Nursing Informatics Research Agenda

The studies (N = 55) found in the literature search represent different WHO world regions: Europe (n = 11), South East Asia (n = 3), and the Americas (n = 41). The number of papers based on publication year are as follows: 2019 (Scott et al. 2017); 2016 (Koivunen and Saranto 2017); 2015 and 2011 (Oh et al. 2005); 2014 (Block et al. 2011); 2017, 2013, and 2012 (Peltonen et al. 2016); 2018 and 2010 (Dowding et al. 2013); and 2020 (Brennan et al. 1998). After exclusion and based on the analysis of the papers (n = 42), the results show that the three highest number of publications in the research topic areas focused on "the development of decision support systems specific to nursing practice decisions" (n = 8), "the evaluation of the impact of HIT systems for nursing care (e.g., EHR) on outcomes for patients (safer care, better patient outcomes)" (n = 6), and "evaluation of the impact of standardized nursing documentation content/meaning on the utility of information for feedback and quality improvement" (n = 6). Table 13.2 describes the state of the art based on the number of papers in each prioritized research category and the ranking in 2013 and 2020 (Table 13.2).

Table 13.2 Research evidence in 2020

Rank 2020	Number of papers 2020 (N = 42)	Research topic areas 2020 based on number of publications	Rank 2013
1	8	The development of decision support systems specific to nursing practice decisions	3
2	7	Evaluation of the impact of HIT systems for nursing care (e.g. EHR) on outcomes for patients (safer care, better patient outcomes)	2
3	6	Evaluation of the impact of standardized nursing documentation content/meaning on the utility of information for feedback and quality improvement	11
4	4	Assessment of if and how decision aids for patients improves shared decision making between patients and nurses	14
5	3	Investigation of the impact of HIT systems for nursing care (e.g. EHR) on nurses' work practices and workflow	4
6	3	Identification of users' (nurses, patients, families) health information needs to inform the design of HIT systems	12
7	3	The development, validation and formalization of nursing language terms, taxonomies and classifications to support interoperability between HIT systems	16
8	2	The role of patient-held electronic records on participation in their care, and quality of care	9
9	2	Evaluation of the impact of HIT systems for nursing care (e.g. EHR) on outcomes for staff (e.g. less documentation, faster documentation)	10
10	1	The development of electronic information systems that can provide real-time feedback to nurses about their practices/ health care delivery to improve safety	1
11	1	Effective ways of training nurses in the use of HIT to support new care delivery models	11
12	1	The role of mobile technology (e.g. use of smart phones, tablet devices) in supporting nurses deliver high quality and safe health care	13
13	1	The development of more advanced methods for measuring the impact of HIT nurses' work and communication patterns	17
14	–	The design and management of nursing information databases for use in patient management, clinical records and research	5
15	–	The identification of outcomes associated with the quality of nursing care that are important to patients, which can be used to evaluate the quality of care provided by nurses	7
16	–	Evaluation of the impact of e-prescribing systems on nursing care, medication safety and patient outcomes	8
17	–	Investigation of how telecommunications technology and telehealth initiatives impact on nursing practice (e.g. in providing care to individuals in remote and rural areas)	15

Table 13.2 (continued)

Rank 2020	Number of papers 2020 (N = 42)	Research topic areas 2020 based on number of publications	Rank 2013
18	–	Investigation of how social media (e.g. twitter, Facebook) may affect the ways patients interact with health care providers including nurses.	18
19	–	Theory development to support the design of HIT that better meets the information and practice needs of nurses	19
20	–	Integrating genomic data (information specific to the genetic makeup of patients) into the HIT systems used by nurses to inform nursing care	20

One paper was identified as focusing on the most import defined topic in 2013, "the development of electronic information systems that can provide real-time feedback to nurses about their practices/health care delivery to improve safety." The three lowest-ranked priorities were the same in this review and in the 2013 priority list. Altogether, seven defined research topic areas had no publications.

13.1.3 What Is This All About?

This paragraph summarizes the findings in relation to the Nursing Informatics Agenda for 2008–2018 published by Bakken et al. (2012). The same structure is used as in the beginning of the chapter to highlight the research gaps that need to be addressed in future studies. The observations proposed here must be interpreted in light of the strengths and weaknesses discussed at the end.

User Needs

In software design, users' needs are the basis of a successful system. Some studies addressed the topic "identification of users' (nurses, patients, families) health information needs to inform the design of HIT systems", focusing on both professionals' and patients' needs (Kneale et al. 2016; Rogers et al. 2012). It was ranked fifth based on the publications. Decision support was of interest from two perspectives— "the development of decision support systems specific to nursing practice decisions" and the "assessment of if and how decision aids for patients improves shared decision making between patients and nurses"(Jeffery et al. n.d.). The nursing practice perspective was ranked as highest based on the number of studies, and shared decision making between nurses and patients was ranked fourth in this review. As the latter was ranked fourteenth in 2013, it seems there is evidence that patients have changed from being passive recipients of care to active users of information technologies (Brennan et al. 1998).

There were no publications on the topic "genomic data integration (information specific to the genetic makeup of patients) into the HIT systems and use by nurses. "Obviously, however, this topic has relevance in the future of nursing informatics research.

Acquisition, Representation, and Storage of Data

Nursing documentation structures and terminology use have been widely studied in the previous decades (Saranto et al. 2013). In this review, the topic "evaluation of the impact of standardized nursing documentation content/meaning on the utility of information for feedback and quality improvement" also ranked as the second research area. Further, there were also publications (Applied Clinical Informatics 2017; Hoonakker et al. 2019; Johnson et al. 2013) on "the development, validation and formalization of nursing language terms, taxonomies and classifications to support interoperability between HIT systems" and the "evaluation of the impact of HIT systems for nursing care (e.g., EHR) on outcomes for staff (e.g., less documentation, faster documentation)". Design issues were represented in this area by the topic "the design and management of nursing information databases for use in patient management, clinical records and research." However, we could not find any publication on this topic. Although economic or resource issues were present in the background of the studies, they were not highlighted in the study design as would have been expected (Koivunen and Saranto 2017). All these topics under this research area must obviously be included among the research priorities in the near future.

Informatics Support for Patients/Families/Consumers

Nursing care is no longer just provided in face-to face appointments; technology is increasingly being used to facilitate remote care (Koivunen and Saranto 2017). Surprisingly, only one study (Ranegger et al. 2014) represents this important evolving service. The topic "role of patient-held electronic records on participation in their care, and quality of care" previously ranked eleventh compared to ninth in 2013 (Dowding et al. 2013). In today's technology-oriented health care, patients' active role in the management of, for example, chronic diseases is increasingly emphasized (Block et al. 2011; Korach et al. 2019; Gartrell et al. 2015). Overall, the role of family is neglected, which is interesting as we found several studies on acute and long-term care where cooperation with families is evident. Further, we did not find any studies in the pediatric context.

Informatics Support for Nursing and Healthcare

In this review, we only found one study (Denecke et al. 2019) focusing on competencies for the topic "effective ways of training nurses in the use of HIT to support new care delivery models". This is surprising, as education and training have been regarded as the main priority in HIT implementation.

Further, as legislation and guidelines to support the confidentiality and privacy of users and care providers was not set as a research topic among the research priorities, we could not identify any studies in the area. However, in previous studies data security has been connected to technology use in health care, especially in secure and more effective communication(Koivunen and Saranto 2017). In our review, communication was often mentioned in the research priorities related to the development of more advanced methods to measure communication patterns.

In many countries, nurses are also involved in e-prescribing(Kannry et al. 2016; European Federation of Nurses Associations (EFN 2015). The topic "the evaluation of e-prescribing systems on nursing care" was internationally ranked eighth in 2013 (Dowding et al. 2013), but we found no papers related to that topic. The changes in roles and responsibilities in providing care call for research from various perspectives. Many studies had a sound theoretical basis. However, we could not identify a single study for the topic "theory development to support the design of HIT that better meets the information and practice needs of nurses."

Use of Telecommunications Technology for Nursing Practice

In the previous survey in 2016, mobile health and data exchange and interoperability were among the 10 research priorities (Peltonen et al. 2016). In this review, the role of mobile technology (e.g., use of smart phones, tablet devices) in helping nurses deliver high-quality, safe health care was addressed in only two studies (Villaseñor et al. 2017; Hayakawa et al. 2013). Surprisingly, there were no papers on topics such as the "investigation of how telecommunications technology and telehealth initiatives impact on nursing practice (e.g., in providing care to individuals in remote and rural areas)" and the "investigation of how social media (e.g., Twitter, Facebook) may affect the ways patients interact with health care providers, including nurses." Bakken et al. (2012) highlighted the importance of focusing research on informatics support for patients, consumers, and families. This would involve future technologies to empower patients and professionals to collaborate more efficiently in various situations. This is also connected to changes in health services, as we need more knowledge about patients' involvement in care processes.

Design and Evaluation Methodologies

Many topics started with the word evaluation (Smith et al. 2019; Bersani et al. 2020), which was connected to the impact of a special focus, such as "evaluation of the impact of HIT systems for nursing care (e.g., EHR) on outcomes for patients (safer care, better patient outcomes)" or the "investigation of the impact of HIT systems for nursing care (e.g., EHR) on nurses' work practices and workflow". These studies focused on usability issues and user satisfaction. As indicated in the phrases, outcome measures are important to prove nurses' input in nursing care. HIT implementation has also been connected to patient safety and, more broadly, to quality of care, which were also focal topics in the publications. The review covered various research designs, not only quantitative and qualitative but also mixed methods. Almost missing was predictive models or hypotheses testing. However, the review contained studies with the secondary use of registered data (Bowles et al. 2016; Holmgren et al. 2016; Westra et al. 2018). In many studies, an interdisciplinary approach could also be discovered, which was also mentioned in the agenda (Bakken et al. 2012). An interdisciplinary approach can open new possibilities for research funding and advance the dissemination of research results (Scott et al. 2017). As mentioned, we only had one paper classified in the topic relating to informatics competencies "effective ways of training nurses in the use of HIT to support new care delivery models." Therefore, we must not forget that nurses also need competencies in research methods to be able to use standardized instruments in research designs and to participate in the development of tools and technologies and new ways of providing services.

This review has some limitations that must be considered. First, this literature search purposefully targeted only one database focusing on applied clinical informatics and eHealth. This naturally results in major bias, but the situation is still described from a certain perspective, thus providing ideas for further research. For the analysis, only papers focusing on nursing or patient care were accepted. Surprisingly, we had to exclude 13 papers, although the term nursing was used as a keyword. These papers were also describing the status of medical informatics or strategy papers. In the strategy papers, the focus was on eHealth in two cases; these were excluded from this review.

The studies in the review represent different WHO world regions—Europe, South East Asia, and the Americas. Studies from the Western Pacific, Eastern Mediterranean, and Africa did not appear in the search, which constitutes a bias. The research topics defined in 1998 were very different in wording compared to those defined in 2013. The topic descriptions in 2013 have nouns such as assessment, development, evaluation, investigation, and identification, which clearly indicate what the research might be about (Peltonen et al. 2016). However, the real focus description—"the identification of outcomes associated with the quality of nursing care that are important to patients, which can be used to evaluate the quality of care provided by nurses"—has many elements that could represent the main aim of a study. Further, the topic "evaluation of the impact of HIT systems for nursing care (e.g., EHR) on outcomes for patients (safer care, better patient outcomes)" was obviously more accurate, as we easily found six studies in this area. There were also studies on this topic published during the whole decade, as there were for the highest-ranked topic, "the development of decision support systems specific to nursing practice decisions." Nevertheless, the structure of in-depth defined topics may have caused problems in interpreting and classifying our review data.

Following are important research topics for the future (slightly re-worded from the previous agenda):

- User needs—from various perspectives (e.g., development of systems, services, usability)
- Acquisition, representation and storage of data from various sources (e.g., registry-data, patient- generated data, data re-use and privacy)
- Informatics support for patients/families/consumers, including empowerment, collaboration, and extension of the scope of health services
- Informatics support for nursing and healthcare, including ethics, economics, and interdisciplinary practice

- Knowledge, skills, and competencies for the evolving care environment
- Use of telecommunications technology for nursing practice and for patient/family participation
- Development and testing of theories in nursing informatics research

In conclusion, the importance of nursing informatics and eHealth research agendas must be stressed because they can be used to find evidence of the state of the art of published research. Nursing informatics research topics are commonly discovered in daily practice routines and address future eHeath research priorities. Research priorities in informatics should be accurate and clearly covering the focus of the research.

Review Questions
1. Reflect on the text in the beginning of the chapter and define the key research priorities for nursing informatics research during the last decade in terms of applied informatics research in nursing for eHealth.
2. How does the research agenda correspond to the publications published during the last decade?
3. How can you define what topics urgently need more research in nursing informatics?
4. What are the limitations of the search results?

Answers
1. The research agenda defined by Bakken et al. (2012) gives guidance, and the list of priorities is presented in Table 13.1.
2. This can be seen in Table 13.2. Almost half of the publications were classified into three research topic areas—the development of decision support systems specific to nursing practice decisions, the evaluation of the impact of HIT systems for nursing care (e.g., EHR) on outcomes for patients (safer care, better patient outcomes), and the evaluation of the impact of standardized nursing documentation content/meaning on the utility of information for feedback and quality improvement. The other half can be classified into 10 research topic areas. Seven research topic areas did not have any publications. Further, several research topics had only a few publications, and the rank based on number was different compared to the early research priority lists.
3. Based on the international priorities for research in nursing informatics, we should focus on those topics not covered in this review. However, we can also use the agenda described by Bakken et al. (2012) and in the paragraphs after the description of the review.
4. The review is based only on the search of one database. The keywords used in the literature search may have been too simple, and more synonyms could have been used.

Glossary

HIT Health Information Technology
NIIRN Nursing Informatics International Research Network

Taxonomy Taxonomy is the process of naming and classifying things such as animals and plants into groups within a larger system, according to their similarities and differences.

References

Applied Clinical Informatics, 2017;8 (3):763–778.

Bakken S, Stone PW, Larson EL. A nursing informatics research agenda for 2008–18: contextual influences and key components. Nurs Outlook. 2012;56:280–90.

Bersani K, Fuller TE, Garabedian P, Espares J, Mlaver E, Businger A, et al. Use, perceived usability, and barriers to implementation of a patient safety dashboard integrated within a vendor HER. Appl Clin Inform. 2020;1:34–45.

Block AD, Car J, Pagliari C, Anandan C, Cresswell K, et al. The impact of eHealth on the quality and safety of health care: a systematic overview. PLoS Med. 2011;8(1):e1000387. https://doi.org/10.1371/journal.pmed.1000387.

Bowles KH, Ratcliffe S, Potashnik S, Topaz M, Holmes J, Shih NW, et al. Using electronic case summaries to elicit multi-disciplinary expert knowledge about referrals to post-acute care. Appl Clin Inform. 2016;7(2):368–79.

Brennan PF, Zielstorff RD, Ozbolt JG, Strombom I. Setting a national research agenda in nursing informatics. Cesnik P et al (Eds) Medinfo IOS Press 1998;9(Pt 2):1188–1191.

Denecke K, Jolo P, Sevinc B, Nüssli S. Creating individualized education material for diabetes patients using the eDiabetes platform. Stud Health Technol Inform. 2019;260. http://ebooks.iospress.nl/volume/dhealth-2019-from-ehealth-to-dhealth-proceedings-of-the-13th-health-informatics-meets-digital-health-conference

Dowding D, Currie LM, Borycki E, Clamp S, Favelae J, Fitzpatrick G, et al. International priorities for research in nursing informatics for patient care. In CU Lehmann, et al. (Eds.), MEDINFO2013 Proceedings. Stud Health Technol Inform. IOS Press, 2013;192:372–376.

European Federation of Nurses Associations (EFN). 2015. Evidence Based Guidelines for Nursing and Social Care on eHealth Services. ePrescribing. http://www.efnweb.be/wp-content/uploads/Final-ENS4Care-Guideline-5-Nurse-ePrescribing-pv.pdf. Accessed March 15, 2020.

Eysenbach G. What is e-health? J Med Internet Res. 2001;3(2):e20. https://doi.org/10.2196/jmir.3.2.e20.

Gartrell K, Trinkoff AM, Storr CL, Wilson ML, Gurses AP. Testing the electronic personal health record acceptance model by nurses for managing their own health: a cross-sectional survey. Appl Clin Inform. 2015;6(2):224–47.

Gassert CA, Salmon M. Setting a national informatics agenda for nursing education and practice to prepare nurses to develop and use information technology. In Cesnik P et al. (Eds) Medinfo. IOS Press 1998;9 (Pt 2):8748–751.

Hayakawa M, Uchimura Y, Omae K, Waki K, Fujita H, Ohe K. A smartphone-based medication self-management system with realtime medication monitoring. Appl Clin Inform. 2013;4(1):37–52.

Holmgren AJ, Pfeifer E, Manojlovich M, Adler-Milstein J. A novel survey to examine the relationship between health IT adoption and nurse-physician communication. Appl Clin Inform. 2016;7(4):1182–201.

Hoonakker PLT, Rankin RJ, Passini JC, Bunton JA, Ehlenfeldt BD, Dean SM, et al. Nurses' expectations of an inpatient portal for hospitalized patients and caregivers. Appl Clin Inform. 2019;10(4):625–33.

Hübner U, Thyea J, Shaw T, Elias B, Egberta N, Saranto K et al. (2019) Towards the TIGER international framework for recommendations of Core competencies in health informatics 2.0: extending the scope and the roles. In Ohno-Machado L, Seroussi B (Eds.) health and wellbeing e-networks for all. International medical informatics association (IMIA) and IOS press, Amsterdam, stud health Technol inform. IOS Press. 264, 1218–1222.

Jeffery AD, Kennedy B, Dietrich MS, Mion LC. Novak LL. (n.d.) A qualitative exploration of nurses' information-gathering behaviors prior to decision support tool design.

Johnson KE, McMorris BJ, Raynor LA, Monsen KA. What big size you have! Using effect sizes to determine the impact of public health nursing interventions. Appl Clin Inform. 2013;(3):434–44.

Kannry J, Sengstack P, Thyvalikakath TP, Poikonen J, Middleton B, Payne T, et al. The chief clinical informatics officer (CCIO): AMIA task force report on CCIO knowledge, education, and skillset requirements. Appl Clin Inform. 2016;7(1):143–76.

Kinnunen UM, Heponiemi T, Rajalahti E, Ahonen O, Korhonen T, Hyppönen H. Factors related to health informatics competencies for nurses-results of a National Electronic Health Record Survey. CIN: Computers, Informatics, Nursing. 2019;37(8):420–9.

Kneale L, Choi Y, Demiris G. Assessing commercially available personal health records for home health: recommendations for design. Appl Clin Inform. 2016;7(2):355–36716.

Koivunen M, Saranto K. Nursing professionals' experiences of the facilitators and barriers to the use of telehealth applications: a systematic review of qualitative studies. Scand J Caring Sci. 2017; https://doi.org/10.1111/scs.12445.

Korach ZT, Cato KD, Collins SA, Kang MJ, Knaplund C, Dykes PC, et al. Unsupervised machine learning of topics documented by nurses about hospitalized patients prior to a rapid-response event. Appl Clin Inform. 2019;10(5):952–63.

Moher D, Liberati A, Tetzlaff J, Altman DG. The PRISMA group. Preferred reporting items for systematic reviews and meta-analyses: the PRISMA statement. PLoS Med. 2009;6(7):e1000097. https://doi.org/10.1371/journal.pmed1000097.

Oh H, Rizo C, Enkin M, Jadad A. What is eHealth (3): a systematic review of published definitions. J Med Internet Res. 2005;7(1):e1. https://doi.org/10.2196/jmir.7.1.e1.

Peltonen LM, Topaz M, Ronquillo C, Pruinelli L, Sarmiento RF, Badger MK, et al. Nursing informatics research priorities for the future: recommendations from an international survey. Stud Health Technol Inform IOS Press. 2016;225:222–6. Available http://ebooks.iospress.nl/volume/nursing-informatics-2016-ehealth-for-all-every-level-collaboration-from-project-to-realization

Ranegger R, Hackl WO, Ammenwerth E. A proposal for an Austrian nursing minimum data set (NMDS): a delphi study. Appl Clin Inform. 2014;5(2):538–47.

Rogers M, Zach L, An Y, Dalrymple P. Capturing information needs of care providers to support knowledge sharing and distributed decision making. Appl Clin Inform. 2012;3:1):1–13.

Saranto K, Kinnunen U-M, Kivekäs E, Lappalainen A-M, Liljamo P, Rajalahti E, et al. Impacts of structuring nursing records: a systematic review. Scand J Caring Sci. 2013;18:1–19.

Saranto K, Ronquillo C, Velez O. Nursing competencies for multiple modalities of connected health technologies. In: Murphy Judy, Goossen William, Weber Patrick (eds.), *Forecasting informatics competencies for nurses in the future of connected health. Stud Health Technol Inform.* IOS Press, 2017;232:172–182.

Scott PJ, De Keizer NF, Georgiou A. Reflecting and looking to the future: what is the research agenda for theory in health informatics. In Scott PJ et al. (Eds.), Applied Interdisciplinary theory in Health Informatics. Stud Health Technol Inform. IOS Press. 2017, 263, 205–218. https://doi.org/10.3233/SHTI190124

Smith CJ, Jungbauer RM, Totten AM. Visual evidence: increasing usability of systematic reviews in health systems guidelines development. Appl Clin Inform. 2019;10(4):743–50.

Villaseñor S, Walker TM, Fetters L, McCoy M. Prescribing in the acute care setting—determining the educational and motivational needs of healthcare providers. CIN: Computers, Informatics, Nursing. 2017;35(8):392–400.

Westra BL, Johnson SG, Ali S, Bavuso KM, Cruz CA, Collins S, et al. Validation and refinement of a pain information Model from EHR Flowsheet data. Appl Clin Inform. 2018;9(1):185–98.

Chapter 14
Knowledge Networks in Nursing

Rosanne Burson, Dianne Conrad, Catherine Corrigan, Katherine Moran, Subhashis Das, Anne Spencer, and Pamela Hussey

Abstract In line with the Nursing Now campaign discussed in Chap. 3 of this edition, we provide an update in this chapter and consider how Communities of Practice and associated action projects within the profession of nursing are evolving. We consider how established nursing networks are trying to adapt to the challenges posed by twenty-first century healthcare.

Underpinned by the core values and principles of the Nursing Now campaign, our goal within this knowledge network is to raise the profile and status of nursing worldwide.

Seeking support from the Fulbright Scholarship programme, the authors of this chapter have embraced an opportunity to advance our understanding of informatics in differing contexts and to learn from one another. Through dedicated Community of Practice action group, we discuss and demonstrate the value of direct and indi-

Electronic Supplementary Material The online version of this chapter (https://doi.org/10.1007/978-3-030-58740-6_14) contains supplementary material, which is available to authorized users.

R. Burson (✉)
University of Detroit Mercy, CHP/MSON, Detroit, MI, USA
e-mail: bursonrf@udmercy.edu

D. Conrad · K. Moran
Grand Valley State University, Grand Rapids, MI, USA
e-mail: conraddi@gvsu.edu; morakath@gvsu.edu

C. Corrigan · S. Das · P. Hussey
School of Nursing Psychotherapy and Community Health, Dublin City University, Dublin, Ireland
e-mail: catherine.corrigan@dcu.ie; subhashis.das@dcu.ie; pamela.hussey@dcu.ie

A. Spencer
St Michael House, Ballymun, Dublin, Ireland
e-mail: anne.spencer@smh.ie

rect activities explaining how we came to focus on advancing nursing into leadership positions and conducting purposeful research to demonstrate how nurses can have the greatest impact for delivery of Sustainable Development Goal (SDG) 3 by 2030.

Keywords Communities of practice · Digital Health · Knowledge networks in nursing · Health and social care · Education

Key Concepts
Communities of practice
Digital health
Knowledge networks in nursing
Health and social care

Learning Objectives for the Chapter
1. Understand the importance of the nursing contribution to eHealth and Digital Transformation.
2. Review in context this contribution through existing Communities of Practice and evolving new paradigms for collaboration such as Open Innovation 2.0 and Ecosystems in Health and Social Care.
3. Consider the importance of global collaboration through education and research and consider their impact in the context of the profession of nursing.

14.1   Introduction

> Education is not the filling of a pail … but the lighting of a fire. W B Yeats (Education is not the filling of a pail 2020)

As was the case in the fourth edition we continue to affirm that education is a catalyst for action and draw on the above quote from Yeats as a gentle reminder that this is the case. We do however consider that in some instances nursing is "stumbling" into practicing in a digital enabled society (see Chap. 16), and for this reason we add an additional quote from Seamus Heaney's Human Chain poem published in 2010. We believe the opening lines of this verse articulates well nursing engagement in digital health transformation. *Had I not been awake, I would have missed it* (Seamus Heaney 2020). Nursing is preoccupied with daily operations of patient care delivery, and patient safety (see Chap. 9), and so for many practitioners the transformation and impact of digital health has occurred in the background. This we believe needs to change. Policy analysts and health leaders are increasingly recognising the untapped potential of nursing and the contribution the profession can make to optimise the impact of digital in health and social care. In this chapter, we provide pragmatic examples of where nursing is contributing to the design of systems through knowledge networks. We illustrate research which is actively shaping the development and implementation of eHealth and policy translation in practice. Selecting examples that have used differing approaches, we describe the tactical deliverables which have been realised through the emergence of new roles and nurses who have taken a path of action to address *the winds of change*. Described in Chap. 11 as wide in variety, nursing positions in informatics can vary in type from the unit-based "nurse super user" to "informatics nurse" or at the organizational executive level nurse executive position such as "Chief Nursing Informatics Officer" (CNIO).

Digital literacy has never been more in demand as national eHealth programmes seek to source new and innovative ways to support a decreasing skilled and aging workforce. We argue the case in this chapter that for advancing the profession of nursing leadership and focused purposeful research, new roles as described in Chap. 11 need to be accelerated and underpinned by targeted education further expanded upon in Chap. 15. This is our first principle: the core drivers of change are education underpinned by targeted informatics knowledge and skills. Such an approach can advance and broaden nursings' adoption and use of digital within the context of health and social care. The State of the World's Nursing Report 2020 from the WHO originally cited in Chap. 1 of this text, affirms that attention to leadership and digital competencies is now needed to support required nurse-led models of care and advanced practice roles, leveraging opportunities arising from digital health (World Health Organization 2020). Informed by the All-Party Parliamentary Group (APPG) report on global health, nursing will improve health, promote gender equality and support economic growth https://www.who.int/hrh/com-heeg/digital-APPG_triple-impact.pdf?ua=1. (All-Party Parliamentary Group on Global Health 2016).

The focus in this chapter is on 'real life' examples of how education and informatics skills are supporting nursing practitioners to become leaders, innovators and educators. It presents a brief summary of established Communities of Practice that are successfully evolving and other examples, which are new. These Communities of Practice are providing tactical deliverables and shaping future leaders within the domain of nursing informing industry and inter-professional teams. Section 14.2 provides a summary overview of the Communities of Practice core mission. It expands the notion of Communities of Practice to include how open Innovation 2.0 as an evolving new paradigm includes ecosystems and networks, which align well with the nursing informatics agenda. In Sect. 14.3, we revisit some examples of Communities of Practice from the fourth edition to demonstrate their progression since 2015. In Sect. 14.4, we introduce new initiatives and explain the importance of global networking.

14.2   Communities of Practice

Communities of Practice (COP) are increasingly demonstrating their effectiveness as educational frameworks. As an organic structure, COP present opportunities for informal knowledge exchange and development of social networks. Formally recognised by WHO as effective network and partnership activities, COP also afford a collaborative approach, which in the current economic downturn is pragmatic and purposeful. A core attribute of COP's is the use of tele networking and digital platforms for knowledge transfer and scholarship. Online webinars for example, can be used by nursing communities to come together to share expertise, experience and knowledge in both a synchronous and asynchronous manner. Examples of the Fulbright Scholars' COP featured later in this chapter, include virtual international classroom discussions on pertinent issues that nurses face across three countries: the U.S., Ireland and Saudi Arabia. This sharing of expertise offers a greater potential for knowledge exchange and cultivates innovation to address shared challenges in health and social care in contemporary society. There is a strong association between COP's and the Open Innovation 2.0 paradigm of ecosystems, particularly when it comes to digital innovation and new modes of care delivery (Curley and Salmelin 2018).

The World Health Organisation Strategic Directions Plan for Nursing and Midwifery for 2016–2020 stresses the importance of community partnerships (WHO 2020). Suggesting that they offer innovative approaches for the uptake and acceleration of new knowledge, COP's are demonstrating their effectiveness particularly as agents of change. Key features include their ability to advance teamwork with health care practitioners, increase health promotion efforts, enhance patient outcomes, and build capacity through knowledge exchange to treat disease and rehabilitation programmes (WHO 2020).

Advances in digital offer practitioners a vehicle to develop and sustain COP's and gradually such groups can act as an enabler for the delivery of education and skills training of nurses. Earlier chapters in this edition explained the progression of generations of computing and discussed how fifth generation computing initially introduced in the 1980's is now established within healthcare (see Chap. 2). Such advances in technology are shaping how we communicate, in particular considering how we can provide health and social care through various modes of delivery. Nurse education is no exception to this approach. Technology in education has moved beyond traditional didactic teaching modes to more established constructivist learning approaches (Hussey et al. 2020; Rodger and Hussey 2017). Whether you are dealing with patients or students, learning is increasingly becoming a participatory process to be conducted in partnerships with the participant. An activated participant believes their role is significant, has confidence and knowledge to act, and takes actions to incorporate change for success. A critical success factor that influences communities of practice development within the profession of nursing is the opportunity to co-construct and share knowledge in both formal and informal ways.

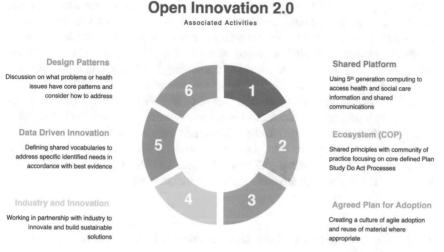

Open Innovation 2.0

Associated Activities

Design Patterns

Discussion on what problems or health issues have core patterns and consider how to address

Data Driven Innovation

Defining shared vocabularies to address specific identified needs in accordance with best evidence

Industry and Innovation

Working in partnership with industry to innovate and build sustainable solutions

Shared Platform

Using 5th generation computing to access health and social care information and shared communications

Ecosystem (COP)

Shared principles with community of practice focusing on core defined Plan Study Do Act Processes

Agreed Plan for Adoption

Creating a culture of agile adoption and reuse of material where appropriate

Fig. 14.1 Open Innovation 2.0 as an overarching paradigm for COP knowledge exchange. (Adapted from OI 2.0 Curley and Salmelin 2018)

New terms such as the Open Innovation 2.0 paradigm describe the impact of the global economic downturn and include the creation of health ecosystems, which can be linked in structure and form to COP. Common denominators between COP and ecosystems include the sharing of expertise and action to address current and priority health issues, such as Covid 19. Open Innovation 2.0 and ecosystems are identified as a core approach to underpin a new mode of technical and societal innovation that presents opportunities to industry, academia and government bodies to work together to achieve a more focused integrated collaboration. This approach involves co-creation, shared values and acceleration of ecosystems, which can unleash potential for solutions that are based on service improvements which are designed for sustainability. Figure 14.1 provides a summary illustration of Open Innovation 2.0 key attributes. The success of Open Innovation 2.0 in Asia has prompted the European Union Framework Programme for Research and Innovation 2021–2027 (Horizon Europe) to identify this paradigm as an important feature in future research agendas (WHO 2020), (European Commission 2020). Activities within Open Innovation 2.0 are strongly linked to COP and informatics research. Some examples include seeking core patterns that occur in a domain in health, for example transition of care, developing a shared purpose, an agreed plan for adoption and testing. In addition, the approach also endorses using agile production underpinned by data driven approaches. The EU considers such groups as coherent networks that can provide test beds for innovation and reduce risk in deployment of services therefore offering a better return on investment (European Commission 2020).

Focusing on the perspective of nursing engagement in COP's, there is an increasing realisation that action must be taken. The profession needs to contribute to the provision of robust structures to protect the citizens during deployment of healthcare systems, which as a consequence of increasing fiscal costs and an increasing and aging population, is under threat. Chapter 7 notes that nurses hold a unique function as they are the only healthcare professionals to interact with individuals, carers and families on a 24 hour, 7 days a week basis. When one considers the scale of skill hours and the overall projected costs of nursing skill mix within healthcare, it is reasonable to suggest that within this emerging health ecosystem nursing as a profession is potentially vulnerable and so too are recipients of health care.

In Sect. 14.3, we revisit some examples of COP from the fourth edition to demonstrate their progression since 2015. On review of the fourth edition it is encouraging to see that the existing COP's developed are evolving and in good shape continuing to progress. In Sect. 14.4, we introduce some new initiatives which have emerged from the existing COP's in Ireland the U.S. and Saudi Arabia which have been funded and are advancing global collaboration.

14.3 Communities of Practice Revisited from Fourth Edition

In the fourth edition of An Introduction to Nursing Informatics, we introduced a number of examples of COP's in Ireland. In this next edition, we revisit some of these networks and consider how they have progressed over the past five years. Table 14.1 provides a summary of the networks and provides an update on their development since then.

14.4 New Research Initiatives Influencing Knowledge Networks Through the Center for eIntegrated Care

Case 1: Nursing Engagement in Health Informatics System Development
Authors Dr Subhashis Das, Ms Anne Spencer and Dr Pamela Hussey

The EHR insight COP identified that there was at the time a pressing need at the European level to have interoperable models, which can provide mechanisms to access or provide EHR data within a distributed record system. Today in 2020, this need prevails and as a consequence a core mission of the CeIC research center is to advance eIntegrated care in order to improve health and wellbeing. The specifics of interoperability are expanded upon well in Chaps. 2, 5 and 6. Here we provide a concrete examples of how CeIC is advancing this agenda through knowledge networks using ontology in partnership with the Adapt Research Center Programme (The Adapt Research Center Ireland 2020). The term ontology in computer science can be described as a formal representation of knowledge by a set of concepts within a domain (in this case health and social care) and the relationships between those concepts. Here we provide a short summary of our work on ontology development, the purpose of which is to advance knowledge on health informatics standards for continuity of care. We also provide a second example of implementation research which responds to the Covid 19 epidemic in progress with our community partners.

Table 14.1 Summary of COP Progression 2015–2020

Network project name 2015	Current progress 2020	Comment and links
Partners CT COP this project focused on development of concepts and terminology for shared assessment tools using participatory action research methods.	The Partners COP has evolved to become a funded research center. An interdisciplinary team launched the Center for eIntegrated Care (CeIC) in 2017. At the time of writing this report there are 19 primary investigators who are researching various projects. Some examples of projects include investigating the use of digital smart devices in the home, creating care transition data catalogues and promoting the use of health informatics standards for terminology and information modelling services.	To review the work of the Center for eIntegrated Care please see the website https://www.dcu.ie/ceic (Hussey 2020). A summary of the work that directly relates to the partners CT project can be accessed from this link https://www.mdpi.com/2227-9709/6/3/37/htm (Hussey and McGlinn 2019)
Mental Health TrialogueThis is a network established to promote and empower communities about mental health	Mental Health TrialogueNetwork continues to grow and has a dedicated website and associated Facebook page. There is also now a dedicated recovery college which provides an empowering and educational approach to mental health and wellbeing.	The link to the Mental Health Trialgoue is available form https://trialogue.co/ (Mental Health Trialogue Ireland [Internet] 2020) The link to Dublin North Recovery College is http://recoverycollege.ie/ (The Recovery College Dublin North Ireland 2020)
Bone Health in the ParkThis is a community of practice led by Ms Daragh Rodger ANP in Dublin North Community Services	Bone Health in the ParCOP has progressed and offers a number of bone health promotion educational resources from the home landing page of the website which has been widely accessed (over 20,000 hits globally a year). The COP also won a national Irish Health Care Award in 2016.	The link is https://www.bonehealth.co/ (Bone Health in the Park 2020). Additional projects in Intellectual Disability Services relating to bone health are also available from www.happybones.ie (Happy Bones 2020)
EHR InsightThis COP was devised in 2013 by academics across a number of institutions in Dublin	Today EHR InsightCommunity of practice has progressed to more formal engagement in Health Informatics Standards Development and individual funded research project. The focus remains the same to advance students understanding of electronic health records.	An example of the research that is currently in flight in this COP is discussed in Sect. 14.4 under research.

Example 1

An ontology for Continuity of Care

The Ontology of Continuity of care (ContSOnto) is an emerging research area consisting of the extension of a healthcare ontology to inform the continuity of care

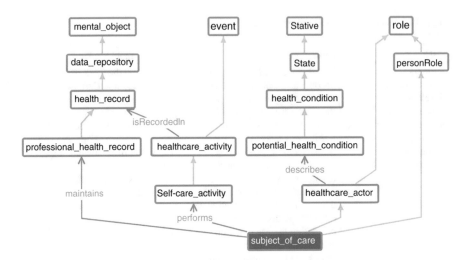

Fig. 14.2 Formal relationships in Webprotégé and ISO 13940 (Systems of concepts for continuity of care 2018)

domain. This field is positioned at the confluence of health informatics, nursing informatics, process modelling, and artificial intelligence.

This research relating to ContSOnto is underpinned by a health informatics standard ISO 13940 Systems of Concepts for Continuity of Care (Systems of concepts for continuity of care 2018). ContSOnto focuses on how information flows from different information systems across and between services for clinical applications and health care professionals to use. Figure 14.2 provides an illustration of how the different classes and relationships in the standard are represented. Subject of care refers to the individual service user and health care actor which can be human or non-human, for example, a health care professional or an organisation.

Example 2

Covid 19 Planning and deployment of Higher Care Area using Technology

The second exemplar we wish to demonstrate is in response to the Covid 19 pandemic and links to ontology development work discussed above and in flight in CeIC. A short description of the clinical issues faced by nursing teams is expanded upon.

COVID 19 as a virus has gripped the world population to reach a Global pandemic status by March 2020. European data has shown older persons, and marginalised groups such as those for example with chronic conditions and an intellectual disability are the most vulnerable populations in terms of impact and mortality. In particular, there are many challenges facing service providers caring for people with an intellectual disability in community residential houses, the reality being faced is that health care resources are finite and the impact of how this virus may impact upon an individual's physical and mental health is still unknown. Many service users have complex pre-existing physical conditions and behavioural problems, which add to the care challenges faced in respect of diagnosing and subsequently caring for them. To pre-empt some of the issues, we are looking to be proactive in two key ways firstly by transforming one of the day service centres into a designated 'higher care area' purposefully designed and managed by their own care team. The aim is to care for service users who are not able to self-isolate or who are displaying symptoms / confirmed as having Covid19. Where possible, the aim is to care for service users in their own home but this may not be achievable for numerous reasons. A diagrammatic overview of the design is available below in Fig. 14.3. Secondly, based on the defined needs and requirements of our partner services, we are now building an ontological conceptual model through which we are able to explicitly connect who are the healthcare actors (i.e. carer, healthcare professional or healthcare organization) collecting, observing and analysing data on which a subject of care i.e. service user and mobile app can collect real time clinical information from the observation of the service users in a timely evidence based and robust manner. One example will take the form of an early warning system. The impact of this initiative will be to assist with clinical decision making and flag service users whose physiological status is changing. This approach in essence leaves the IoT (inanimate entities) to record observations of service users and support medical and nursing practitioner's clinical decision making in a timely way.

Case 2: International Collaboration: Nursing Engagement in Health Informatics in Ireland
Authors Dr Dianne Conrad, Dr Rosanne Burson, and Dr Katherine Moran

This exemplar outlines the abilities of a scholarship team as a community of practice to advance and share nursing knowledge between countries. A scholarship team is defined in this context as a network of scholars coming together, either in person or virtually with technology, sharing expertise for a common purpose, to promote scholarly work to advance the nursing profession. Communities of practice can be expanded globally with the use of technology and can impact the local and global context. Our scholarship team developed a unique approach to international work via a group process with the support of the Fulbright Scholarship Program, to promote advanced nursing practice education in Ireland. This exemplar community of practice includes a network of scholars from Grand Valley State University (GVSU), University of Detroit Mercy (UDM), George Washington University (GWU) in the U.S. and Dublin City University (DCU) in Ireland. The team used digital technology to conduct meetings and connect colleagues across the world. Dr. Dianne Conrad and Dr. Rosanne Burson were awarded Fulbright Scholarships to Ireland for academic year 2019–2020, assisted by this international scholarship team.

The scholarship team model consists of core components to assure that the community of practice thrives and includes members who:

(a) use a relationship-based approach,
(b) intentionally select a diverse group of team members who contribute their unique talents and perspectives,
(c) trust each other,
(d) have willingness to embrace critique,
(e) have a desire to develop a work environment that focuses on systems-level thinking, innovation, and synergy, and

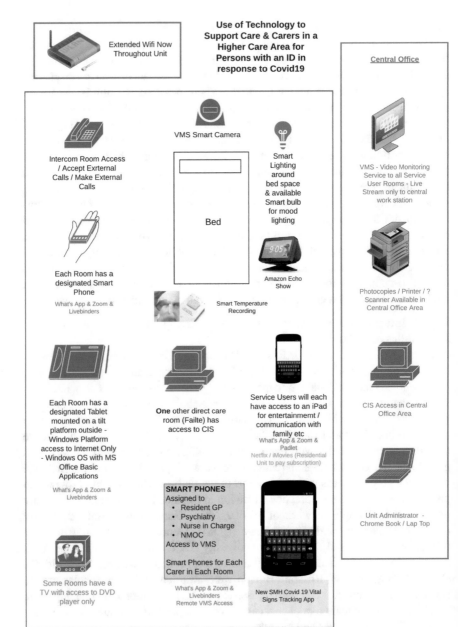

Fig. 14.3 Covid 19 higher care area overview

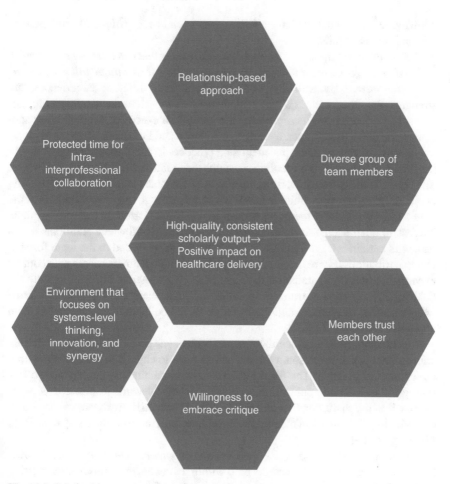

Fig. 14.4 Scholarship team components

(f) prioritize protected time for intra- interprofessional collaboration. (See Fig. 14.4, Scholarship Team Components)

By addressing the critical components identified within this model, one can reasonably expect to *experience high-quality, consistent scholarly output that collaboratively addresses the complexities of healthcare delivery.*

The scholarship team is *relationship-based* with an emphasis on shared, intentional communication to enhance the connection between team members. There is a sense of support that permeates the team. All members are focused on optimal results as a team, rather than the success of the individual. With this attitude in mind, all work critiques are honest, thoughtful, and non-political. Each individual is valued for their contributions and their particular view and expertise. Over time, this approach creates an environment of *trust* that continues to build and deepen, allowing team members to have a *willingness to embrace critique* to grow personally and professionally.

An important component of the scholarship team is that it is *intentionally formed*, with a *diverse group of team members who contribute their unique talents and varied perspectives*. By utilizing team members with different experiences and strengths, the group creates a very wide lens to view each topic of scholarship. For example, our core team incorporates the views of an executive, clinical nurse specialist, and nurse practitioner, as well as academics and informatics experts to incorporate various aspects of advanced nursing practice. In addition, each team member has personal writing and presenting strengths that contribute to the team as a whole. The team is semi-permeable, meaning that team members work together depending on the project and opportunity at hand. For some projects, only two members of the core team are required; members choose to participate based on availability, topic interest, or other needs. At times, project support is required where additional members with certain intra or interprofessional expertise are added to the team for specific contributions. For example, certain projects require team members with content expertise in finance or statistics; their experience and interest bring strength to the final product. Feedback from these additional team members have demonstrated understanding, excitement and appreciation of the collaborative scholarship team approach.

A scholarship team comes together with planned, periodic meetings, virtually with technology or in-person, with the unique need to engage in scholarship within the context of practice. The team generates and disseminates scholarship work—through presentations, publishing, and other scholarly work in practice. A team approach to the dissemination and publication of scholarly work can enhance productivity by allowing team members with unique expertise to collectively contribute (Tschannen et al. 2014).

The fertile *relationship-based team creates an environment that invites innovation and synergy*. Ideas bud and develop within team conversations and the writing process that contributes to the final product in a way that creates more impact than any individual contribution. There is an excitement and an energy that is released as the team interacts and creates new ideas. The collaboration required in these sessions further builds both the quality of the product and feeds the team relationship.

The intentional work within a scholarship team results in a very high quality and consistent level of scholarship output. Our team has noted that the individual tends to experience an ebb and flow to work output that can lead to a variability in scholarly product output. The ebb and flow phenomenon can be attributed to environmental factors, such as other work and family responsibilities or personal factors, such as fatigue and motivation. The scholarship team approach accommodates for these naturally occurring inconsistencies in scholarly output experienced by the individual. For example, team members share the workload by taking the lead on projects on a rotational basis. This occurs in both planned and unplanned situations. The lead team member initiates the development of the product and is responsible for dissemination activities. The team meets periodically *with planned, protected time for collaboration* to assess needs and direction of topics for presentation, writing, and consultation and sets timetables for review and team input. In this way, each team member contributes to the development of the project. A variety of methods are used to edit and further refine work, such as a round-robin approach to review a presentation or manuscript prior to submission. The goal is to continue the high output of the group, with each individual contributing to their highest level of ability at the time.

The scholarship team composed of *intra and interprofessional members has the potential to impact not only the profession of nursing but improve healthcare delivery of organizations with innovations that facilitate timely translation of evidence to practice.* Moreover, the scholarship team can impact the Quadruple Aim (Bodenheimer and Sinsky 2014) goals of improving the patient experience of care, improving the health of populations, reducing the per capita cost of health care, and optimizing the clinician experience, by supporting team members in their efforts to improve evidence-based healthcare delivery. The scholarship team evolves the singular and perhaps lonely act of scholarly activities, such as writing, into an exciting, interactive, and collegial experience that positively impact academia and practice. Teams need to use 'overall big picture' thinking that incorporates the needs of the system and individual patient. The healthcare environment of today requires a diverse scholarship team that can collaboratively address the complexities of healthcare delivery.

Technology has opened up an opportunity to network and collaborate with just a touch of a digital link. Use of these digital tools increases the reach in academia, practice and education. For example, our team began with monthly digital meetings to discuss global health. The team included colleagues from two universities in Michigan (GVSU and UDM), one in Washington, DC (GW), and another in Ireland (DCU) and Saudi Arabia. The group developed a mission statement and purpose to stay focused in our discussions. Review of the current evidence around the need for health system change and population health ensued. As time evolved, an understanding of the similarities and differences in healthcare delivery and graduate nursing education between the USA and Ireland emerged as a topic of interest.

The scholarship team members provided a network of contacts internationally, which facilitated a request for a letter of support from Dr. Pamela Hussey at Centre for eIntegrated Care (CeIC) at DCU. The group identified two members who had the time-based ability to function on the ground in Ireland through a sabbatical leave of absence from their roles in academia. It was determined that the two members would apply for a sabbatical and work together consecutively. One member started in Fall of 2019 and second member continued the work in the Winter 2020. Both members participated in project progress through the entire experience. This occurred via participation in DCU team meetings and developmental work through digital meetings that occurred irrespective of who was physically present in Ireland. Monthly Global Scholarship Team meetings continued with the aid of digital technology to keep the team informed and solicit input of team members on activities. For example, the team reviewed institutional review board (IRB) documentation, as well as abstracts and literature review progress from the graduate assistant student who was brought into the group to learn from the experience of international scholarship work.

Both sabbatical participants were able to secure Fulbright Scholarship grants to support the sabbatical work. Shortly after World War II, U. S. Senator J. William Fulbright sponsored the legislation that laid the foundation for the Fulbright Program. The Fulbright basic objective is *to promote mutual understanding between the people of the United States and the people of other countries. Senator Fulbright believed that, through educational exchange, people would better understand citizens and cultures of other nations.* Fulbright scholarships are competitive individual applications. Within this endeavour, the sabbatical members of the team applied individually, but included objectives in their applications that built on each other's proposed work and highlighted the team approach. Through Fulbright support, both team members were able to implement the plan as envisioned (Fulbright 1. US Awards 2020).

The use of the digital environment was extensively used during the implementation phase. The global team was tapped for input on an IRB application related to the environmental assessment of practitioners, academics, and policy experts in Ireland. Additionally, virtual classroom education sessions, linking graduate nursing students from Ireland and the U.S. were accomplished. Global experiences for students will be a sustainable opportunity through the use of digital environments. Finally, after assessing policy makers in Ireland's needs to promote nursing informatics, a project was initiated to develop informatics competencies with the Health Service Executive of Ireland and a national leadership team. This work was accomplished through the aid of the virtual environment to produce scholarly output and enlist the continued support of the scholarship team members.

During the second half of the sabbatical experience, the Coronavirus (COVID-19) pandemic evolved and affected the ability to remain as visiting scholars to Ireland. However, because of digital capabilities that had been developed previously, the team was able to continue with the planned projects. This included presentations in the classroom to students, work on informatics competencies, and ongoing relationship development for future nursing scholarship opportunities.

This exemplar identifies the strengths of working together, even over distances, and through unforeseen difficulties, to maintain relationships, continue projects and develop new potentials for nursing, patients and healthcare utilizing digital tools and technology. In this way, global communities of practice with a focused agenda and scholarship team-based structure can assist in the delivery of progressing the nursing profession and improve healthcare delivery.

Case 3: Nursing Informatics and Progression of Nursing Informatics Skills in an ANP Programme in Saudi Arabia
Authors Dr Catherine Corrigan and Dr Pamela Hussey

In 2017, Dublin City University in collaboration with Princess Nourah Bint Abdul Rahman University in Saudi Arabia implemented a post graduate programme of study for Nursing in a public women's university located in Riyadh, the capital of

Saudi Arabia (Princess Nourah 2020). Princess Nourah Bint Abdul Rahman University is the largest women's university in the world. The university registered 38 students in the first cohort that graduated in the Autumn of 2019. A key focus for the educational programme was to educate women to become advanced nurse practitioners.

Fast-paced changes in the cultural, economic and political arenas are occurring in Saudi Arabia. This movement can be greatly attributed to the *2030 Saudi Vision* that has the overarching goal for the country to be an 'exemplary and leading nation' (Saudi Vision 2030). *The National Transformation Program* that is part of the *Saudi Vision 2030* has 'transforming healthcare' as its first goal. This led to a critical focus on the education of healthcare workers and aligns with Sustainable Health Goal No. 4 *Quality Education* (United Nations Sustainable Development Goals). This applies to Saudi nursing nationals in particular, who currently occupy 50% of the nursing workforce (Alboliteeh et al. 2017). The opportunity to expand the nursing profession to the advanced practice level in collaboration with the largest women's university in the world presented itself.

Assessing the service need in the community is paramount to align the meaningful contribution of advanced practice nursing education. The impetus for introducing an advanced nursing practice programme was to progress primary care that is currently used principally for screening and immunizations. The advanced practice nursing program is a broad-based knowledge curriculum that equips nurses to practice in the community—identified as one of the key areas most in need of healthcare improvement in Saudi Arabia. Secondly, Saudi nurses who are relatively inexperienced and with variable levels of education (Alboliteeh et al. 2017), were in need of clinical leaders equipped with the knowledge, skills and attitudes necessary to engage in leadership activities such as process improvement initiatives, policy change and research. Additionally, nurse leaders are required to work with multiple stakeholders to include those who struggle with change (O'Rourke and Higuchi 2016).

Nursing in some cases is not viewed positively in Saudi Arabia because of gender desegregation, family and cultural values (ALYami and Watson 2014). Although somewhat aware of the challenging landscape, nursing academics ventured to Saudi Arabia from Ireland to begin the advanced practice nursing programme—the first of its kind in the country. Programme competencies and clinical hours aligned with international nurse practitioner standards affording graduates eligibility to apply for registration in other countries. Although the advanced nursing practice concept is spreading globally, it is still relatively new. Programme delivery was unique in that there is not an abundance of doctorate prepared, female, advanced practice nurses with academic experience (required attributes) in the world, available to travel to and reside for defined periods in Saudi Arabia. Nevertheless, with an understanding that 'flexibility is key' a team of highly experienced academics, most of them practicing nurse practitioners, was created to deliver the programme.

Face-to-face is the prescribed method of delivery of education in Saudi Arabia, which meant that intense delivery of modules over a three-week period was warranted. Students were financially supported to take off work for the entire 2-year

duration of the programme enabling them to focus solely on their scholarly obligations. On the ground personnel included Dublin City University faculty that taught
modules and managed the clinical component (two 9-week long modules) in collaboration with the local university. Additionally, adjunct professors that included
doctoral prepared advanced practice nurses from Ireland and America flew to Saudi
Arabia for intense delivery of modules. Obtaining clinical preceptors was particularly challenging because of the lack of understanding of the role of advanced practice nurses amongst the nursing and medical professionals as well as other members
of the interdisciplinary team. We sought out clinical partner organizations with an
interest in participating and being part of the student experience and instructed the
students to request to join healthcare teams during rounds and ask questions. Their
presence was quickly noticed, and physicians began to facilitate a variety of learning experiences for the students.

Although face-to-face was the preferred method of delivery with the majority of
instructors flying in from the US to deliver content, information technology was
incorporated into the programme. Remote communication included a presentation
by the Librarian at the university in Ireland and a team member graded remotely
from New York. Some students completed clinical hours in a 'digital hospital' that
was entirely paper free and the government in Saudi Arabia is emphasising the need
to incorporate information technology to the healthcare sector (Al Kuwaiti et al.
2018). In addition, student proposals were supervised remotely by a team of doctor-
ally prepared advanced practice nurses. This adjunct faculty worked completely
online with the students from their home countries. Student proposals were developed using digital tools that included the Google Classroom, and a digital platform
to facilitate teleconference meetings to discuss progress. The student shared the
written proposal on a Google Document where the supervisor could then review and
make comments prior to meeting through teleconference meetings. In this way,
communication was enhanced and students developed their proposals with significant verbal and written guidance. These factors and the recent Coronavirus pandemic forced a decision to convert the programme (except for clinical evaluations)
to an online format in the spring of 2020. The programme team also identified the
need for an *Informatics in eHealth* module to be incorporated into the future delivery of the programme. Telehealth was a particular interest of one of the students
who expressed a need to improve the health and well-being of people living in
remote areas in the desert along the Yemen border. The student joined with a Global
Team from the U.S. to discover the possibilities for her innovative plan that aligns
with the Sustainable Development Goal No. 3 *Good Health and Well-Being* (United
Nations Sustainable Development Goals).

The Arab world is lagging in nursing education; nevertheless, there is an obvious
starvation for knowledge to positively impact health outcomes. Despite the many
challenges, the programme has survived and is thriving; albeit within a steep learning curve while both cultures strived to understand each other and deliver a rigorous
programme that upheld best international standards. The rewards to date have been
great as faculty staff see the motivation inspired by the female students who
expressed feelings of empowerment with knowledge gained; not only from an

academic perspective, but personally and professionally as well. Over time we believe that graduates of the programme will positively impact on health outcomes within the country.

Navigating unknown waters requires some knowledge of support systems, for instance fiscal support; certain personality traits; flexibility, and a willingness to become culturally aware within a predominately male-orientated society. Transformational leadership can be applied to primary care setting; it has the potential to motivate Nurse Practitioners (NPs), and promote NP practice to achieve the collective purpose of ensuring better care for patients and improved health outcomes (Poghosyan and Bernhardt 2018).

Advanced practice nurses are positively effective from patient care to policy change, as the drive toward population health initiatives evolves. In a vision for the future, the advanced practice nurse working in Saudi Arabia will have the attributes to function as change agents with a solution-orientated approach, especially within the community care setting where they will be equipped to develop new models of care, using digital tools (Nursing Now 2020) to meet the service needs of local and national populations with the support of a globally dedicated community of practice group.

14.5 Conclusion

Nursing and its future use of technology within the scope of healthcare delivery needs to be managed carefully and strong leadership is now required. The WHO State of the World's Nursing Report 2020 (World Health Organization 2020), emphasizes the importance of nursing education regarding both leadership and digital competencies to promote the improved quality of healthcare delivery worldwide. In this edition Chaps. 3, 11, and 15 identify the importance of education on informatics, and the training of nurses on *digital literacy and leadership skills*. Delivery of such skills and understanding their value will enable nurses to protect not only the profession of nursing, but also the health Ecosystem that is increasingly under threat and the individuals who use this ecosystem. Much is written reporting nurses as knowledge workers in eHealth care who through a process of assimilation convert data to information—information to knowledge and with experience, convert knowledge in context to progress the profession (Matney et al. 2010). By considering health as an ecosystem and embracing Open Innovation 2.0 methods, it offers the profession of nursing opportunities to innovate and provide new ways of working in a digital enabled health care setting.

Education, particularly in nursing informatics is a key requirement and should underpin all undergraduate and postgraduate programmes. It is however critical that the impact of educated nurses is seen and recognised in the wider context. Forming knowledge networks in nursing, utilizing leadership and digital tools, enable communities of practice with teams of nurses not only to deliver high quality, evidence-based care, but also generate timely, practice-based knowledge to promote the profession of nursing. We finish this chapter on a cautionary note revisiting the poem by Seamus Heaney from the beginning of the chapter which the authors consider holds an important message for the profession at this time.

> Had I not been awake I would have missed it,
> It came and went too unexpectedly
> And almost it seemed dangerously,
> Hurling like an animal to the house,
> A courier blast that there and then
> Lapsed ordinary. But not ever after.
> And not now. (Seamus Heaney 2020)

Questions

1. Discuss the role of the COP in the accelerating service improvements for technology adoption in Health and Social Care.
2. Do you think the feature of the Open Innovation 2.0 paradigm and COP are aligned? Discuss the key features on where there is overlap between them?
3. Learning activity—Select one of the COP websites listed in Table 14.1. After reviewing the resources on this website, consider how you would create a community of practice within your own practice domain. Identify the topic what resources you would need and who you would ask to join your knowledge network.

Answers

1. The role of COP primarily offers an opportunity for knowledge exchange and the sharing of innovative solutions through collaboration and team work. COP's provide a pragmatic and purposeful approach using tele networking and digital platforms for knowledge transfer and scholarship. Online webinars for example, can be used by nursing communities to come together to share expertise, experience and knowledge in both a synchronous and asynchronous manner.
2. Yes, Open Innovation 2.0 and COP are primarily focused on knowledge exchange team work and innovation. Innovation 2.0 is particularly suited as a paradigm to underpin digital and data driven solutions underpinned by a developed Ecosystem that includes both industry academia and government agencies.

Glossary

ANP Advanced Nurse Practitioner
APPG All-Party Parliamentary Group
Asynchronous A term used in association with communication online the term refers to data which is transmitted intermittently rather than in a simultaneously in real time
Community of Practice An informal network of individuals who share a concern or passion for something and who usually need to advance their own knowledge, experience and skills with each other

ContSOnto A research initiative engaged in the development of an Ontology of Continuity of care based on an ISO Standard ISO 13940 Systems of Concepts for Continuity of Care

DNP Doctorate of Nursing Practice

Enabling technologies Equipment or method that allows the user to combine or use stand alone technologies to enhance performance and capabilities

OI 2.0 Open Innovation 2.0, a core approach to underpin a new mode of technical and societal innovation that presents opportunities to industry, academia and government bodies to work together to achieve a more focused integrated collaboration

PAHO Pan American Health Organization

Synchronous A term used in association with communication online the term refers to data which is transmitted in real time simultaneously

Trialogue A dialogue or meeting between three people or groups

Web 2.0 The second stage of development of the Internet, includes the migration from static web pages to dynamic or user-generated content and the growth of social networking.

References

Al Kuwaiti A, Al Muhanna FA, Al Amri S. Implementation of digital health technology at academic medical centers in Saudi Arabia. Oman Med J. 2018;33(5):367–73.

Alboliteeh M, Magarey J, Wiechula R. The profile of Saudi nursing workforce: a cross-sectional study. Nursing Research and Practice. Hindawi. 2017;2017:1–9.

All-Party Parliamentary Group on Global Health: Triple impact—how developing nursing will improve health, promote gender equality and support economic growth; London, 17 October 2016. http://www.appg.globalhealth.org.uk/.

ALYami MS, Watson R. An overview of nursing in Saudi Arabia. Journal of Health Specialties. 2014;2(1):10–2.

Bodenheimer T, Sinsky C. From triple to quadruple aim: care of the patient requires care of the provider. Ann Fam Med. 2014;12(6):573–6. https://doi.org/10.1370/afm.1713.

Bone Health in the Park [Internet]. [cited 2020 May 8]. http://www.bonehealth.co.

Curley M. Salmelin B. Open Innovation 2.0 A New Paradigm. Switzerland: Springer 2018.

Education is not the filling of a pail, but the lighting of a fire [Internet]. Psychology Today. [cited 2020 May 8]. http://www.psychologytoday.com/blog/dont-delay/200805/education-is-not-the-filling-pail-the-lighting-fire.

European Commission I Choose your language I Choisir une langue I Wählen Sie eine Sprache [Internet]. [cited 2020 May 8]. https://ec.europa.eu/; Orientations towards the first Strategic Plan for Horizon Europe. https://ec.europa.eu/info/sites/info/files/research_and_innovation/strategy_on_research_and_innovation/documents/ec_rtd_orientations-he-strategic-plan_122019.pdf.

Fulbright 1. US Awards [Internet]. Fulbright. [cited 2020 May 8]. https://www.fulbright.ie/coming-to-ireland/us-awards/.

Happy Bones [Internet] [cited 2020 May 8]. www.happybones.ie.

Hussey P. Center for eIntegrated care. Online Resource [cited 2020 May 8]. https://www.dcu.ie/ceic.

Hussey P, McGlinn K. The role of academia in reorientation models of care—insights on eHealth. Informatics. 2019;6(3):37.

Hussey, P.; Corbally, M; Rodger, D.; Kirwan, A.; Adams, E.; Kavanagh, P; Matthews, A. ICNP® R&D Centre Ireland Defining requirements for an intersectoral digital landscape informatics MDPI Special Issue Edition Nursing Informatics n.d.;4(2):7. https://doi.org/10.3390/informatics4020007-http://www.mdpi.com/2227-9709/4/2/7/htm.

Matney S, Brewster P, Sward K, Cloynes K, Staggers N. Philosophical approaches to nursing informatics data-information-knowledge-wisdom framework. Adv Nurs Sci. 2010;34(1):6–18.

Mental Health Trialogue Ireland [Internet]. [cited 2020 May 8]. http://www.trialogue.co/.

Nursing Now. 2020. https://www.icn.ch/what-we-do/campaigns/nursing-now.

O'Rourke T, Higuchi KS. Activities and attributes of nurse practitioner leaders: lessons from a primary care system change. Nurs Leadersh. 2016;29(3):46–60.

Poghosyan L, Bernhardt J. Transformational leadership to promote nurse practitioner practice in primary care. J Nurs Manag. 2018;(8):1066. https://0-doi-org.aupac.lib.athabascau.ca/10.1111/jonm.12636

Princess Nourah Bint Abdul Rahman University—Home [Internet]. [Cited 2020 May]. https://www.pnu.edu.sa/ar/Pages/home.aspx.

Rodger D, Hussey P. From entry to practice to advanced practitioner—the progression of competencies and how they assist in delivery of eHealth Programmes for healthy ageing. In: Muphy J, Goosen W, Weber P, editors. Forecasting informatics competencies for nurses in the future of connected health. Amsterdam: IOS Press; 2017. http://ebooks.iospress.nl/ISBN/978-1-61499-738-2.

Saudi Vision 2030. http://vision2030.gov.sa/en.

Seamus Heaney—'Had I not been awake I would have missed it' [Internet]. Genius. [cited 2020 May 8]. Accessed https://genius.com/Seamus-heaney-had-i-not-been-awake-i-would-have-missed-it-annotated.

Systems of concepts for continuity of care (ISO 13940:2015) [Internet]. 2018. https://www.iso.org/standard/58102.html.

The Adapt Research Center Ireland [Internet] [cited 2020 May 8]. https://www.adaptcentre.ie/.

The Recovery College Dublin North Ireland [Internet]. [cited 2020 May 8]. http://recoverycollege.ie/.

Tschannen D, Anderson C, Strobbe S, Bay E, Bigelow A, Dahlem C, et al. Scholarly productivity for nursing clinical track faculty. Nurs Outlook. 2014;62(6):475–81. https://doi.org/10.1016/j.outlook.2014.05.006.

United Nations Sustainable Development Goals. 2015. https://www.un.org/sustainabledevelopment/sustainable-development-goals/.

WHO | Global strategic directions for strengthening nursing and midwifery 2016–2020 [Internet]. WHO. [cited 2020 May 8]. http://www.who.int/hrh/nursing_midwifery/global-strategy-midwifery-2016-2030/en/.

World Health Organization. (2020). State of the world's nursing report 2020. https://www.who.int/publications-detail/nursing-report-2020?utm_source=National+League+for+Nursing&utm_campaign=9939e27e43-EMAIL_CAMPAIGN_2020_04_06_06_19&utm_medium=email&utm_term=0_2b4a0f0e05-9939e27e43-355357485.

Chapter 15
Technology Enabled Learning in Nursing

Diane J. Skiba

Abstract Over the last decade, technology enabled learning has thrived in the health care professional education arena. This is particularly true as the rise of disruptive technologies has greatly impacted not only education but also the delivery of health care across the globe. Thus, it is immensely important that nurses use a variety of digital tools to provide learning experiences that will best prepare for health care professionals to practice in a digital health ecosystem. In this chapter, the goal is to highlight examples of technology-enhanced learning and to prepare nurses for a technology-enhanced practice within a digital health ecosystem.

Keywords Computer based simulations · Immersive virtual simulations · Virtual reality · Online learning · Connected health digital tools · Virtual visits

Over the last decade, technology enabled learning has thrived in the health care professional education arena. This is particularly true as the rise of disruptive technologies has greatly impacted not only education but also the delivery of health care across the globe. Thus, it is immensely important that nurses use a variety of digital tools to provide learning experiences that will best prepare for health care professionals to practice in a digital health ecosystem. In this chapter, the goal is to highlight examples of technology-enhanced learning and to prepare nurses for a technology-enhanced practice within a digital health ecosystem.

Electronic Supplementary Material The online version of this chapter (https://doi.org/10.1007/978-3-030-58740-6_15) contains supplementary material, which is available to authorized users.

D. J. Skiba (✉)
College of Nursing, University of Colorado, Aurora, CO, USA
e-mail: Diane.Skiba@CUAnschutz.edu

© Springer Nature Switzerland AG 2021
P. Hussey, M. A. Kennedy (eds.), *Introduction to Nursing Informatics*, Health Informatics, https://doi.org/10.1007/978-3-030-58740-6_15

Learning Objectives for the Chapter
1. Identify technology tools that will enable you to learn about nursing and health care.
2. Describe the use of virtual clinical simulations to master nursing knowledge, skills and attitudes.
3. Describe the concept of connected health and its impact on the healthcare environment.
4. Identify digital health care tools that patients, families, consumers and caregivers will use now and in the future.
5. Assess your current and future role as a nurse in the digital health ecosystem.
6. Understand that as a nurse, professional development, particularly in the area of informatics, is important.
7. Understand that consumers are becoming more engaged in their care and are using many digital tools to manage their health.
8. Understand that clinical practice requires collaboration with nursing informatics specialists to provide safe quality patient centric care.
9. Consider that digital health tools will continue to influence your nursing practice now and in the future.

15.1 Introduction

The term technology enhanced learning has various definitions. "The term, Technology-enhanced learning (TEL), is used to describe the application of technology to teaching and learning. It is a broad category that isn't particularly defined, but, in short, TEL is any technology that enhances the learning experience." (Cullen 2018). In some instances, digital education is "the innovative use of digital tools and technologies during teaching and learning, and is often referred to as Technology Enhanced Learning (TEL) or e-Learning." (University of Edinburgh Institute for Academic Development 2018). The bottom line is how technology can foster learning.

The use of technologies to facilitate and enhance the learning experience is the focus of this chapter. The exploration includes both existing and emerging technologies. As a learner, you may be exposed to some of these technologies in your formal educational program or you may experience these technologies as part of your professional development opportunities. Regardless, it is important for all nurses to have a broad understanding of the various digital tools as they will be part of your nursing practice now and in the future.

15.2 Simulations

The use of simulation is a predominate method of teaching nurses. In the beginning, simulation consisted of the use of a manikin. The original manikin, Mrs. Chase, was developed in 1911 and was first used by Hartford Hospital Training School in

Connecticut (Hermann 1981). Mrs. Chase and her accompanying family were fixtures in numerous nursing schools across the globe for over 60 years. These simulation manikins were incorporated into nursing education as a major teaching method to prepare students for clinical practice in a safe learning environment. In the late 1950s and 1960s, new manikins such as Resusci-Anne and Sim One were introduced. New dimensions, such as heartbeats, breathing and patient responses to intravenous drugs, were now included in the simulation manikins. "With improvements in technology, more tasks and clinical skills could be simulated." (Harder 2009).

High fidelity simulators, that mimic human responses, continue to be used in nursing schools across the globe. In addition, standardized patients has been introduced into nursing curriculum. "Standardized patients (SPs) are trained actors who portray patients in realistic clinical interview and physical examination scenarios used in health professions education." (Brender et al. 2005, p. 1172). SP are used to teach a variety of nursing clinical competencies. Here are a few examples. Andrea and Kotowski (2017) have used SPs to teach undergraduate nursing health assessment skills that included interviewing a patient and taking their health history. Sarmasoglu, Dinc and Elcon (2016) used SPs for nurses' psychomotor skill development taking blood pressures and subcutaneous injections. At the graduate level, SPs have been used in nurse practitioner education (Gibbons et al. 2002). According to Shin et al. (2019, p. 19) "high fidelity simulators and standardized patients have a demonstrable impact on enhancing learner's performance skills and metacognitions." However, labor time and costs associated with high fidelity simulations, SPs development and implementation (Shaikh et al. 2017) and growth of online education has prompted the need to find alternative simulation strategies. Technological advances, including the rise of the Internet have served as a catalyst for these alternative simulation strategies.

15.3 Computer-Based Virtual Simulations

According to Cant et al. (2019, p. 27) "Computer-based simulation may include virtual worlds, virtual environments, virtual patients, virtual reality task trainers, and serious games." In some cases, the term virtual reality is used to describe learning experiences. Bell (2008, p. 2) uses the term, virtual reality simulations to mean "a synchronous, persistent network of people, represented as avatars, facilitated by networked computers." In this section, examples of various types of virtual simulations are given. The goal is to familiarize you with various technologies as they are not only used for education of nurses but are also being used to educate and engage patients.

One of the most common computer based simulations are virtual patients. Virtual patients "are interactive computer simulations of real-life clinical scenarios for the purpose of healthcare and medical training, education, or assessment." (Ellaway et al. 2008, p. 170). Padilha et al. (2019) described the use of virtual patients on a computer touchscreen for nursing students in Portugal. In this particular case, students used a clinical virtual simulator called Body Interact. This simulator program uses physiologic algorithms as a basis of the virtual patient. The student is able "to interact with the virtual patient through dialogues, monitoring of physiological parameters, observation and physical examination, the prescription and/or analysis of complementary examinations, and the prescription of intervention and/or pharmacological treatment." (Padilha et al. 2019, p. e11529). At the end, there are two options for closure of the case: successful resolution or amount of time that has lapsed. The student's performance in terms of clinical reasoning is assessed and feedback is provided.

In Sweden, virtual patients were used to assess clinical reasoning for nursing students. Fosberg et al. (2011) conducted a pilot study to assess student feedback about using virtual patients as a part of their distance-based classes. Virtual patients were designed using Web-SP (Web-based Simulation of Patients). This particular software program "was initially developed at Karolinska Institutet (Zary et al. 2006) and used worldwide at several universities in health care educations. Based on the feedback from students as they interacted with the virtual patients, it was determined that virtual patients alongside self-evaluations provided an assessment of their clinical reasoning skills development. This team continued the development and use of virtual patients for their undergraduate students. Most recently, Forsberg et al. (2019) conducted a qualitative study to train nursing students to develop clinical reasoning and support active students participation. Student received lectures and then were assigned virtual patients to assess, identify health problem and the nursing care needed. Based on their analyses, the team concluded "that use of the VP cases helped the students to broaden their thinking, which improved their ability to draw conclusions and their problem-solving ability when obtaining a comprehensive view of the patient." (Forsberg et al. 2019, p. 1480).

Peddle et al. (2016) conducted an integrative review of virtual patients and nontechnical skills of undergraduate health care professionals. In their study, nontechnical skills were defined as "the cognitive, social and personal resource skills that complement technical skills and contribute to safe and efficient task performance." (Flin et al. 2008, p. 1). Twenty eight studies met their criteria and were deemed of sufficient quality. The majority of the studies were from the United States with other studies emanating from Australia, Sweden, United Kingdom, Iran and the Netherlands. Studies were examined using a thematic analysis. The first theme indicated that virtual patients were used in a variety of ways to teach, reinforce, practice, build confidence with communication skills. It was also noted that it was useful in developing verbal and non-verbal communication skills. A second theme centered on teamwork. This included developing team skills and team communication skills. It was also used to clarify roles and promote interaction plus collaboration with team members. There were a smaller number of studies that represented the following themes: decision-making, socialization into professional role, transfer of knowledge to clinical setting, and authenticity.

Virtual patients are important technology enabled learning experiences for not only nursing students but would be beneficial to practicing nurse who may be taking care of patients. This could be particularly true for nurses who may be practicing in new nursing units or transitioning from a medical surgical unit to oncology care.

Another example was the development of a virtual gaming simulation (VGS). Verkuyl, Romaniuk, Atack and Mastrilli (2017) developed a computer based game where students were asked to provide care for a pediatric post-appendectomy recovery. Video clips of the patient and their mother provided a background for the case. Students were able "to collect assessment data, make intervention decisions, and experience the consequences of their choices as they care for the child and his mother." (Verkuyl et al. 2017, p. 240). Students were assessed using a pediatric Skills Self-Efficacy tool.

15.4   Immersive Virtual Simulations

These simulations allowed learners to become immersed in a health care environment and interact with avatars. The avatars represented patients, family members and in some cases other health care professionals. According to Shin et al. (2019) integrative review, Second Life was the most common platform used for virtual reality simulations. One example is the use of a virtual pediatric primary care clinic in Second Life used to teach family nurse practitioners (Cook 2012). This system allowed learners to practice clinical decision making by interacting with avatars representing child and their parent. Learners could access the patient's medical and family history, medication and allergies list as well as other pertinent patient information.

Schaffer et al. (2016) used Second Life to teach public health to RN degree completion students. Faculty created several different virtual environments for their students. One was an opportunity for students to triage victims of a plane crash at a chemical plant. They were also able to visit a Women's & Children Clinic & Adolescent Health Clinic to conduct family assessments and to visit an elderly woman in her home to conduct a home safety assessment.

At the University of Kansas, a virtual assisted living center, Jayhawk Community Living Center (JCLC), was created to allow informatics students to create a fall-risk management system (Manos and Modaress 2020). Learners were given a request for a proposal to develop the system. Their first task was to meet with the Director of Nursing avatar (a faculty member) to determine system requirements. The learners were responsible for taking a tour of the clinic to process system requirements and generate any questions. The learners were responsible for several deliverables such as use cases, storyboards and workflow diagrams. Learners in their database theory course also used the JCLC to create a database for the fall-risk assessments.

At the University of Colorado, Second Life was used by a variety of graduate students who were enrolled in online courses. As part of their interprofessional education, students in nursing and pharmacy were engaged in assessing and treating patients in the CU Virtual Health Hospital/Clinic. Virtual Clinic/Hospital consists of: "clinical exam rooms for observation and interaction; medical surgical unit patient rooms; a psychiatric unit with sound proof walls; pharmacy; medical records room; patient registration; a nursing station; an auditorium for grand rounds; numerous administrative offices; and conference rooms complete with whiteboards for brainstorming, poster board for presentations, a presentation wall for PowerPoint slides or streaming videos, and web access for students to use during their clinical conferences." (Skiba et al. 2014, p. 59). Learners created their own avatars and interacted with avatar patients and other health care professionals. For example, psychiatric nurses interacted with an adolescent and her mother. The adolescent suffered from a bipolar disorder and was having difficulties with the side effects of her medication. In this case scenario, the nurse practitioner did a video consult with a pharmacist to adjust the medication regime (Figs. 15.1 and 15.2).

The University of Colorado also used Second Life In the graduate nursing informatics program. Graduate students used Virtual Hospital/Clinic to complete a

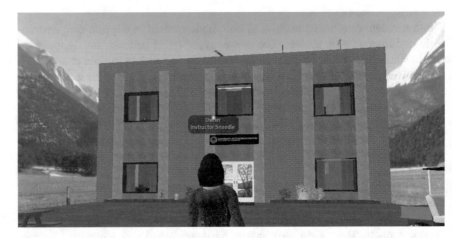

Fig. 15.1 This is a picture of the entrance to the University of Colorado Virtual Hospital in Second Life

Fig. 15.2 This picture shows an Interprofessional Team meeting with patient in University of Colorado Virtual Hospital in Second Life

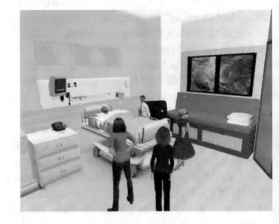

system life cycle project. Students were assigned to teams and were required to select and implement either a bar code medication administration system or a decision support system. As a collaborative team assignment, students used Second Life to meet together, interview key health care professionals and to assess system environments. In one year, students from Colorado, Lebanon and New Zealand, met in Second Life to make decisions about project planning, system analysis tasks, writing a Request for Proposal, making a final system selection and designing an implementation and evaluation plan for their project (Danforth et al. 2012).

15.5 Virtual Reality Devices

For some learning, it was necessary to have virtual reality devices to become immersed in the environment. There are several different types of virtual reality devices. The most common is a head mounted device or VR headset. There is also a headset that is available for use with a smartphone. These devices allow one to become immersed in the environment and are sometimes accompanied by other devices such as haptic tools or treadmills. The popularity of VR headsets used by gamers has helped to make devices affordable for not only academic environments but also for use of VR in clinical settings. VR is used in various clinical setting for: pain management, minimizing fear and anxiety for children in the hospital, provide a distraction for certain procedures such as injections or for chemotherapy infusions. What follows are some examples of VR devices being used in nursing education.

For a graduate course in nursing leadership, virtual reality experience was designed to allow a team to summit Mount Everest. The immersive environment, Everest 2, required a computer based simulation and a VR headset. Students selected various roles in the simulation: "team leader, team doctor, photographer, marathoner, environmentalist, and an optional observer." (Aebersold et al. 2020, p. 2). In their evaluation of this experience, students feedback was categorized into three themes: communication, team dynamics and success or failure. The authors concluded that there was potential to use immersive virtual reality to provided realistic simulated experiences for students.

Jenson and Forsyth (2012) described the use of a virtual reality device along with a haptic arm device to teach nurses how to insert and intravenous catheter. The students used a computer based program to select items such as equipment, cleaning the site and starting the insertion. The haptic arm device was connected to the computer and the student could palpate the arm and then virtually insert the catheter. This experience made use of three dimensional graphics and provided students with a simulated environment to feel vascular access.

At Vanderbilt School of Nursing, nurse practitioners students use a virtual headset to "master competencies in the use of ultrasound technologies."(Weiner et al. 2019, p. 893). The team developed this virtual reality using a immersive VR authoring system called Cenario VR. The software creates both photo and videos into an immersive learning environment. The learner wears a VR headset which allows them to participate directly in the experience. The study concluded that "VR offers one solution to expand the teaching-learning environment." (Weiner et al. 2019, p. 896).

A recent study, Ball and Hussey (2020) examined the effects of augmented reality on anxiety level of nursing students. According to the Interaction Design Foundation (2020), "Augmented reality (AR) is a view of the real, physical world in which users find elements enhanced by computer-generated input. Designers create inputs ranging from sound to video, to graphics to GPS overlays and more, in digital content that responds in real time to changes in the user's environment, usually movement." In their study (Ball and Hussey 2020) used a type of AR, 360 degree photosphere, to orient students for their first clinical site before they began their clinical practicum at maternal child clinical setting. The goal was to prepare students for this rotation and to lower their anxiety about this first clinical experience. With cooperation from the clinical site, the university team built this 360 degree photosphere. This augmented reality experience was uploaded to a secure web site for all students to access prior to their clinical rotation. In this study, student were randomly assigned to either a control group (instructor-led orientation) and the experimental group (AVR). Students were given pre and post tests to measure their anxiety using the State Trait Anxiety Test. Although no statistically significant differences were found between the two groups on the anxiety measure, the team concluded there was still value in using this technology. The value was that it presented a consistent orientation to the clinical setting whereas there could be differing faculty presentations about the clinical setting.

Another example of augmented reality device is the use of Google Glasses to teach nursing students. At Duke University, students using Google Glass watched a video of a car accident in which the victim was having difficulty breathing. As the student watched the video, they had to deliver care to a manikin representing this victim. "The video of the patient was played in each student's field of vision to augment the clinical changes the manikin was programed to display. The intent was for the patient in the video to show in real time what the manikin was displaying." (Chaballout et al. 2016, p. 2). At the University of Miami, faculty could use their laptop and telehealth software to watch a student perform an intubation. According to Foronda et al. (2020), "The software synced the telehealth glasses to the computers so that faculty could see in real time the vantage of the student on their laptops. The faculty directly observed the students performing the intubation and provided verbal instruction to guide and assist students through the simulated intubation of a manikins."

15.6 Online Learning

A major component of TEL is the availability of online learning. Over the past twenty years, online learning has evolved from a novel experience to a standard in higher education. The growth of online learning has increased yearly and offers nurses formal education and professional development learning opportunities, formal education. Early examples of online learning typically mimicked the classroom environment. Early online courses were fairly passive learning consisted of: recorded lectures, quizzes and tests and a discussion board.

As the technology for offering online course progressed and course management systems were designed, there were many schools experimenting with different learning strategies in the online environment. Faculty began to minimize lectures and begin to engage the student in their own learning. The shift was from a passive learning to a more active learning environment. In these early days, some faculty followed principles designed to foster learning. These principles, *Seven Principles for Good Practice in Undergraduate Education* (Chickering and Ehrmann 1996) were adapted for use in web-based courses. Billings et al. (2001) adapted these principles and established a benchmarking project, Evaluating Educational Uses of the Web in Nursing (EEUWIN). This project spanned three different universities and was focused on graduate education being offered for nurse practitioners, acute care clinical specialists and informatics students. As part of this benchmarking project, teaching and learning strategies were shared to increase the overall effectiveness of individual courses. As a member of this project, the University of Colorado College of Nursing enhanced their online graduate healthcare informatics Master's degree program.

In the last decade, online learning flourished with the introduction of emerging technologies to allow both synchronous and asynchronous learning. Nursing education has embraced online learning and offered many online learning degree programs for RN-BSN completion learners, graduate students earning their master's or doctoral degree.

As new technologies became available, more online learning incorporated technology tools to foster:

- communication (blogs, twitter, video conferencing, real time discussion groups)
- teamwork and collaboration (google docs, Slack, BaseCamp, Dropbox)
- data visualization (Tableau, Google Charts, Infogram)
- knowledge creation (whiteboards, mind maps)
- social interactions (Facebook journal clubs, Instagram, Vimeo)
- animation (Adobe Character, Animaker, Moovly, Polygon)

Online learning was not limited to text only content materials with web link but now incorporates a variety of multimedia such as You Tube videos, podcasts, animations and infographics. Students were now using these multimedia tools to complete homework assignments.

15.7 New Models of Education

Also in the last decade, society entered into the Connected Age with development of the Internet of Things (IOT) and more connectivity via mobile technologies. The IOT "is the latest evolution of network-aware smart objects that connect the physical world with information." (Johnson et al. 2012, p. 30). As a result of this evolution, two transformations occurred in academia and in health care. The first was the development of new models of education for the connected age. In health-care, there was a subsequent transformation to an era of connected health. What does connected mean?

> Connecting is about reaching out and bringing in, about building synergies to create a whole that is greater than the sum of its parts. Connecting is a powerful metaphor. Everyone and everything—people, resources, data, ideas—are interconnected: linked and tagged, tweeted and texted, followed and friended. Anyone can participate. (Oblinger 2013, p. 3)

Online learning had now new models to guide the development of courses and program. Connected learning fostered new ways for connecting people with resources, experiences and communities.

> With connected learning, the idea is to connect-the-dots: to connect learning with life." Connected learning is engaging, customized, flexible, affordable, accessible, and lifelong. The connections enable the construction of pathways that can guide learners and institutions. (Oblinger 2013, p. 4)

Online learning no longer was promoting a passive learning environment but an active learning environment. Learners were now given opportunities to create their own learning pathways in an online course. At the University of Colorado, we created learning guides for students in their online courses. Courses were designed in a modular format and each module focused on an in depth guide to a particular content area. The learning guides was tailored for those students new to the field of informatics and those that were already practicing in the informatics field. Thus, based on your existing knowledge and experience with the topic at hand, learners created their own learning pathway to achieve learning outcomes.

Other universities also created online learning opportunities that incorporated social media such as Facebook for journal clubs and twitter and blogs for student discussion groups. Other schools of nursing experimented with online polling via smartphones. Kouri et al. (2017) highlighted examples of the use of social media in health education. They noted that tools such as Google Scholar were useful for nursing research, YouTube for creating multimedia presentations for class assignments and LinkedIn to begin to establish a professional nursing network. They also described how Savonia University used student blogs. Each student created their own personal learning environment using both a blog to document their learning experiences and the WhatsApp for communication and collaboration within their learning environment. Procter (Proctor et al. 2016) shared an example of their virtual exchange designed to provide learning opportunities across three countries (United Kingdom, United States and New Zealand). In this project, a closed Facebook group was established and undergraduate students participated in discussions related to population health.

During this transformation time, higher education also witnessed the development of the Massively Open Online Courses (MOOCs) movement. According to Educause (2020), a MOOC "**is a model for delivering learning content online to virtually any person**—and as many of them—who wants to take the course".

MOOCs can involve thousands of students. The structure tends to be asynchronous and flexible to accommodate the varying levels of participation. Anyone can participate for free in any or all of the course's learning activities (e.g. discussions, blogs, video lectures, other social media tools). While there may not be feedback from the instructor, chances are there will be lots of discussion form all open participants. (Skiba 2012, p. 416)

Throughout the next few years, numerous MOOCs were developed by many universities in a variety of disciplines including health care. Learners from across the globe participated in MOOCs. "Like most innovations, MOOCs passed through Gartner's (2017) hype cycle … and fell into Gartner's trough of disillusionment. With interest in creating MOOCs subsiding, some universities did not reap the benefits of offering the free online courses they developed." (Skiba 2017, p. 291). To renew the interest in MOOCs, the model was adapted to move toward sustainability and profitability. There still exists some free MOOCs but other business models have evolved and include charges for grading and certificates of completion or a subscription model with fees.

The major MOOC providers include:

- Coursera (https://www.coursera.org/)
- EdX (https://www.edx.org/)
- FutureLearn (https://www.futurelearn.com/).

15.8   Connected Health

With the advent of the connected age, higher education was not alone in their transformation. The connected age also impacted health care and spurred the development of Connected Health. Caulfield and Donnelly (2013, p. 704) were one of the first to define it as

Connected Health encompasses terms such as wireless, digital, electronic, mobile, and telehealth and refers to a conceptual model for health management where devices, services or interventions are designed around the patient's needs, and health related data is shared, in such a way that the patient can receive care in the most proactive and efficient manner possible. All stakeholders in the process are 'connected' by means of timely sharing and presentation of accurate and pertinent information regarding patient status through smarter use of data, devices, communication platforms and people.

Their position was that it was not just technology that was promoting connected health but it was the rise of consumerism. More and more people were engaging in their healthcare through the use of mobile applications, access to patient portals and consumer products like blood pressure monitoring equipment. Connected health represented a transition from telemedicine and e-health concepts.

More recently as the digital world became more popular in society, the term has evolved into Digital Health. In 2019, The World Health Organization noted that

The term digital health is rooted in eHealth, which is defined as "the use of information and communications technology in support of health and health-related fields". Mobile health (mHealth) is a subset of eHealth and is defined as "the use of mobile wireless technologies for health". More recently, the term digital health was introduced as "a broad umbrella term encompassing eHealth (which includes mHealth), as well as emerging areas, such as the use of advanced computing sciences in 'big data', genomics and artificial intelligence. (WHO 2019)

More recently, the Health Information Management Systems Society (HIMSS) on 2 March 2020 published the following definition of digital health as

Digital health connects and empowers people and populations to manage health and wellness, augmented by accessible and supportive provider teams working within flexible, integrated, interoperable and digitally-enabled care environments that strategically leverage digital tools, technologies and services to transform care delivery. (Snowden 2020) (https://www.himss.org/news/himss-defines-digital-health-global-healthcare-industry).

Given the rise in digital health, it is incumbent on nursing education to ensure future and current nurses are prepared to practice in this digital health era. Numerous countries have recognized the need to prepare nurses to practice in a digital health ecosystem. In some countries, the nursing association were responsible for setting the agenda to prepare nurses for the digital era. In other cases, individual schools of nursing were preparing the nursing workforce through both formal education or professional development programs. Here are a few examples across various countries.

- In Finland, The Finnish Nursing Association developed the *eHealth Strategy of the Finnish Nurses Association 2015–2020* (https://sairaanhoitajat.fi/wp-content/uploads/2020/01/eHealth_RAPORTTI-_ENGLANTI.pdf).
- In the United States, the National League for Nursing released a statement, *A Vision for The Changing Faculty Role: Preparing Students for the Technological World of Health Care* (http://www.nln.org/docs/default-source/about/nln-vision-series-(position-statements)/a-vision-for-the-changing-faculty-role-preparing-students-for-the-technological-world-of-health-care.pdf?sfvrsn=0). In this document, they made recommendations to Administrators, Faculty and to their organization on how to incorporate more teaching and clinical experiences to prepare current nursing students about digital health, in particular tools related to consumer engagement, data analytics/visualization and virtual health.
- The Royal College of Nursing in the United Kingdom developed a campaign, *Every nurse an e-nurse*, to prepare nurses for their digital health roles (https://www.digitalhealth.net/2017/08/nhs-digital-endorses-every-nurse-an-e-nurse-campaign/) and in 2017, there was the launch of the NHS Digital Academy (https://digital.nhs.uk/about-nhs-digital/careers/the-academy-at-nhs-digital) in 2017 to prepare leaders to promote the NHS's digital transformation.
- In Canada, a national survey was conducted to describe the current state of the inclusion of digital health content in the nursing education curriculum. It also identified exemplars of digital health integration (https://www.casn.ca/wp-content/uploads/2019/06/SoN-Final-Report-EN.pdf). The study identified there was a gap in teaching nurses about digital health across schools of nursing. They also found educators taught "about the use of technology for teaching and learning as

opposed to the technologies used specifically in the delivery and management of health care services." (Nagel et al. 2018, p. 6). Another interesting finding was that educators felt because students were computer literate, they were therefore also digital health literate.

- In New Zealand, Honey et al. (2020) conducted a study to develop nursing informatics competencies specific within the context of their country. The result was the development of Guidelines for Nursing Informatics Competencies for Undergraduate Nurses in New Zealand (https://auckland.figshare.com/articles/ Guidelines_Informatics_for_nurses_entering_practice/7273037)
- More recently, The Australian Digital Health Agency (ADHA) conducted a survey to "identify the necessary digital health capabilities for nurses and midwives to further improve the quality, safety and efficiency of care (https://www.hisa. org.au/nurses-and-midwives-framework/).

Here are some examples of schools of nursing incorporating digital health education in their curriculum.

- Drake and Leander (2013) described the use of a social network (NING) to engage community health students across 11 different nursing schools in an online assignment. The assignment was for students to watch a video, "In Sickness and in Wealth" and engage in guided discussions related to their understanding of health disparity.
- Jackson, Getting and Metcalfe (2018) described how nursing students at the Florence Nightingale Faculty of Nursing, Midwifery & Palliative Care at King's College London were encouraged to use Twitter to share the most pertinent and key messages from presentations given at a nursing conference. The exercise helped students to engage in the appropriate use of social media to share ideas within the nursing community.
- Ross and Myers (2017) described a social networking project in which students from two countries connected with each other to learn about cultural competence. The students were given opportunities to connect via Facebook, wikis, blogs and Skype.

The University of Colorado has implemented various learning activities for all graduate students to learn more about digital health. These learning opportunities provide them with experiences to use and evaluate various digital health tools. Here is an example:

Patient Portal Exercise: Students are sent a patient portal email asking for help in seeking a website, a social network to join and a mobile application to manage their new diagnosis of epilepsy. Student received the email and access to the patient's electronic health record and their last two health visit summaries. The student must use evaluation criteria to assess an appropriate web page, social network and a mobile application. They then response to the patient's email.

Students may also take a course, Digital Tools for Connected Health

- Emoji assignment: Students are asked to propose a plan to facilitate the use of emojis to interact and monitor students with a particular chronic disease.

- Evaluation of a mobile app: Students are asked to select a mobile application from the Veterans Administration Mobile Applications Store (https://www. mobile.va.gov/appstore/). They download the free m-app and then using evaluation criteria to assess the application.
- Visit different web sites (such as https://aflacchildhoodcancer.org/ or https:// www.ces.tech/Topics/Health-Wellness/Digital-Health.aspx) related to innovative consumer digital tools and determine their potential in clinical environments and for consumer engagement.
- Digital Health Campaign-Create a video campaign that highlights the benefits and challenges of a digital health tool for a designated patient population or nursing staff.

15.9 Virtual Visits with Patients

As health care institutions begin to embrace digital health, there has been a greater acceptance of virtual patient visits. The coronavirus pandemic served as a catalyst to offer patients the opportunity to have a virtual patient visit. Using secure video conferencing system available for desktop, tablets or smartphones serve as the platform for these virtual visits. In some cases, the virtual visit may be initiated by a virtual assistant (chatbot) that will seek pertinent information from the patient before connecting the patient to their health care professional. Here are some different examples of how faculty are preparing nurses to participate in virtual patient visits.

Grady (2011) was a pioneer in the development of a virtual practicum for nursing students. Students enrolled in an Associate degree program course on the management of adult patients with complex health needs. Students from this rural area conducted patient visits via telehealth video conferencing. The patients were at a military base hospital in another state. The telehealth connection allowed for visits with the patients and joining with the health care team as they discussed the particular patient and their health care needs.

Merritt, Brauch, Bender and Kochuk (2018) developed a web-based simulation to teach nurse practitioner student to conduct an e-visit. Students were introduced to virtual patients and had the ability to interact with the patients by selecting questions. Responses to their questions were recorded voice over patient responses. The student conducted the e-visit by identifying the appropriate diagnosis and documenting a management plan including prescriptions and pertinent patient education.

Erickson, Fauchald and Ideker (2015) created a telehealth experience for their nurse practitioner students. The students first received training in conducting a telehealth visit and were then assigned a 4 hour clinical to conduct telehealth visits. Using a video conferencing system, students connected with off-site telehealth provider and with their patients. Students were allowed to observe and interact with the patient and the provider during the visit.

At the University of Colorado, family nurse practitioners students teamed with a pharmacy student to conduct a virtual visit with a standardized patient (Skiba

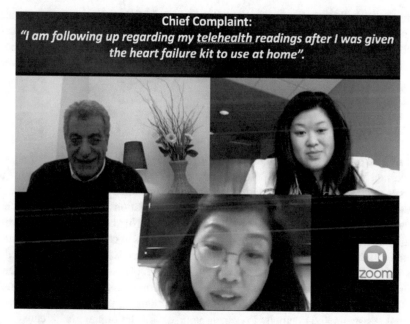

Fig. 15.3 A three-way virtual patient visit with a nurse practitioner student, a pharmacy student and a standardized patient

et al. 2016). The standardized patient was trained to use the video conferencing system and also how to use a variety of digital health tools. The standardized patient was a 74 year old man who has a follow up visit with his health care team after being discharged from the hospital with his heart failure kit for use at home. This heart failure kit included the following digital health tools: Digital Stethoscope, Pulse Oximeter, Wireless Blood Pressure Monitor & Smart Body Weight Analyzer. Students evaluated the experience as being valuable and it prepared them to participate in virtual visits in their professional roles (Estes et al. 2016) (Fig. 15.3).

15.10   On the Horizon

As we look to the future, the digital ecosystem will continue to expand with the use of more smart tools. As Sarasohn-Kahn noted "the new front door for healthcare will be the patients' home front door." (Sarasohn-Kahn 2018). Patients will have access to numerous digital health tools and massive amounts of data to facilitate their health care decisions (Skiba 2018a). These digital tools will include wearable smart devices, mobile apps, robots and virtual assistants. Healthcare will witness the intersection of data, devices and artificial intelligence that will lend itself to the concept of an invisible health care professional (Skiba 2018b). This invisible health care professional may be a virtual chatbot using artificial intelligence to determine a diagnosis or help with the management of chronic health conditions. As these technologies become commonplace in our health care ecosystem, nurses will need additional preparation to interact and care for future patients, families and caregivers.

15.11 Summary

As a nurse either starting their career or currently a nurse in practice, it is of utmost important for you to become a technology enabled nurse. There is a need for all nurses to develop competencies that allow them to practice in a digital health ecosystem. Nurses will encounter the use of virtual simulations in their practice when they are introduced to new or complicated patients. Nurses will be using virtual reality devices with their patients and assigning patients to complete virtual simulations to understand more about their particular health care issue. Nurses will need to manage a deluge of patient data from digital health tools and understand data analytics and data visualization. Nurses will need new communication and engagement skills to provide virtual care to patients in their homes as well as interacting with virtual assistants and chatbots. Preparing yourself for the digital health ecosystem will enable the technology enabled nurse will become a valuable asset within the digital health ecosystem.

Review Questions
1. In your clinical practice, how might you/a health care team use immersive clinical simulations to continue to develop your clinical expertise?
2. You are serving on a hospital quality improvement committee, you are interested in increasing your knowledge about quality improvement. What online learning opportunities are available to you?
3. To gain a better understanding of the responsibilities of a technology enabled nurse, this video lecture will introduce you to a patient, Josephine, recently discharged from the hospital and how digital tools are helping her recovery at home (https://youtu.be/EjletAiz1_8). The video starts with the description Internet of Things (IOT) and the concept of connected care. You will meet Josephine and see how she was using digital health tools through her inpatient care and also when she was discharged. Here are some questions:

   (a) What digital health tool was being used when she was receiving inpatient care? How was she using this tool during her inpatient stay? How will this tool going to impact your nursing role?
   (b) What digital health tools was she given upon discharge? What are the pros and cons of these tools?
   (c) Where can you seek advice for recommending digital health tools for your patients?

Answers

1. Here are some examples of how your health care team might use a virtual simulation. You are providing care for a Covid-19 patient who has underlying conditions such as pulmonary hypertension. Your education program can program a virtual case scenario and your team could interact with this virtual patient to develop a plan of care. You could also use a virtual reality device to practice your skills in preparing yourself with Personal Protective Equipment (PPE). Using a virtual reality device to better understand the process of intubation and Ventilation to explain to your patient's family.

2. Here are some examples of how you can increase your professional knowledge. You can do a google search and find the Institute for Healthcare Improvement and see they have open courses as well as a wealth of online resources. You can go to Coursera and find the following MOCCs that are available: Leading Healthcare Quality and Safety (George Washington University), Take the lead on healthcare quality improvement (Case Western Reserve University) Patient safety and quality improvement: Developing s systems review (Johns Hopkins University) or go to FutureLearn and find Quality Improvement in Healthcare: The case for change (University of Bath) and Making Change in a healthcare environment (University of East Anglia)

3. Here are the responses for the case study

   (a) Josephine is given a tablet in the inpatient setting. This tablet provides here with access to her interprofessional health care team, view her health assessment, patient goals and treatment plan. She is also able to develop her own personal health goals and can access health care educational materials.

   (b) Josephine is given a digital stethoscope, pulse oximeter, blood pressure monitor and digital weight scale. The advantages are the patients will be able to monitor herself in between virtual visits with her health care provider. Her family will also be able to see her progress. Data can also be transmitted to her health care provider to alert them if there is a health issue that needs attention. Some issues may be that the patient lacks access to the Internet, does not have the digital literacy to use the tools and issue of who pays for the access to these digital health tools. Security and privacy issues may also be of concern.

   (c) I can contact the nursing informatics specialists at my hospital or the health care informatics office.

Glossary

Computer-based simulations Virtual environments, created digitally, in which students can engage in scenarios to mimic real life situations and complete tasks designed to enhance their learning

Connected health Healthcare that is inclusive and utilizes digital health technologies

Enhanced learning Teaching and learning using a variety of digitally-mediated technologies

Online learning Active learning using digital technologies to engage with course content, peers, and faculty in a dynamic manner

Virtual visits Health care encounter between a provider and client using digital or virtual platforms

References

Aebersold M, Rasmussen J, Mulrenin T. Virtual Everest: immersive virtual reality can improve the simulation experience. Clin Simul Nurs. 2020;38:1–4. https://doi.org/10.1016/j.ecns.2019.09.004.

Andrea J, Kotowski P. Using standardized patients in an undergraduate nursing health assessment class. Clin Simul Nurs. 2017;13:309–13. https://doi.org/10.1016/j.ecns.2017.05.003.

Ball S, Hussey L. The effects of augmented reality on prelicensure nursing students' anxiety levels. J Nurs Educ. 2020;59:142–8.

Bell MW. Toward a definition of "virtual worlds". J Virtual Worlds Res. 2008;1:1–5.

Billings D, Connors H, Skiba D. Benchmarking best practices in nursing web-based courses. Adv Nurs Sci. 2001;23:41–52.

Brender E, Burke A, Glass RM. Standardized patients. JAMA. 2005;294:1172.

Cant R, Cooper S, Sussex R, Bogossian F. What's in a name? Clarifying the nomenclature of virtual simulation. Clin Simul Nurs. 2019;27:26–30. https://doi.org/10.1016/j.ecns.2018.11.003.11.

Caulfield B, Donnelly S. What is connected health and why will it change your practice? QJM. 2013;106:703–7. https://doi.org/10.1093/qjmed/hct114.

Chaballout B, Molloy M, Vaughn J, Brisson R III, Shaw R. Feasibility of augmented reality in clinical simulations: using google glass with manikins. JMIR Med Educ. 2016;2:e2. https://doi.org/10.2196/mededu.5159.

Chickering AW, Ehrmann SC. Implementing the seven principles: technology as lever. Amer Assoc High Educ Bull. 1996;49:3–6.

Cook MJ. Design and initial evaluation of a virtual pediatric primary care clinic in second life. J Am Acad Nurse Pract. 2012;24:521–7. https://doi.org/10.1111/j.1745-7599.2012.00729.x.

Cullen E. What is technology enhanced learning. Interactive blog. 10 September 2018. https://www.mentimeter.com/blog/interactive-classrooms/what-is-technology-enhanced-learning-and-why-is-it-important. Accessed 5 April 2020.

Danforth C, Condon T, Deforest R, Marini A, Al AZ. Informatics students across the globe learn to collaborate in second life. In: Abbott P, Hullin C, Nagle L, editors. Studies in informatics: advancing global health through informatics. Proceedings of the NI2012. The 11th international congress of nursing informatics. American Medical Informatics Association: Bethesda, MD; 2012. p. 376–80.

Drake M, Leander S. Nursing students and Ning: using social networking to teach public health/community nursing in 11 baccalaureate nursing programs. Nurs Educ Persp. 2013;34:270–2.

Educause. MOOCs: seven things you should know about MOOCs. https://library.educause.edu/resources/2011/11/7-things-you-should-know-about-moocs. Accessed 5 April 2020.

Ellaway R, Poulton T, Fors U, McGee J, Albright S. Building a virtual patient commons. Med Teach. 2008;30:170–4. https://doi.org/10.1080/01421590701874074.

Erickson C, Fauchald S, Ideker M. Integrating telehealth into the graduate nursing curriculum. J Nurs Pract. 2015;11:e1–5.

Estes K, Gilliam E, Knapfel S, Lee C, Skiba D. Discovering eHealth technology: an innovative interprofessional graduate student learning experience. In: Weber P, Seremus W, Proctor P, editors. The 13th international nursing informatics congress. Leiden: IOS Press; 2016.

Flin R, O'Connor P, Crichton M. Safety at the sharp end: training non-technical skills. Cornwall: Ashgate Publishing; 2008.

Foronda C, Crenshaw N, Briones L, Snowden K, Griffin M, Mitzova-Valdinov G. Teaching and learning the skill of intubation using telehealth glasses. Clini Sim Nurs. 2020;40:31–5.

Forsberg E, Georg C, Ziegert K, Fors U. Virtual patients for assessment of clinical reasoning in nursing—a pilot study. Nurs Educ Today. 2011;31:757–62. https://doi.org/10.1016/j.nedt.2010.11.015.

Forsberg E, Bäcklund B, Telhede EH, Karlsson S. Virtual patient cases for active student participation in nursing education—students' learning experiences. Creat Educ. 2019;10:1475–91. https://doi.org/10.4236/ce.2019.107108.

Gartner. Gartner hype cycle. 2017. www.gartner.com/technology/research/methodologies/hypecycle.jsp. Accessed 5 April 2020.

Gibbons S, Adamo G, Padden D, Ricciardi R, Graziano M, Levine E, Hawkins R. Clinical evaluation in advanced practice nursing education: using standardized patients in health assessment. J Nurs Ed. 2002;41:215–21. https://doi.org/10.3928/0148-4834-20020501-07.

Grady J. The virtual clinical practicum: an innovative telehealth model for clinical nursing education. Nurs Educ Persp. 2011;32:189–94.

Harder N. Evolution of simulation use in health care education. Clin Simul Nurs. 2009;5:e169–72.

Hermann E. Mrs. chase: a noble and enduring figure. Am J Nurs. 1981;81:1836.

Honey M, Collins E, Britnell S. Education into policy: embedding health informatics to prepare future nurses—New Zealand case study. JMIR Nurs. 2020;3:e16186. https://doi.org/10.2196/16186.

Interaction Design Foundation. Augmented reality. https://www.interaction-design.org/literature/topics/augmented-reality. Accessed 5 April 2020.

Jackson J, Gettings S, Metcalfe A. "The power of twitter:" using social media at a conference with nursing students. Nurs Educ Today. 2018;68:188–91. https://doi.org/10.1016/j.nedt.2018.06.017.

Jenson CE, Forsyth DM. Virtual reality simulation: using three-dimensional technology to teach nursing students. Comput Inform Nurs. 2012;30:312–8.

Johnson L, Adams S, Cummins M. The NMC horizon report: 2012 higher education edition. Austin, TX: New Media Consortium; 2012.

Kouri ML, Rissanen P, Weber P, Park H. Competencies in social media use in the area of health and healthcare. In: Murphy J, Goossen W, editors. Forecasting informatics competencies for nurses in the future of connected health. Leiden: IOS Press; 2017.

Manos E, Modaress N. A paradigm shift in simulation: experiential learning in virtual worlds and future use of virtual reality, robotics and drone. In Saba V, McCormick, K (editors). Essentials of nursing informatics. 2020,

Merritt L, Brauch A, Bender A, Kochuk D. Using a web-based e-visit simulation to educate nurse practitioner students. J Nurs Educ. 2018;57:304–7.

Nagle L, Kleib M, Furlong K. Study of digital health in Canadian schools of nursing: curricular content and nurse educator capacity. A report of the findings-2018. Canada Health Infoway and Canadian Association of Schools of Nursing. 2018. https://www.casn.ca/wp-content/uploads/2019/06/SoN-Final-Report-EN.pdf. Accessed 5 April 2020.

Oblinger DG. The connected age for higher education is here. Are we ready for the future? EDUCAUSE Rev. 2013;48:4–5.

Padilha JM, Machado PP, Ribeiro A, Ramos J, Costa P. Clinical virtual simulation in nursing education: randomized controlled trial. J Med Internet Res. 2019;21:e11529. https://doi.org/10.2196/11529.

Peddle M, Bearman M, Nestel D. Virtual patients and nontechnical skills in undergraduate health professional education: an integrative review. Clin Simul Nurs. 2016;12:400–10. https://doi.org/10.1016/j.ecns.2016.04.004.

Proctor P, Brixey J, Honey M, Todhunter F. Social media and population health virtual exchange for senior nursing students: an international collaboration. In: Weber PW, Seremus W, Proctor P, editors. The 13th international nursing informatics congress. Leiden: IOS Press; 2016.

Ross J, Myers S. The current use of social media in undergraduate nursing education: a review of the literature. Comput Inform Nurs. 2017;35:338–44.

Sarasohn-Kahn J. Healthcare comes home at CES. 2018. https://www.huffpost.com/entry/health-care-comes-home-at-ces-2018_b_5a553760e4b0e3dd5c3f8cec. Accessed 5 April 2020.

Sarmasoglu S, Dince L, Elcon M. Using standardized patients in nursing education: effects on Students' psychomotor skill development. Nurs Ed. 2016;41:e1–5.

Schaffer M, Tiffany J, Kentack K, Anderson L. Second life virtual learning in public health nursing. J Nurs Educ. 2016;55:536–40.

Shaikh F, Inayat F, Awan O, Santos M, Choudhry A, Waheed A, Tuli S. Computer-assisted learning applications in health educational informatics: a review. Cureus J Med Sci. 2017;9:e1559.

Shin H, Rim D, Kim H, Park S, Shon S. Educational characteristics of virtual simulation in nursing: an integrative review. Clin Simul Nurs. 2019;37:18–28. https://doi.org/10.1016/j.ecns.2019.08.002.

Skiba D. Disruption in higher education: massively open online courses (MOOCs). Nurs Educ Persp. 2012;33:416–7.

Skiba D. What has happened to massively open online courses? Nurs Educ Persp. 2017;38:291–2.

Skiba D. Consumer electronic show 2018: a focus on digital health tools. Nurs Educ Persp. 2018a;39:194–5.

Skiba D. The invisible health care professional: exploring the intersection of data, devices and artificial intelligence. Nurs Educ Persp. 2018b;39(4):264–5.

Skiba D, Barton A, Knapfel S, Moore G, Trinkley K. Infusing informatics into Interprofessional education: the iTEAM (interprofessional technology enhanced advanced practice model) project. In: Saranto K, Weaver C, Chang P, editors. East meets west: eSMART. Proceedings of the 12th international congress on nursing informatics. Leiden: IOS Press; 2014.

Skiba D, Barton A, Estes K, Gilliam E, Knapfel S, Lee C, Moore G, Trinkley K. Preparing the next generation of advanced practice nurses for connected care. In: Weber P, Seremus W, Proctor P, editors. The 13th international nursing informatics congress. Leiden: IOS Press; 2016.

Snowden A. Health information management systems society (HIMSS). HIMSS defines digital health for the global healthcare industry. 2020. https://www.himss.org/news/himss-defines-digital-health-global-healthcare-industry. Accessed 5 April 2020.

University of Edinburgh Institute for Academic Development. What is digital learning? 2018. https://www.ed.ac.uk/institute-academic-development/learning-teaching/staff/digital-ed/what-is-digital-education. Accessed 5 April 2020.

Verkuyl M, Romaniuk D, Atack L, Mastrilli P. Virtual gaming simulation for nursing education: an experiment. Clin Simul Nurs. 2017;13:238–44. https://doi.org/10.1016/j.ecns.2017.02.004.

Weiner E, Gordon J, Rudy S, McNew R. Expanding virtual reality to teach ultrasound skills to nurse practitioner students. In: Ohno-Machado L, Seroussi B, editors. Health and wellbeing e-networks for all. Proceedings of the 17th world congress on medical and health informatics; 2019.

WHO. WHO guideline: recommendations on digital interventions for health system strengthening. Geneva: World Health Organization; 2019.

Zary N, Johnson G, Boberg J, Fors UG. Development, implementation and pilot evaluation of a web-based virtual patient case simulation environment-web-SP. BMC Med Educ. 2006;6:10. https://doi.org/10.1186/1472-6920-6-10.

Chapter 16
The Future of Nursing Informatics in a Digitally-Enabled World

Richard Booth, Gillian Strudwick, Josephine McMurray, Ryan Chan, Kendra Cotton, and Samantha Cooke

Abstract The nursing profession has a history of embracing novel technologies that support the delivery of compassionate, person-centred care. The emergence and rapid adoption of 'intelligent' technologies that have the ability to act autonomously, but that are often embedded and 'invisible' to users, is challenging the nursing profession to reconsider their role in the health system of the future. Using a socio-technical lens the authors examine artificial intelligence and process automation technologies because of their significant potential to become much further embedded into nursing work and disrupt the healthcare system as we know it. Opportunities for nurses to transform their role in the healthcare value chain, will arise from the profession's proactive reconceptualization of the nursing role in an era where technology is moving from discrete transaction processing and monitoring applications to pervasive computing. But the nurse's traditional patient and family advocacy role will remain important, as policy, regulatory and ethical challenges arise from the development and use of these emergent digital technologies. The rapidly changing healthcare ecosystem demands nursing involvement in the research, design, adoption and use of emergent digital technologies. The subtle normalization of these technologies into the nursing role will require new nursing knowledge and skills, and different relationships between nurses (i.e., practice, education, research, leadership) and other actors (i.e. patients, physicians, technologies) in the healthcare ecosystem of the future.

R. Booth (✉) · R. Chan · K. Cotton · S. Cooke
Arthur Labatt Family School of Nursing, Western University, London, ON, Canada
e-mail: rbooth6@uwo.ca; rchan228@uwo.ca; kcotton4@uwo.ca; scooke28@uwo.ca

G. Strudwick
Centre for Addiction and Mental Health, Toronto, Ontario, Canada

Institute of Health Policy, Management and Evaluation, University of Toronto, Toronto, ON, Canada
e-mail: gillian.strudwick@camh.ca

J. McMurray
Business Technology Management/Health Studies, Wilfrid Laurier University, Waterloo, ON, Canada
e-mail: jmcmurray@wlu.ca

© Springer Nature Switzerland AG 2021
P. Hussey, M. A. Kennedy (eds.), *Introduction to Nursing Informatics*, Health Informatics, https://doi.org/10.1007/978-3-030-58740-6_16

Keywords Nursing informatics · Digital health · Emergent digital technology ·
Health information technology · Nursing · Artificial intelligence · Robotics ·
Socio-technical · Future · Nursing

Learning Objectives for Chapter
1. Understand emergent digital technology, as related to nursing practice, education, research, and leadership.
2. Explore new social and technical (socio-technical) relationships that are beginning to emerge between humans and technology in all areas of nursing practice.
3. Understand philosophical and conceptual inquiry as it relates to the use of artificial intelligence and robots/robotics within nursing practice and future models of care.
4. Evaluate the ethical, social justice, and nursing care implications of emergent digital technology like artificial intelligence and robotics upon various aspects of the nursing role.

16.1   Introduction

The nursing profession has witnessed significant technological and societal change over the last few decades. With the increased adoption of all forms of electronic and communication innovations and increasing diffusion of emergent digital technologies like artificial intelligence across all areas of society, the nursing profession is currently entering a critical point in its history. How will the emergent technological forces of today *shape* the nursing profession, and the role and function of nursing in the future? How can the profession differentiate itself from other caring professions? How do emergent technologies complement current nursing value(s) and reveal entirely new ones? The profession as we know it, may be facing a subtle existential crisis - what will the nursing role *look like* and *be like*, in the future?

In this chapter, we will explore the rapid growth and adoption of emergent digital technologies and the impact, growth and relevance to the nursing profession now and into the future. While nursing has a long track record of using innovation in both proactive and creative fashions, the exponential growth of disruptive emergent digital technologies has resulted in uncertainty around how best to align current-state nursing roles and knowledge with approaches to health(care) in the not-too-distant future. Although it is has been predicted that many of the roles and skills currently fulfilled by nurses will continue to exist in the foreseeable future (Frey and Osborne 2017), remaining static as a profession in this quickly evolving environment will likely be incompatible with a productive or prosperous future (Booth et al. 2019). To help practitioners plan for this future, the chapter will also help identify strategic opportunities and practical suggestions as to areas where nursing can evolve in meaningful and proactive ways that leverage emergent digital technologies to advance the profession and remain relevant to the goal of improved patient care. The chapter will conclude with a range of strategic planning considerations and exemplars to help guide practitioners to reconceptualize aspects of their nursing role in light of emergent digital technology, and reflect on how the profession can differentiate itself and generate new and innovative ways to contribute to the healthcare value chain in a digitized and automated world. While not always comfortable, with this level of discussion and candour we hope to stimulate timely and important reflection of the nursing profession.

16.2   Current State

The current state of the nursing profession in relation to informatics and other digital technologies is both extensive and multi-dimensional. Recent societal and global events (i.e., COVID-19 pandemic, climate change induced diseases and disasters) have reinforced the importance and potential of modern information and communication technology. It would be redundant to enter into a discussion here about what the nursing profession uses *now* in terms of technology (as of writing in April 2020) or to provide a list of current state technologies that are important within contemporary nursing. For that we encourage readers to consult other chapters of this book and the numerous other resources available on the topic (Booth et al. 2019; Risling 2017; Morse et al. 2019; Frazier et al. 2019; Huston 2013).

Instead we intend to explore nursing's current-state interpretation of *emergent* digital technologies. Over the decades, numerous scholars and practitioners have presented their ideas regarding the state and value of all forms of technology used within the nursing profession. Taken as a collective, there appears to be an underlying notion across much of the nursing discourse that the impressive growth and diversity of technology adoption happens around or adjacent to the nursing profession. That is, the nursing profession possesses the ability to remain largely unchanged in the types of traditional roles and activities for which its known, despite an ever-increasing variety and complexity of emergent digital technologies used in and for nursing work. Although there are a variety of reasons the nursing profession commonly elects to discuss informatics and emergent digital technology from a socially-grounded and human-centric perspective, for the remainder of this chapter, we will adopt a more balanced conceptual lens that balances the *social* aspects of action (e.g., nursing roles, their relationships with patients, etc.) with the complementary *technical* aspects of reality (e.g., emergent digital technology and the processes they facilitate, etc.). We believe this *socio-technical* (Berg et al. 2003; Sittig and Singh 2010) approach to conceive and generate recommendations for future practice offers a more balanced theoretical perspective from which to generate implications for future practice. As we progress in this fashion, it will become quickly apparent that the digital healthcare ecosystems of the future will challenge the nursing profession's conception of the nursing role and necessitate a move to leverage the best elements of *what is human* and *what is technology*. It must engage in discussion that privileges both social and technical features as equally powerful, important, and essential to the generation of realistic recommendations for the future of nursing as it relates to emergent digital technology.

16.3   Nursing's Contemporary Relationship with Technology

The dominance of discourse in nursing about advantage or disadvantage of technology exemplifies a profession struggling to come to terms with the phenomenon. (Barnard, 2016, p. 9)

As described by Barnard (2016), throughout nursing discourse *technology* (of all types) is often characterized as an object or tool which, through the act of being used by a nurse, can generate outcomes that are potentially beneficial to practice. While a seemingly accurate characterization, the role, presence, and potential value of technology within the profession has been largely reduced to discussions about the explicit advantages and disadvantages brought by the presence or functionality of a specific technology (Barnard 2016). The nursing informatics literature has a long tradition of discussing and examining various technologies used by nurses in practice, leadership, research and education, commonly through a lens that assesses benefits and/or drawbacks. Although this approach to conceptualizing the role and merits of technology is valuable, these high-level assessments fall short when applied to newer forms of emergent digital technologies many of which invisibly shape models of practice and nursing activities.

For instance, there is a long lineage of health and nursing informatics research that describes how traditional health technology (e.g., electronic medical records, bar code medication administration systems, etc.) used by practitioners can sometimes (re)shape actions of people in both intended and unintended fashions (Koppel et al. 2005; Gephart et al. 2015; Novak et al. 2013). As both Sandelowski (1999) and Barnard (2002) describe, nursing discourse has privileged the notion that technology sometimes possesses an overt ability to direct the actions of people, and to be "everywhere we practice, yet we are not always aware of it" (Barnard 2002, p. 19). These seemingly invisible forces acting upon and between the relationship of nurses and technology continues to accurately depict the contemporary reality faced by many nurses, especially as related to emergent technologies that use advanced functionality like artificial intelligence. Recently, concerted efforts have been undertaken within informatics research to synthesize how emergent digital technology using artificial intelligence and other self-learning functionalities *can* and *do* influence their human clinician counterparts in both intended and unintended fashions (Shortliffe and Sepúlveda 2018; Lynn 2019; Cresswell et al. 2020). Given the increasing embeddedness of many newer technologies and an individual's inability to consistently be "aware of it" (Barnard 2002, p. 19), we propose that the rapid evolution of many modern-day technologies has superseded the abilities of many nurses to remain situationally aware of their presence in health(care) practice. In the span of less than a decade, all forms of mobile technology, digital communications infrastructure, robotics, and innovations using artificial intelligence which were once the narratives of science fiction, have become fixed realities in many western societies and health(care) practices. Although technology has evolved significantly, nursing's conceptualization and descriptions of technology and the new human-technical relationships it can stimulate are still constrained by a range of traditional semantic and cultural factors. As described by Sandelowski (1999), the nursing profession has historically utilized a "traditional western binary distinction…" (p. 204) between what is conceived to be *human* and what is *technology*. Further, Sandelowski (1997) suggests that "English language customs make it difficult to convey the human-technology relation as other than one of us/it and cause and effect" (p. 222). While written over 20 years ago, the desire to discuss the function of humans and technology separately persists today. While it would seem that the semantic division of humans and technology is still commonly preferred in nursing discourse, the rapid integration of emergent digital technology in the profession and across society is making it increasingly difficult to ignore how interdependent the relationships between humans and technology have become. For instance, with a range of wearable Internet of Things (IoT) devices now available (e.g., FitBit, biometric trackers, modern smartphones) that connect humans to devices and to larger networks of devices (e.g., 5G cellular internet, home automation technology, social media platforms), that also possess varieties of potentially human (e.g., real-time chat for product consultations, multi-person webinar and teleconference technology) and non-human interaction points (e.g., internet bots, personalized marketing, artificial intelligence bots for journalism, news articles, and publications, blockchain), we are entering a new paradigm where it is almost impossible to discuss the modern-day activities of humans in the absence of technology. With the blurring boundaries between embedded digital technology and many activities of daily life, it is increasingly difficult, if not impossible, to conceptualize nursing actions in the absence of some form of modern digital technology (and vice versa). Although it is appreciated that nursing is not technology and technology is not nursing, the challenge for practitioners and scholars moving into the future is to embrace and better understand the socio-technical relationships that have become normalized (either consciously or unconsciously) over the last decade.

16.4 Conscious and Unconscious Normalization

As described by Agar (2015), *hedonic normalization* is the tendency for people to form "goals and experiences … [as] appropriate to the environments experienced as an individual comes to maturity." Simply put in reference to technology, experience of using technology by an individual is normalized through use of the specific technology. Over time, an individual can add to their baseline of experiences, and subsequently normalize the use, function, and existence of the innovation as being commonplace or necessary for action. If the technology is useful and beneficial to individuals, they continue to draw hedonic gains from its use, which can eventually result in treating the innovation as *normal* or potentially requisite in everyday life.

As an extension to Agar's interpretation of hedonic normalization, we suggest that the rate of change and innovation has become so rapid in recent times, that most individuals no longer have adequate time to consciously understand or realize which digital technologies they normalize into everyday life. Thus, we propose that hedonic normalization of technology occurs at a rate faster than individual generations of people now realize, and commonly occurs unconsciously, stimulated by the nature and subtle embeddedness of many modern-day digital technologies in daily life. Insomuch as we have entered a new time period in nursing history where the life cycles of technology occur so quickly, we suggest that conscious awareness of the role, function, and even presence of many innovations is never fully realized by users of the technology. For instance, there are over 100 million artificially-intelligent, cloud-computer connected, natural language conversational Amazon Alexa smart devices that have been sold to date (Bohn 2019). A decade ago, a device like the modern-day Alexa would have been described as a primordial prototype of a future voice-enabled smart device; two decades ago, a device like Alexa would have been viewed more of an artifact arising from science-fiction, than an easily obtainable piece of digital technology that is currently sold globally. From a nursing perspective, we have entered a new domain where the profession is having to evolve in response to many types of emergent digital technology, and awareness of this evolution and intended [or unintended] consequences may not be present or appreciated. To our original point, we have stumbled into a reality where the socio-technical blurring of human and technological roles, knowledge, and action occurs on a daily basis in nursing, commonly without conscious awareness. In the coming sections, we provide explicit examples where blurring is happening between the nursing role and emergent digital technology, and explore the new roles, actions, and knowledge possible from this reconceptualized human-technical relationship. Furthermore, we expand upon how nursing must position itself to impact healthcare and patient outcomes in the technology-normalized future.

16.5   Conceptualizing the Future of Nursing

Across society, many types of emergent digital technologies have been used to stimulate new patterns of human behavior, models of economy, and approaches to knowledge sharing and dissemination. With the generation of new approaches to human action, new relationships between humans and technology are formed, refined, and evolved as necessary. While nursing and healthcare have begun to leverage many of these emergent digital approaches in support of nursing work and knowledge generation, further discussion of how nursing can leverage the best parts of human presence, knowledge, and abilities augmented by the power of emergent digital technology must be conducted. To do this, deeper exploration and reconceptualization of nursing roles and knowledge in health(care) activities of the future is required. Through theorization of the future roles and knowledge requirements, this chapter aims to provide practitioners with a blueprint from which to begin reconceptualizing all aspects of nursing practice, education, research, and leadership.

16.5.1   Future Roles and Knowledge Required by Nurses

In light of the advances in novel technologies, there is a substantive amount of scholarly literature exploring the future trajectory of the profession (Tanioka et al. 2019; Buchanan et al. 2020; Nagle et al. 2017; Topaz et al. 2016; Strudwick et al. 2020; Remus and Kennedy 2012a; Remus and Donelle 2019; Fridsma 2018). Within the nursing informatics domain, experts have speculated on various competencies and trends that will be important over the coming decade. For instance Nagle et al. (2017) suggest that a future nursing informatics specialist will function within virtual models of care, complemented by a range of knowledge related to data analytics, and leverage new care delivery approaches enabled by IoT and other technologies. Topaz et al. (2016) completed a large cross-sectional survey of 272 international nursing informatics researchers and practitioners and uncovered a desire within the discipline to expand the roles of nurses related to digital technologies by: (1) increasing leadership opportunities for nurses (i.e., chief nursing informatics officer); (2) integrating informatics more deeply into nursing education; and, (3) demonstrating clear linkages between the use of nursing data and related health outcomes, including its impact on clinical decision-making, interprofessional collaboration, and increasing research opportunities for practitioners. They note that as consumers have progressively more access to their own health records, the role of nurses will expand to include that of digital knowledge broker and system navigator. More recently, Strudwick et al. (2020) propose that the nursing role within future digital healthcare ecosystems supported by artificial intelligence and process automation technologies, will require the profession to reconsider how compassionate, person-centred care is conceptualized and enacted. Through an extensive review of literature and expert panel consultations, the authors conclude that difficult decisions will need to be made including: (1) reconsidering traditional roles and tasks conducted by nurses that may not contribute value or be valued in future healthcare ecyosystems; and, (2) how the profession can better position itself to direct future health(care) processes in relation to critical issues such as ethics, social justice, and humanistic practice, in light of technological advances.

As introduced by Strudwick et al. (2020), the ability of nurses to provide compassionate, person-centred care in the future will be contingent on a deep understanding of not only the mechanical skills needed to use the technology, but an evolved appreciation of the ethics and social justice issues associated with its use. Nagle et al. (2017) and Topaz et al. (2016) both describe nursing in the future as requiring receptivity toward various virtual and digital care models that may look significantly different than approaches used in the past. Taken together, these scholars have suggested that future nursing roles will require an evolved understanding of various processes (and their related implications) stimulated by new opportunities generated by digital technology. Two such emergent digital technologies that have been projected to significantly influence the nursing profession include artificial intelligence and process automation (Booth et al. 2019; Buchanan et al. 2020; Strudwick et al. 2020; Pepito and Locsin 2019; Archibald and Barnard 2018; Erikson 2016; Frith 2018; Booth 2016). While there are other innovations that will likely have material influence on the role and knowledge used by nurses, artificial intelligence and process automation technologies have been targeted for deeper exploration due to their significant potential to become much further embedded into nursing work. In the following section we conduct a detailed discussion and analysis related to the use of artificial intelligence and process automation technologies in nursing and within the nursing role.

16.5.2   *Artificial Intelligence*

As with much technology discourse in the past, *artificial intelligence* has become a monolithic term within the nursing discourse and refers to many different forms of machines or digital systems that mimic the cognitive functions of a human, including actions like problem-solving, decision-making, and learning (Stuart and Peter 2016). While the domain of artificial intelligence is wide and diverse, for the purposes of simplicity, this chapter will use the term to describe technology that has the ability to perform actions or tasks (e.g., decision-making) which would normally require some degree of human intelligence (Buchanan et al. 2020). As described previously, over the last decade the use of artificial intelligence in society has become both ubiquitous, but also commonly invisible. Applications using artificial intelligence underpin numerous processes and activities that support contemporary life and economies (West and Allen 2018). Virtually every device connected to the Internet now uses some form of artificial intelligence, either through its embedded decision-support functionalities, or its connectivity with larger intelligent systems that can generate personalized or predictive information for a user. While it is beyond the scope of this chapter to provide a fulsome discussion of the pervasiveness of artificial intelligence within contemporary society, it is sufficient to say that many aspects of modern life have been transformed through the use of these forms of technology. One common feature of artificial intelligence in a system is its use of complex algorithms to execute actions. Unlike traditional computerized systems that are unable to evolve the algorithms pre-programmed into the system, technology using artificial intelligence generally possesses the ability to improve upon preexisting algorithms through self-learning and exploration of new or existing data. *Machine learning* is a subset of techniques in artificial intelligence, that helps systems receive, process and analyze data then change their embedded algorithms as they learn more about the data they're processing; in essence they improve their predictive capabilities and accuracy in semi- or autonomous fashions without human intervention (Kwon et al. 2019).

The increased penetration of artificial intelligence into computerized and digital systems used by humans, has generated concerns amongst privacy and ethics proponents regarding the use of systems that can self-learn with limited human oversight. According to Vayena et al. (2018) one of the primary concerns about the use of machine learning systems in healthcare is that "algorithmic bias" (p. 3) in the machine learning process may reinforce inequity, stigma, and imbalanced representations of people or populations. AI's blackbox problem, caused by our inability to always fully understand how algorithms work the way they do, means that many machine learning processes particularly those that teach themselves to make predictions on datasets, are unable to be reverse engineered leaving clinicians with outcomes they are unable to interpret or justify.

While artificially intelligent systems using machine learning can interrogate massive data sources and generate important recommendations and predictions to optimize outcomes, they may be susceptible to algorithmic biases, with unintended consequences. *Automating inequalities* is the term used to describe the outcomes of algorithmic decision-making approaches that are applied uncritically and amplified through the use of digital technology (Bullock 2019; Eubanks 2018). There are reports in both the media and scholarly literature that suggest the uncritical use of digital technology underpinned by self-evolving algorithms can sometimes reinforce inequities found in society due to over or under representation of various population traits in data sets used to train the machine learning systems (Vayena et al. 2018; Gianfrancesco et al. 2018). From a nursing practitioner's perspective, the potential amplification and reinforcement of inequities should be of significant concern. With a long history of social justice advocacy in the profession (Woods 2012), we envision an equally important role for nurses in future digital health(care) ecosystems (Sensmeier 2020). It is predicted that investments in artificial intelligence and machine learning technologies related to healthcare will eclipse $36 billion by 2025 (Brenswick 2018), further reinforcing that nurses must continue to play a role in advocacy and oversight to ensure algorithmic biases within these systems are both detected and addressed. As outlined by a number of nursing scholars (Nagle et al. 2017; Strudwick et al. 2020; Frith 2018; Booth 2016; Kwon et al. 2019; Brennan and Bakken 2015; Remus 2016), the profession needs to become more embedded in data sciences in order to act as a steward for patients and their families who might suffer inequities due to the inappropriateness of automated algorithms or its underlying data. Further, the nursing profession must become more adept at understanding the purpose or value of applying artificial intelligence to various care processes; the various latent biases that may exist within the algorithms or data sets; and, the clinical appropriateness of applying predictions generated by these systems to real-life practice and clinical workflows (Frith 2018; Kwon et al. 2019).

To date, the existing nursing discourse addressing algorithmic bias and the automation of inequities has focused on healthcare-centric models of care, or data sources used or generated by nurses (Remus 2016; Hansen et al. 2014; Bakken and Reame 2016; Brennan and Bakken 2015). Although this is a logical starting point, we suggest that a more pervasive view of algorithmic bias across all areas of society and its interface with health(care) would be beneficial (e.g., digital economy; information manipulation; online personalization-marketing; education; civil and societal governance). As champions of social justice, nurses must acquire not only the skills and knowledge to participate in the development of predictive analytics, but also advocate on behalf of marginalized populations who stand to suffer the most from the automation of inequalities. Therefore, along with developing professional skills and expertise in data analytics, nurses must conceptualize equity-based and social justice nursing theories, and develop complementary and mutually synergetic skills sets. It will not be enough in the future for nurses to learn data science and artificial intelligence methods; rather, nurses will also need to contemporaneously generate evolved understandings and theoretical interpretations of ethics and social justice in a world underpinned by artificially intelligent entities. As previously described, in the healthcare ecosystems of the future, the blurring of human and technological entities will become increasingly difficult to tease apart – equally, so will the intertwined ethical and social justice implications generated from this emergent human-technical relationship. Therefore, we recommend that the use of advanced data analytics such as artificial intelligence and machine learning in health care, include the contributions and refined understanding of the nurse as advocate for the values of compassion and social justice. Clearly, without reconceptualizing nursing's role as advocates for ethics and social justice in light of technological advances (Risling 2017), the profession will not possess the robust moral and philosophical heuristics from which to accurately assess, advise, or help develop artificial intelligence systems to support practice and patient care into the future.

16.5.3   Robotic Process Automation

Humans have been using various forms of automation technology for thousands of years in an effort to reduce human labour needed to complete various procedures, processes, or tasks. In contemporary terms, the use of automation technology has been observed in many industries, including manufacturing, food production, and other domains where activities that require the completion of repetitious, predictable tasks or necessitate certain levels of production consistency that humans have difficulty replicating (Peruffo et al. 2017). Although there are many types of automation technologies used currently, for the purpose of this chapter we focus on *process automation technologies* that seek to re-engineer large scale business operations (Khodambashi 2013; Martinho et al. 2015). Currently, there are many kinds of process automation technologies that are embedded and largely invisible within nursing activities and workflow. While many healthcare practitioners would not generally conceive technologies like electronic medical records, Lean process optimization activities, and other inventory and/or supply chain devices (e.g., medication dispensing cabinets) as a form of explicit process automation, these innovations have all been designed to standardize the replication of various procedures and tasks and capture process efficiencies if and where possible. Since the domain of process automation has not been well studied within the nursing literature (Lu et al. 2018), the profession currently only possesses limited conceptual and philosophical understanding regarding the use, function, and potential implications of this form of technology upon the nursing role.

As a profession that has historically prided itself on the delivery of therapeutic care through a range of well-developed knowledge and skills, the development of robotic-enabled process automation technologies has stimulated scholars to question *how*, *where*, and *why* these sorts of devices might be used to support care. While *robotic process automation* is essentially a new topic to the profession (Kangasniemi et al. 2019; Syed et al. 2020), a long lineage of theorization related to the use of robots in care, cyborg ontology, and other hybridized human-machine approaches to supporting the nursing role have been published over the last few decades (Sandelowski 1999; Maalouf et al. 2018; de Almeida Vieira Monteiro APT 2016; Lapum et al. 2012). Much of this preliminary theorization related to robotics in the profession demonstrates invaluable historical thought-leadership and visioning by nursing scholars and has generated situational awareness to the topic and potential for robotics within nursing practice. That said, most of this work was completed when nursing-centric robotics and their corresponding functionalities were still largely primordial or prototypical. Until recently, many of the robotic process automation technologies used within healthcare did not influence the nursing role in a direct fashion; rather, these technologies served in largely invisible ways, supporting providers to complete their respective clinical tasks and activities, including lab specimen processing, medication dispensing, and other ancillary supply chain logistics. With the improved functionality of robotics and advancements in artificial intelligence, robotic process automation that directly influences aspects of the nursing role have become reality. To date, there is increasing use of robotics to support or augment tasks once completed almost exclusively by humans in health(care) settings (Schwab 2019; Whitesell 2017). For instance, collaborative robotics (cobots) are a growing type of robotic process automation technology that are specifically designed to work in close proximity with humans to complete shared tasks (Bendel 2020). Unlike previous automation technology that was largely mechanistic and potentially dangerous to be those nearby, cobots are a type of service robot that can be used in a range of settings (e.g., healthcare, domestic) to assist in the co-completion of various tasks, activities, and procedures (Bendel 2020; Marr 2018). Healthcare has begun experimenting and testing the use of cobots in a range of clinical and service applications. For instance, the use of humanoid supportive robots in the care or recovery of patients; drone robotics to assist or support supply and transportation logistics within a facility; and, an ever-increasing variety of semi-autonomous robotics that assist nurses in stocking shelves and other non-patient facing tasks (Schwab 2019; Whitesell 2017; Bendel 2020).

The growing presence and availability of robotics like cobots to support and augment aspects of the nursing role has engendered deep philosophical discussions within the profession (Strudwick et al. 2020; Maalouf et al. 2018; de Almeida Vieira Monteiro 2016). To date, most contemporary nursing discourse has cautiously viewed the rise of cobots and other robotic process automation as being potentially beneficial to the profession, in the way that these innovations can support the nursing role and generate nursing efficiencies that can be applied back to important human-centred roles (e.g., more time with patients; free nursing time to complete more important therapeutic and knowledge activities; etc.). While there is significant interest in the use of robotics within the nursing profession, there also remains a great deal of hesitation and qualification by nursing scholars regarding the presence and function of these non-human entities. Speculation about the potential *replacement* of nurses by robots and other computerized devices remains a perennial topic of discussion by the profession over the years (Pepito and Locsin 2019; Rinard 1996; Almerud et al. 2008; Wollowick a 1970), however the general consensus by scholars is that the direct displacement of nurses by robotics and other process automation is not foreseeable, Instead, wider scale augmentation of nurses and their roles by artificially intelligent, robot process automating technologies like cobots is more likely to occur as these forms of innovation become increasingly available within healthcare environments (Booth et al. 2019; Pepito and Locsin 2019; Erikson 2016).

Although the profession appears cautiously optimistic regarding the role and value of robotic process automation technologies (Pepito and Locsin 2019; Archibald and Barnard 2018), the augmentation and evolution of traditional nursing roles by these forms of collaborative robotics requires immediate thought-leadership and scholarship. Much like the unintended consequences generated by artificial intelligence, we propose that the increasing desire within healthcare settings to enable and scale the use of robotic process automation technologies should also be met with both theoretical development and empirical research to guide practice. To date, work on theoretical and empirical assessment of robotics used in/for nursing roles has generally revolved around two central themes: (1) examining the proposed or actual impacts of robotics upon some aspect of the nursing role and specific tasks (e.g., Frazier et al. 2019; Tuisku et al. 2019); and/or, (2) conceptual or synthesis discussions regarding the implications of using robots as related to traditional values structures of the nursing profession, including caring, patient-centred care, and therapeutic relationships (e.g., Archibald and Barnard 2018; Maalouf et al. 2018; Carter-Templeton et al. 2018). Although the evidence in this domain is still nascent, there appears to be general, theoretical and empirical consensus in nursing discourse that aspects of robotic process automation have a high likelihood of significantly disrupting certain traditional roles and workflows conducted by nurses.

As new robots are developed for healthcare, the profession of nursing must become more present and active in this domain. To date, there are promising glimpses of nursing professionals becoming involved in the development, design, and evaluation of robotics that can be used within practice settings (Frazier et al. 2019; Glasgow et al. 2018); regardless, we believe more can and must be done. Similar to preceding discussion regarding the intended and unintended consequences of artificial intelligence, the use and adoption of robotic process automation in the profession must be met with increased theoretical and empirical interrogation by nursing scholars and practitioners. As with emergent digital technologies, the nuanced socio-technical relationships that process automating innovations can engender with humans is an area of inquiry nearly absent in nursing literature. Drawing from work in other disciplines that have experienced significant investments in robotic process automation, there are currently many important ethical and labour policy implications from the adoption of these forms of innovations that have yet to be explored by nursing. For instance, Theodore et al. (2019) conducted a large scale workplace policy analysis examining the use of automation and optimization technologies within warehouse and storage facilities. They concluded that while newer process automation technologies like robotics "promise to alleviate the need for the most arduous activities... [their use] will be coupled with attempts to increase the pace of work and productivity in other tasks, with new methods of motivating and monitoring workers." (Theodore et al. 2019, p. 52). Although there are material differences between warehouse and health(care) work environments and related roles, tasks, and knowledge needed to operate in each respective domain, Theodore et al.'s (2019) conclusions are striking and worthy of deeper consideration. From a nursing perspective, much of the discourse related to robotic process automation has avoided explicit discussion of the potential policy implications that might arise from adoption and use of these technologies. While many of these process automating technologies may be designed or branded as possessing the ability to increase productivity by alleviating or assisting humans with mundane tasks, rarely is there deeper discussion of *where* or *how* this realized efficiency will be reapplied to the nursing role or patient care. Commonly, the underlining assumption of robotic process automation is that when productivity gains are generated, these derived benefits will be altruistically reinvested in aspects of the nursing role, including the reduction of workload; will afford clinicians the opportunity to seek higher level cognitive or value activities; or to provide nurses *more time* with the patient (Kachouie et al. 2014; Katsuya and Kelemen 2011; Vänni and Salin 2019). Drawing from conclusions proposed by Theodore et al. (2019), we suggest benefits realized from automation may not be equitably reapplied to proactively amplify nursing activities, without nursing profession's advocacy and stewardship of policy development to protect these emergent gains. The use of robotic automation technology which can augment or displace traditional human activities is a perfect storm of social versus technological friction. The nursing profession must proactively explore its adoption in relation to labour policy and contractual agreements. Further, entirely new domains of nursing inquiry exploring the human-robotic relationships developed by the increasing presence of robotic process automation innovation is needed to afford the profession guidance into the future. It is proposed that new areas of inquiry should be undertaken, including deeper theoretical and empirical analysis related to: (1) nursing activities and tasks through which humans and robotics can co-collaborate to achieve higher and more robust outcomes; (2) exploration of specific nursing roles and tasks related to robotic process automation that can be successfully and safely amplified in semi- or autonomous fashions; (3) re-examination of traditional nursing informatics topics like technology usability and user-centred design, in light of robotic technology that potentially possesses self-intelligence and the ability to learn and meaningfully respond to human interaction; and, (4) other future-forward policy, practice guidance, and legal frameworks related to the delegation of complex and regulated tasks to artificially-intelligent robotics. Although the profession is still likely years away from seeing robotic process automation en masse within work environments, without this sort of theoretical and empirical grounding, nursing may miss a significant opportunity in its history to expand and evolve the nursing profession in ways previously unimaginable.

16.6 Implications for Nurse Educators

Globally, nurse educators represent an important group in shaping the nursing profession as they prepare tomorrows nurses for the realities of the practice world and beyond. However the current challenge is that nurse educators at the entry-to-practice level are not well equipped to tackle future-focused topics such as artificial intelligence, robotics, and implications of innovative technologies on the nursing profession (Risling 2017; Nagle et al. 2014). In fact, this group is at times not well prepared or comfortable teaching some of the basic nursing informatics topics present today (Nagle and Furlong 2019). Since the future of nursing informatics is constantly evolving, nurse educators will need to understand and be comfortable teaching concepts that supersede individual technologies, and that can be applied to a variety of novel technologies that nursing students may interact with in their clinical practicum environments. Nurse educators must do so while still recognizing the implications of specific technologies (e.g. automation, sensors, voice activated technologies) on practice, and at times incorporate these innovative technologies into their usual teaching methods like simulations, skill development, lectures and beyond. One crucial opportunity that nurse educators must be equipped for and embrace is to engage students in important discussions about the privacy, regulatory and legal implications when new technologies are developed for healthcare contexts. Numerous countries have developed entry-to-practice competencies for nursing informatics (CASN/Infoway 2012; O'Connor et al. 2017); while these initiatives are an important start, they should be assessed for relevancy in the context of future-forward topics and technologies.

16.7 Implications for Nurse Leaders

Similar to nurse educators, nurse leaders in influential roles today can have a significant impact on shaping the nursing profession of the future. These nurse leaders are often in the position to support procurement, selection, budgeting, implementation, optimization, evaluation and other critical processes common to the lifecycle of technology in healthcare organizations, regions or authorities, or even countries. Nurse leaders should work towards the inclusion of nursing input at all levels of the technology adoption lifecycle, influencing decision-making to ensure that technologies support nursing professional practice, and in turn, positively impact the recipients of their care. In doing so, if done consistently, there are tremendous opportunities for improvements to the profession and more importantly for patients. However, several challenges exist. In many cases nurses in senior leadership positions have not had informatics-related topics discussed or taught during their entry-to-practice education, and therefore the knowledge may be unfamiliar to them (Collins et al. 2017; Remus and Kennedy 2012b). In addition, informatics competencies that are unique to the nurse leader level may not be well developed (Strudwick et al. 2019).

Nurse leader informatics competencies have been uniquely identified in several countries (Strudwick et al. 2019; Westra and Delaney 2008). The uptake of these competencies at the present time is low but growing, as more opportunities for professional development and advanced degrees in nursing informatics is offered. The shortage of nurse leaders skilled in informatics frustrates the professions' ability to generate positive benefits from technology implementation and use in nursing practice.

16.8   Implications for Nurse Researchers

Nursing informatics applications of the future offer a significant opportunity for nurse researchers. The breadth and volume of health-related data available to nurse researchers to ask and answer important profession-related questions are unprecedented. Data sources include electronic health record systems, wearables from both patients and nurses themselves, voice-activated and voice-recognition technologies, sensors, active and passive data collection from mobile phones, biometrics, and other remote patient-monitoring systems in the home. Advanced statistical methods such as text mining using natural language processing and social media analytics, and predictive analytics using data mining techniques such as decision tress and artificial neural networks are increasingly used by nurse researchers. These new tools allow them to ask new and different questions that have been impossible in past clinical and health services research (Strudwick et al. 2020; Kwon et al. 2019; Brennan and Bakken 2015). Nurse researchers also play an important role in conceptualizing the changing role of nurses in our tech-enabled future. The opportunities for nurses studying and researching in this domain is limitless.

16.9   Differentiating Nursing *Now* and into the Future

As described in the previous sections, nursing is at a significant inflection point in its history and evolution as a profession. Advanced technologies that were once the topics of science fiction mere decades ago are now real-life considerations that influence and shape nursing practice. In order to fully leverage this new and emerging reality the nursing profession must act quickly and decisively to communicate its vision for the future. While collective action is sometimes difficult, given the exponential gains made by emergent digital technology over the last few years and the creeping *skill-mix* augmentation of the nursing role with lower-skill healthcare providers (Aiken et al. 2017), difficult questions will need to be addressed to help differentiate the profession *now*, and into the future. In short, the nursing profession will need to clearly delineate its competitive advantage moving into the next few decades, that will likely be underpinned in fundamental ways by artificial intelligence and other robotic process automation that will continue to challenge modern day nursing activities and value-structures. As outlined in previous sections, the socio-technical blurring of roles, action, and behavior related to the presence of emergent technology like artificial intelligence and robotics are variables that need to be considered in all future conceptualizations of the profession. Partaking in deeper discussions related to how nursing and emergent digital technologies can work *together* in new ways to deliver care that is both human-centric but also receptive to nursing role, knowledge, and activity evolution, is of utmost importance. The nursing profession needs to view the growing presence and importance of these technologies not as a barrier; instead, as an antecedent force that will allow the profession to amplify its future value proposition to health(care), by allowing the nursing role to evolve in meaningful ways to interact in and within virtual and digital models of care that are currently primordial or uncontested by other healthcare professionals (Booth 2016). In order to move forward into this future as a unified and valued profession, nursing needs to explore how it will synergize with various emergent technologies, and amplify the new roles, behaviours, and knowledges these newfound relationships can enable. Without approaching future visioning for the profession using this socio-technical mindset, the profession will miss a significant opportunity to differentiate itself from the roles of other healthcare providers and capabilities of emergent health technology – both of which, purposefully or not, will begin to augment the traditional nursing role in ways that may not be compatible with aspects of professional longevity or autonomy.

16.10 Conclusion

Throughout this chapter, we explore the future of the nursing profession in an era where technology is moving from discrete transaction processing and monitoring applications to pervasive computing where "intelligent" systems are used for problem analysis, prediction, decision support, and the autonomous performance of tasks in the healthcare setting. While this chapter provides, at times, a critical interpretation of the technologies currently or foreseeably used within the nursing role, we advocate for the nursing profession to adopt a more proactive stance. The rapidly changing clinical environment demands nursing involvement in the research and design of these tools, as well as in developing the necessary policies and regulations that will govern their adoption and use. The subtle normalization of these technologies into the nursing role engenders new and different relationships between nurses (i.e., practice, education, research, leadership) and other actors in the clinical theatre. Without critical reflection and proactive future visioning, the profession will miss the opportunity to establish consistent professional structures, messaging and guidelines that appropriately differentiate nursing value(s) that are strengthened by emergent technologies, from those of other human care providers. The nursing profession has long understood the value of data, tools, and technology in regards to patient and client care; it is now time to fully actualize these attendant skillsets towards revisioning the future of the nurse-technology relationship and strengthening the role of nursing into the future.

Review Questions

1. Compare and contrast the approach that the nursing profession has historically taken to examine the impact of new technology on its role in healthcare with the socio-technical approach used here to explore the role of emerging digital technology.
2. Define artificial intelligence, and its sub-domain machine learning. Artificial intelligence is being used in the detection of disease, management of chronic conditions, delivery of health services and drug discovery. Describe one example of a nursing tool, that you think could improve patient outcomes if it included different data and the capacity for advanced analytics such artificial intelligence.
3. Why might nurses' role in ethical oversight, and as patient and social justice advocates be *more* important with the introduction of advanced analytic techniques and embedded artificial intelligence in healthcare technologies?

Answers

1. The historic notion is that technology should be viewed primarily from a socially grounded and human-centric perspective. The nursing discourse suggests that the impressive growth and diversity of technology adoption happens around or adjacent to the nursing profession. That is, the nursing profession has the ability to remain largely unchanged in the types of traditional roles and activities for which its known, despite an ever-increasing variety and complexity of emergent digital technologies used in/for nursing work. The socio-technical approach is presented as a more balanced conceptual lens that balances the social aspects of action (e.g., nursing roles, their relationships with patients, etc.) with the complementary technical aspects of reality (e.g., emergent digital technology and the processes they facilitate, etc.). It is suggested that the socio-technical approach provides a more balanced theoretical perspective from which to generate implications for future practice, will help leverage the best elements of what is human and what is technology, and privileges both social and technical features as equally powerful, important, and essential to the generation of realistic recommendations for the future of nursing.
2. Artificial intelligence describes technology that has the ability to perform actions or tasks (e.g., decision-making) which would normally require some degree of human intelligence. One common feature of artificial intelligence in a system is its use of complex algorithms to execute actions. Machine learning is a subset of

techniques in artificial intelligence, that helps systems receive, process and analyze data then change their embedded algorithms as they learn more about the datum they are processing; in essence they improve their predictive capabilities and accuracy in semi- or autonomous fashions without human intervention.

Students responses will vary to the question of nursing practice tools that might be improved through the inclusion of more data and advanced AI functionality. Instructors might prompt students with an example:

Think about the type of information that might usually be collected in a suspected coronavirus (e.g., COVID-19) intake form at public health. While an EMR will automatically collate information such as name, date of birth, gender, address, and co-morbidities, an AI enabled application that could access a database with historic geolocation data from the person's phone, and was connected to an exposed population database of similar information, could quickly cross-check possible exposure to infected individuals, and based on morbidity data predict the statistical risk of the person contracting the virus. While this would not possibly change the nursing intake, when tests are in short supply, nurses could use the system to prioritize those who received the actual test, and could advise the patient on quarantine protocols appropriate to their risk.

3. Students responses will vary. However, they should mention the unintended consequences of algorithmic bias when AI is used uncritically in decision-making. The potential for amplification of social inequities related to race, income, gender and disability when using AI have been widely reported in the media and scholarly literature. In one seminal case in the U.S. an algorithm was used by health care providers to screen patients to receive *high-risk care management* intervention (Obermeyer et al. 2019). Patients who had especially complex medical needs based on their treatment history are automatically flagged by the algorithm to receive additional care resources. However, due to unequal access to treatment and affordability, black patients were much less likely to have a history of interventions, and so were much less likely to receive the additional care.

Glossary

Artificial intelligence Technology that has the ability to perform actions or tasks (e.g., decision-making) which would normally require some degree of human intelligence

Big Data A term used to describe the extensive volume of both structured and unstructured data generated in the healthcare system

Collaborative robotics (cobots) Robotics process automation that work in close collaboration with humans to complete shared tasks

Dialectical learning An approach to learning through examination and discussion

Disruptive technologies Technologies that provoke change and innovation, resulting in new or unanticipated opportunities

Emergent digital technologies Technologies that are developing and evolving to become useful or impactful in a variety of settings across society, including healthcare

External modality Factors impacting change and adaptation that the organization can try to influence but not control

Inertial conflict Resistance to change

Internal modality Factors impacting change and adaptation that are within the scope of influence or control of the organization

Intrapreneur An individual that provokes or supports transformative change within an organization

Lifecycle The phases of a specific process from beginning to conclusion, commonly reflecting software development or project management

Marginal analysis An approach to options analysis by calculating the incremental impacts of change on cost and revenues

Mind mapping Graphical representation of the connection between concepts and ideas

Nanorobotics An emerging field of research focused on microscopic robots used to target specific diseases such as cancer

Non-repudiation A security authentication with a high degree of confidence

Normalization The process of becoming accustomed to a specific concept or process, such as the use of technology to perform a specific task, so that it this is perceived to be part of a normal routine.

NRO Non-repudiation of Origin, which documents evidence of origin of the message, and prevents denial of the message by the originating party

OODA loop An approach to decision making that involves Observing information, Orienting or interpreting information, Deciding on a course of action, and Action

Operational management The day to day management of the healthcare system, which includes a variety of departments or services such as human resources, administrative, finance, and inventory

Organizational ambidexterity Two approaches to change reflecting both adaptability and alignment

Performance indicators Specific criteria that are measured at specific points in time to evaluate performance and/or change

Process automation technologies Automation that reengineers processes to minimize human effort and increase both efficiency and productivity

Rose diagram Nightingale's visualization depicting mortality causes

Service management plan Plan to provide oversight or resolution to an issue related to a specific service or product provision

Socio-technical Refers to the relationship between technology and the social aspect of actions that are influenced by the inclusion of technology in activities

References

Agar N. The sceptical optimist: why technology isn't the answer to everything. Oxford: Oxford University Press; 2015.

Aiken LH, Sloane D, Griffiths P, Rafferty AM, Bruyneel L, McHugh M, et al. Nursing skill mix in European hospitals: cross-sectional study of the association with mortality, patient ratings, and quality of care. BMJ Qual Saf. 2017;26:559–68. https://doi.org/10.1136/bmjqs-2016-005567.

de Almeida Vieira Monteiro APT. Cyborgs, biotechnologies, and informatics in health care - new paradigms in nursing sciences. Nurs Philos. 2016;17:19–27. https://doi.org/10.1111/nup.12088.

Almerud S, Alapack RJ, Fridlund B, Ekebergh M. Beleaguered by technology: care in technologically intense environments. Nurs Philos. 2008;9:55–61. https://doi.org/10.1111/j.1466-769X.2007.00332.x.

Archibald MM, Barnard A. Futurism in nursing: technology, robotics and the fundamentals of care. J Clin Nurs. 2018;27:2473–80. https://doi.org/10.1111/jocn.14081.

Bakken S, Reame N. The promise and potential perils of big data for advancing symptom management research in populations at risk for health disparities. Annu Rev Nurs Res. 2016;34:247–60. https://doi.org/10.1891/0739-6686.34.247.

Barnard A. Philosophy of technology and nursing. Nurs Philos. 2002;3:15–26.

Barnard A. Radical nursing and the emergence of technique as healthcare technology. Nurs Philos. 2016;17:8–18. https://doi.org/10.1111/nup.12103.

Bendel O. Co-Robots as Care Robots. 2020.

Berg M, Aarts J, Van der Lei J. ICT in health care: sociotechnical approaches methods. Inf Med. 2003;42:297–301.

Bohn D. Amazon says 100 million Alexa devices have been sold—what's next? The Verge. 2019.

Booth R. Informatics and nursing in a post-nursing informatics world: future directions for nurses in an automated, artificially-intelligent, social-networked healthcare environment. Can J Nurs Leadersh. 2016;28:61–9. https://doi.org/10.12927/cjnl.2016.24563.

Booth RG, Strudwick G, McMurray J, Morse A, Chan R, Zhang T. The best way to predict the future is to [co]create it: a technology primer for healthcare leaders. In: Weberg D, Davidson S, editors. Leadership for evidence-based innovation in nursing and health professions. 2nd ed. Burlington, MA: Jones & Bartlett Learning; 2019. p. 261–83.

Brennan PF, Bakken S. Nursing needs big data and big data needs nursing. J Nurs Scholarsh. 2015;47:477–84. https://doi.org/10.1111/jnu.12159.

Brenswick J. Artificial intelligence in healthcare spending to hit $36B. Health IT Analytics. 2018.

Buchanan C, Howitt ML, Wilson R, Booth RG, Risling T, Bamford M. Nursing in the age of artificial intelligence: protocol for a scoping review. JMIR Res Protoc. 2020;9:e17490. https://doi.org/10.2196/17490.

Bullock JB. Artificial intelligence, discretion, and bureaucracy. Am Rev Public Adm. 2019;49:751–61. https://doi.org/10.1177/0275074019856123.

Carter-Templeton H, Frazier RM, Wu L, HW T. Robotics in nursing: a bibliometric analysis. J Nurs Scholarsh. 2018;50:582–9. https://doi.org/10.1111/jnu.12399.

CASN/Infoway. Nursing informatics entry-to-practice competencies for registered nurses. Ottawa: CASN; 2012.

Collins S, Yen P-Y, Phillips A, Kennedy MK. Nursing informatics competency assessment for the nurse leader: the Delphi study. J Nurs Adm. 2017;47:212–8. https://doi.org/10.1097/NNA.0000000000000467.

Cresswell K, Callaghan M, Khan S, Sheikh Z, Mozaffar H, Sheikh A. Investigating the use of data-driven artificial intelligence in computerised decision support systems for health and social care: a systematic review. Health Informatics J. 2020;26(3):2138–47. https://doi.org/10.1177/1460458219900452.

Erikson H. Future challenges of robotics and artificial intelligence in nursing: what can we learn from monsters in popular culture? Perm J. 2016;20:15–7. https://doi.org/10.7812/TPP/15-243.

Eubanks V. Automating inequality: how high-tech tools profile, police, and punish the poor. New York, NY: St. Martin's Press; 2018.

Frazier RM, Carter-Templeton H, Wyatt TH, Wu L. Current trends in robotics in nursing patents - a glimpse into emerging innovations. CIN - Comput Informatics Nurs. 2019;37:290–7. https://doi.org/10.1097/CIN.0000000000000538.

Frey CB, Osborne MA. The future of employment: how susceptible are jobs to automation? Technol Forecast Soc Chang. 2017;114:254–80.

Fridsma DB. Health informatics: a required skill for 21st century clinicians. BMJ. 2018:k3043. https://doi.org/10.1136/bmj.k3043.

Frith KH. Artificial intelligence: what does it mean for nursing? Nurs Educ Perspect. 2018;40:261. https://doi.org/10.1097/01.NEP.0000000000000543.

Gephart S, Carrington JM, Finley B. A systematic review of nurses' experiences with unintended consequences when using the electronic health record. Nurs Adm Q. 2015;39:345–56. https://doi.org/10.1097/NAQ.0000000000000119.

Gianfrancesco MA, Tamang S, Yazdany J, Schmajuk G. Potential biases in machine learning algorithms using electronic health record data. JAMA Intern Med. 2018;178:1544–7. https://doi.org/10.1001/jamainternmed.2018.3763.

Glasgow MES, Colbert A, Viator J, Cavanagh S. The nurse-engineer: a new role to improve nurse technology interface and patient care device innovations. J Nurs Scholarsh. 2018; https://doi.org/10.1111/jnu.12431.

Gutelius B, Theodore N. "The future of warehouse work: technological change in the U.S. logistics industry" (UC Berkeley Labor Center; Working Partnerships USA, October 2019), http://laborcenter.berkeley.edu/future-of-warehouse-work/.

Hansen MM, Miron-Shatz T, Lau a YS, Paton C. Big data in science and healthcare: a review of recent literature and perspectives. Contribution of the IMIA social media working group. Yearb Med Inform. 2014;9:21–6. https://doi.org/10.15265/IY-2014-0004.

Huston C. The impact of emerging technology on nursing care: warp speed ahead. Online J Issues Nurs. 2013;18:1.

Kachouie R, Sedighadeli S, Khosla R, Chu MT. Socially assistive robots in elderly care: a mixed-method systematic literature review. Int J Hum Comput Interact. 2014;30:369–93. https://doi.org/10.1080/10447318.2013.873278.

Kangasniemi M, Karki S, Colley N, Voutilainen A. The use of robots and other automated devices in nurses' work: an integrative review. Int J Nurs Pract. 2019:1–14. https://doi.org/10.1111/ijn.12739.

Katsuya K, Kelemen A. A systematic review of intelligent patient care assistive technology. CIN - Comput Informatics, Nurs. 2011;29:441–2. https://doi.org/10.1097/NCN.0b013e3182305d5a.

Khodambashi S. Business process re-engineering application in healthcare in a relation to health information systems. Procedia Technol. 2013;9:949–57. https://doi.org/10.1016/j.protcy.2013.12.106.

Koppel R, Metlay JP, Cohen A, Abaluck B, Localio a R, Kimmel SE, et al. Role of computerized physician order entry systems in facilitating medication errors. JAMA. 2005;293:1197–203. https://doi.org/10.1001/jama.293.10.1197.

Kwon JY, Karim ME, Topaz M, Currie LM. Nurses "seeing forest for the trees" in the age of machine learning: using nursing knowledge to improve relevance and performance. CIN - Comput Informatics Nurs. 2019;37:203–12. https://doi.org/10.1097/CIN.0000000000000508.

Lapum J, Fredericks S, Beanlands H, Mccay E, Schwind J, Romaniuk D. A cyborg ontology in health care: traversing into the liminal space between technology and person-centred practice. Nurs Philos. 2012;13:276–88.

Lu SF, Rui H, Seidmann A. Does technology substitute for nurses? Staffing decisions in nursing homes. Manag Sci. 2018;64:1842–59. https://doi.org/10.1287/mnsc.2016.2695.

Lynn LA. Artificial intelligence systems for complex decision-making in acute care medicine: a review. Patient Saf Surg. 2019;13:1–8. https://doi.org/10.1186/s13037-019-0188-2.

Maalouf N, Sidaoui A, Elhajj IH, Asmar D. Robotics in nursing: a scoping review. J Nurs Scholarsh. 2018;50(6):590–600. https://doi.org/10.1111/jnu.12424.

Marr B. The future of work: are you ready for smart cobots? Forbes. 2018.

Martinho R, Rijo R, Nunes A. Complexity analysis of a business process automation: case study on a healthcare organization. Procedia Comput Sci. 2015;64:1226–31. https://doi.org/10.1016/j.procs.2015.08.510.

Morse A, Chan R, Booth R. eHealth, ePatient. In: Charnay-Sonnek F, Murphy A, editors. Principle of nursing in oncology. Springer: Cham; 2019. p. 427–39. https://doi.org/10.1007/978-3-319-76457-3_27.

Nagle LM, Furlong K. Digital health in Canadian schools of nursing part a: nurse educators. Qual Adv Nurs Educ - Avancées En Form Infirm. 2019;6:1–17.

Nagle LM, Crosby K, Frisch N, Borycki E, Donelle L, Hannah K, et al. Developing entry-to-practice nursing informatics competencies for registered nurses. Stud Health Technol Inform. 2014;201:356–63.

Nagle L, Sermeus W, Junger A. Evolving role of the nursing informatics specialist. Stud Health Technol Inform. 2017;232:212–22. https://doi.org/10.3233/978-1-61499-738-2-212.

Novak LL, Holden RJ, Anders SH, Hong JY, Karsh BT. Using a sociotechnical framework to understand adaptations in health IT implementation. Int J Med Inform. 2013;82:e331–44. https://doi.org/10.1016/j.ijmedinf.2013.01.009.

O'Connor S, Hubner U, Shaw T, Blake R, Ball M. Time for TIGER to ROAR! Technology informatics guiding education reform. Nurse Educ Today. 2017;58:78–81. https://doi.org/10.1016/j.nedt.2017.07.014.

Obermeyer Z, Powers B, Vogeli C, Mullainathan S. Dissecting racial bias in an algorithm used to manage the health of populations. Science. 2019;366:447–53. https://doi.org/10.1126/science.aax2342.

Pepito JA, Locsin R. Can nurses remain relevant in a technologically advanced future? Int J Nurs Sci. 2019;6:106–10. https://doi.org/10.1016/j.ijnss.2018.09.013.

Peruffo E, Schmidlechner L, Contreras R, Molinuevo D. Automation of work: literature review. 2017.

Remus S. The big data revolution: opportunities for chief nurse executives. Can J Nurs Leadersh. 2016;28:18–28.

Remus S, Donelle L. Big data: why should Canadian nurse leaders care? Can J Nurs Leadersh. 2019;32:19–30. https://doi.org/10.12927/cjnl.2019.25964.

Remus S, Kennedy M. Innovation in transformative nursing leadership: nursing informatics competencies and roles. Nurs Leadersh. 2012a;25:14–26. https://doi.org/10.12927/cjnl.2012.23260.

Remus S, Kennedy MA. Innovation in transformative nursing leadership: nursing informatics competencies and roles. Nurs Leadersh (Tor Ont). 2012b;25:14–26. https://doi.org/10.1177/0894318413500313.

Rinard R. Technology, deskilling, and nurses: the impact of the technologically changing environment. Adv Nurs Sci. 1996;18:60–9.

Risling T. Educating the nurses of 2025: technology trends of the next decade. Nurse Educ Pract. 2017;22:89–92. https://doi.org/10.1016/j.nepr.2016.12.007.

Sandelowski M. (Ir)reconcilable differences? The debate concerning nursing and technology. J Nurs Scholarsh. 1997;29:169–74. https://doi.org/10.1111/j.1547-5069.1997.tb01552.x.

Sandelowski M. Troubling distinctions: a semiotics of the nursing/technology relationship. Nurs Inq. 1999;6:198–207.

Schwab K. A hospital introduced a robot to help nurses. They didn't expect it to be so popular. Fast Company. 2019.

Sensmeier J. Achieving health equity through use of information technology to address social determinants of health. CIN Comput Informatics, Nurs. 2020;38:116–9. https://doi.org/10.1097/CIN.0000000000000622.

Shortliffe EH, Sepúlveda MJ. Clinical decision support in the era of artificial intelligence. JAMA - J Am Med Assoc. 2018;320:2199–200. https://doi.org/10.1001/jama.2018.17163.

Sittig DF, Singh H. A new sociotechnical model for studying health information technology in complex adaptive healthcare systems. Qual Saf Health Care. 2010;19(Suppl 3):i68–74. https://doi.org/10.1136/qshc.2010.042085.

Strudwick G, Nagle LM, Morgan A, Kennedy MA, Currie LM, Lo B, et al. Adapting and validating informatics competencies for senior nurse leaders in the Canadian context: results of a Delphi study. Int J Med Inform. 2019;129:211–8. https://doi.org/10.1016/j.ijmedinf.2019.06.012.

Strudwick G, Wiljer D, Inglis F. Nursing and compassionate care in a technological world: a discussion paper. Toronto, Canada. 2020.

Stuart R, Peter N. Artificial intelligence: a modern approach. 3rd ed. New York: Pearson; 2016.

Syed R, Suriadi S, Adams M, Bandara W, Leemans SJJ, Ouyang C, et al. Robotic process automation: contemporary themes and challenges. Comput Ind. 2020;115:103162. https://doi.org/10.1016/j.compind.2019.103162.

Tanioka T, Yasuhara Y, Dino MJS, Kai Y, Locsin RC, Schoenhofer SO. Disruptive engagements with technologies, robotics, and caring: advancing the transactive relationship theory of nursing. Nurs Adm Q. 2019;43:313–21. https://doi.org/10.1097/NAQ.0000000000000365.

Topaz M, Ronquillo C, Peltonen LM, Pruinelli L, Sarmiento RF, Badger MK, et al. Advancing nursing informatics in the next decade: recommendations from an international survey. Stud Health Technol Inform. 2016;225:123–7. https://doi.org/10.3233/978-1-61499-658-3-123.

Tuisku O, Pekkarinen S, Hennala L, Melkas H. Robots do not replace a nurse with a beating heart. Inf Technol People. 2019;32:47–67. https://doi.org/10.1108/ITP-06-2018-0277.

Vänni KJ, Salin SE. Attitudes of professionals toward the need for assistive and social robots in the healthcare sector. In: Social robots: technological, societal and ethical aspects of human-robot interaction. Cham: Springer; 2019. p. 205–36. https://doi.org/10.1007/978-3-030-17107-0_11.

Vayena E, Blasimme A, Cohen IG. Machine learning in medicine: addressing ethical challenges. PLoS Med. 2018;15:e1002689. https://doi.org/10.1371/journal.pmed.1002689.

West D, Allen J. How artificial intelligence is transforming the world. 2018.

Westra BL, Delaney CW. Informatics competencies for nursing and healthcare leaders. AMIA Annu Symp Proc. 2008;2008:804–8.

Whitesell AA. Robot-human collaboration for improving patient care in infectious disease environments. In: Proceedings of the companion 2017 ACM/IEEE international conference on human-robot interaction - HRI '17. New York, NY: ACM Press; 2017. p. 385–6. https://doi.org/10.1145/3029798.3034805.

Wollowick a. Will the nursing profession become extinct? Nurs Forum. 1970;9:408–13.

Woods M. Exploring the relevance of social justice within a relational nursing ethic. Nurs Philos. 2012;13:56–65. https://doi.org/10.1111/j.1466-769X.2011.00525.x.

Index

© Springer Nature Switzerland AG 2021   419
P. Hussey, M. A. Kennedy (eds.), *Introduction to Nursing Informatics*, Health
Informatics, https://doi.org/10.1007/978-3-030-58740-6

Printed in the United States
by Baker & Taylor Publisher Services